MW01317442

Neuro-Developmental Treatment Approach

Theoretical Foundations and Principles of Clinical Practice

by Janet M. Howle
in collaboration with the NDTA Theory Committee

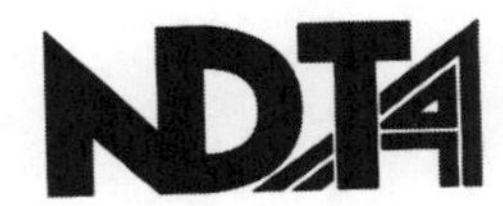

Neuro-Developmental Treatment Association
1540 S. Coast Hwy., Suite 203
Laguna Beach, CA 92651

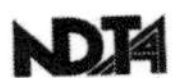

The North American Neuro-Developmental Treatment Association

The North American Neuro-Developmental Treatment Association (NDTA) is a nonprofit professional organization of physical therapists, occupational therapists, speech-language pathologists, and other interested persons who are dedicated to promoting the theory and practice of the Neuro-Developmental Treatment Approach conceived and developed by Berta and Karel Bobath. The NDTA furthers the development of this unique approach for infants, children, and adults with central nervous system pathology and resulting neural and body system impairments by offering continuing education to members and nonmembers, maintaining a lending library of books and videotapes, sponsoring professional conferences, supporting a regional network, providing grants for clinical research, publishing a newsletter containing clinical studies and organizational information, maintaining a website, and promoting client and family advocacy. The North American NDTA was incorporated in 1987 and currently has over 2,000 active members. For information about membership or services provided by the NDTA, contact the NDTA office or visit the website:

Neuro-Developmental Treatment Association
1540 S. Coast Hwy., Suite 203
Laguna Beach, CA 92651
1-800-869-9295
www.ndta.org

ISBN 0-9724615-0-7

1 2 3 4 5 6 7 8 9 10 11 12 A B C D E

Printed in Canada

Dedication

This book is dedicated to Berta and Karel Bobath, Mary Quinton, and Elsbeth Köng, our teachers and mentors, who taught us to ask questions and question the answers.

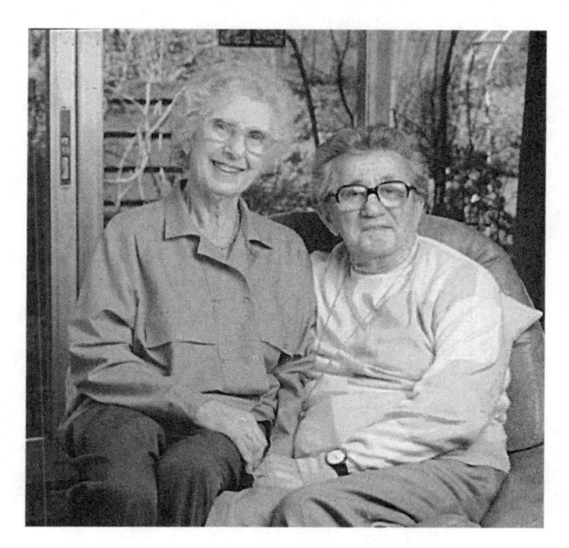

Berta and Karel Bobath

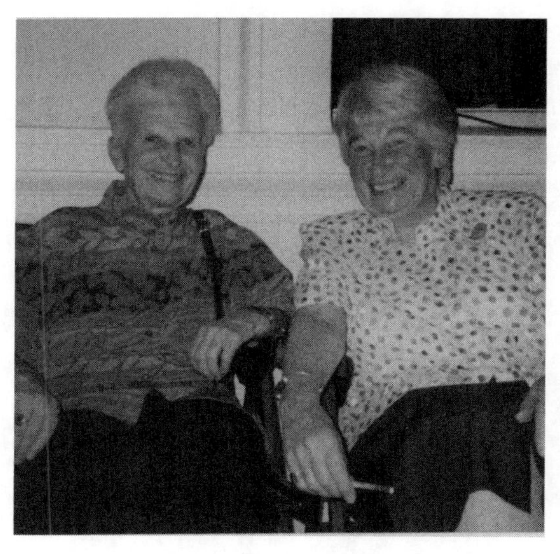

Elsbeth Köng and Mary Quinton

Acknowledgments

I've read that books are joint ventures and this one is perhaps more so than many others. This publication is the product of the collaboration of many people over a long period of time, and I cannot finish it without thanking those individuals who have been such a vital part of the process.

I wish to acknowledge the members of the task force and theory committee who, during their tenure in the past 12 years, provided ideas, insights, expertise, and interest. These clinicians and academicians willingly volunteered their time to develop the documents that served as the foundation for this manuscript. Under the chairmanship of Lois Bly, the task force originally included Lezlie Adler, Jan Allaire, Georgia DeGangi, Girard DeMauro, and Susan Ryerson. Over the years membership changed as other commitments took priority and the committee has included Zahava Alon, Judi Bierman, Linda Caldwell, Barbara Cupps, Suzanne Davis, Monica Diamond, Beth Fisher, Ann Guild, Jan Utley, Evangeline Yoder, and Laura Vogel.

Along the way, the task force received valuable direction and information from Suzann Campbell, Jim Gordan, Margaret Schenkman, and Cathy Tencza. Each of these consultants provided state-of-the-art expertise in various areas of current theory and models of practice.

Currently the theory committee, under co-chairs Judith Bierman and Lois Bly, includes Rona Alexander, Loren Arnaboldi, Barbara Cupps, Suzanne Davis, Monica Diamond, Clare Giuffrida, Mary Hallway, Cathy Hazzard, Helene Larin, Gail Ritchie, Marcia Stamer, and Shirley Stockmeyer. This is the committee that has collaborated with me and has my greatest respect for the commitment each has shown while working full-time as clinicians, NDT instructors, academicians, and family members. These people have dug through their files for references, copied articles, sent books from their professional libraries, thoughtfully responded to uncountable e-mails, redirected me when necessary, read and reread drafts of various chapters, shared their knowledge and experience, and gave liberally of their time and enthusiasm for the final project. I could not have done this without them.

Lois and Judi deserve special mention, Lois for her unconditional encouragement and guidance when my brain imploded or my lack of knowledge precipitated writer's block; for her words of wisdom as an author, colleague, and friend; and the many timely "smiley faces" she sent that I taped to the wall above my computer. She is far too modest about recognizing the contributions she makes to others. I didn't begin to tap the depth of her knowledge and expertise is so many areas.

If one person deserves credit for keeping this project alive, it is Judi Bierman, and for this, the entire committee thanks you. I find it impossible to recognize all of Judi's abilities and contributions. No other person contributed as much on a continuing basis as she has, providing much-needed emotional support, knowledge, and insights. My thank you to Judi for her many telephone consultations–sometimes almost daily–meetings, unfailing interest, and critiques of every draft of every chapter. I think she has read this manuscript as thoroughly as I have.

I also wish to recognize all the NDT instructors who were not on the theory committee but responded to my request for help and who had the interest and took the time to read and critique various chapters at various stages of development: Isabelle Bohman, Linda Caldwell, Lyndelle Owens, Joan Mohr, Pam Mullens, Mechthild Rast, and Mary Ann Sharkey.

I wish to acknowledge the families who participated in the photo case studies. I hope each family sincerely recognizes the importance of their contribution to improving the clinical practice by all professionals who read this book and to all the families who will benefit from their willingness to share their experiences: Mr. and Mrs. Ronald Winkler, Anna and Chaira Pride, and Caitlyn and her family. Thank you to Monica Diamond and Judi Bierman, their colleagues, and their facilities for their many hours photographing, assembling, and writing the case studies that so clearly illustrate the contributions that these families made.

I wish also to thank the NDTA board of directors and the NDTA office for their financial support and patience as this project continued so much longer than expected. Their belief that this project would enhance the standing of NDT in the scientific community was the backbone of it all. Our conference calls and committee meetings would not have taken place without their confidence in the end product, and the book would not be finished without opportunities for the committee and me to get together. E-mail just isn't enough.

I am indebted to Peggy Lang, my editor, and to Lois for directing me to her. I could not have asked for anyone with more skills, knowledge, or a better sense of humor than she has. I now understand those mushy remarks that authors make in the beginning of books regarding their relationship with their editor. This has certainly grown into a special one. I am a better person and this is a better book because Peggy shares herself and her expertise. Not only does she have editing skills, but considerable background and interest in scientific theory and therapeutic approaches to clients with CNS dysfunction. I would like to think this made the reading of this text more enjoyable or at least less frustrating for her. I know I benefited from her knowledgeable reading. My special thank you to you, Peggy, for your careful work with the many details of the text and all the references and your support of my new-author ego, as you politely and patiently managed my mangled verb tenses, run-on sentences, and excessive use of passive voice. If ever the insanity of writing another book overtakes me, I would do it only if you are available to work with me again.

This book would be less interesting without the efforts of graphic artist Claire Wenstrom. She willingly took on this project outside her normal workload with only a little pressure from her sister and committee member, Gail Ritchie. I particularly appreciate her interest in precise representation and her patience with me.

A special thank you to Becky North for pursuing those really hard-to-find references, obscure journals, and books, all while completing her PT studies at MUSC in Charleston. Becky, you saved me valuable time and frustration. I just wish I had hired you earlier.

Finally, I wish to give my personal mention to two very special persons, both of whom have contributed to the person I am today. I thank Suzann Campbell, who, since my graduate school days, has been my mentor and friend. On this project, she offered her expert advice on various aspects of writing and publishing, reading many drafts and providing timely feedback without hesitation. She did this solely based on interest, fitting this into a schedule that puts me constantly in awe. Sue, I can't thank you enough. Your words of support are also taped above my computer. I just hope in a small way I can mentor other professionals with the support you have always provided for me.

The other person who deserves special mention is my husband, Ed Howle. He was excited and proud of me when I was asked to take on this project. He helped me keep my life in balance and reminded me of my capabilities as a person and partner when I was consumed by this task. This support, respect and love has been the foundation of our relationship for more than 26 years, but I am reminded again just how special it is, as this project grows to a close. Now it is time to go sailing.

In Memory
Barbara A. Cupps
1948-2003

As we go to press with this book, it is with great sadness that we acknowledge the death of Barbara A. Cupps who contributed so much to the NDT approach by applying her knowledge and skills in teaching, and her intuition and problem-solving skills in clinical practice. In addition to these full time professional activities, Barb was an active member of the NDT theory committee, and contributed significantly and consistently to the writing and editing of this publication, particularly in the areas of postural control and principles of clinical practice. Our profession has lost a creative, insightful physical therapist. We will all miss her ability to balance reason with enthusiasm for the NDT approach in the same way that she balanced being a wife, a mother and energetic professional.

Contents

Foreword

As I write in April of 2002, the Neuro-Developmental Treatment Approach (NDT) is facing the challenge of defending its position as the primary approach to the treatment of motor dysfunction of cerebral palsy (CP) and as one of several preferred methods for the management of movement dysfunction following a cerebrovascular accident (CVA). Much of the controversy involving NDT over the past few years has been engendered by confusion about what NDT is and what about it is unique. The approach has been changing over time, as new theory is incorporated into the continuing education teaching of its advocates, but change has not been accompanied by regular publications in peer-reviewed journals and presentations at scientific meetings to which critics can easily gain access. This document is, therefore, a timely and welcome description of the theory behind NDT as it has evolved since its origins under the Bobaths in 1940s England. Janet Howle, working with the NDT theory committee of NDT instructors, clinicians, and academicians, has compiled not only current theory and the development of the theory, but also clarifies what remains from the Bobaths' original approach and what is unique to NDT among various current approaches to management of movement dysfunction. Her description of NDT concepts and theory takes into account contemporary motor control, motor development, and motor learning theory, as well as how the motor problems of clients with CP or CVA are viewed from the perspective of NDT. This publication makes it clear that NDT is first and foremost an approach to managing the impairments of these conditions, especially execution of motor synergies, postural control, and alignment. Additionally, individual chapters illustrate the problem-solving process that is basic to NDT and incorporates the treatment of impairments into intervention strategies designed to improve functional activities and participation in family and community life.

This document provides much food for thought. In addition to describing the clinical assumptions and principles of intervention, it provides information that can lead directly to a plan of action to examine the efficacy of NDT. First, because it clarifies what is currently considered unique to NDT, the publication allows one to identify those components of the treatment approach that should be documented as part of any intervention protocol under study that claims to test NDT against control or comparison conditions (which should not contain such elements). Second, it describes the outcomes expected from successful NDT treatment, including the ability to reduce primary impairments in postural alignment and anticipatory postural control, balance during dynamic movement activities, ineffective motor synergies during functional skills, and NDT's ability to reduce secondary musculoskeletal impairments that lead to contractures or deformities that hamper functional activities and cause painful orthopedic conditions later in life. Although progress has been made, problems related to measuring such outcomes must still be solved for such research to produce noncontroversial results. Controlled clinical trials with an untreated control group and blind assessment of outcomes are essential to proving the effectiveness of this approach.

I congratulate the NDTA on its publication of this contribution to the literature on NDT and urge that the Association use it to promote and support further research on the outcomes of NDT.

Suzann K. Campbell, PT, Ph.D.
Professor and Head
Department of Physical Therapy
University of Illinois at Chicago
Chicago, IL 60612

Preface

For the past 50 years, the Neuro-Developmental Treatment (NDT) approach has had a profound impact on managing the sensorimotor impairments of adults and children with neuropathology. NDT, first known as "The Bobath Approach," was originated and developed by Mrs. Berta Bobath, physiotherapist, and her husband, Dr. Karel Bobath, and was first described in the scientific literature in 1948 (B. Bobath, 1948).

The staying power of this approach is in the problem-solving analysis of posture and movement and the correlation of functional activities with underlying impairments. The Bobaths wrote, "Since we began our treatment in 1943 we have been learning constantly, and experience has taught us to change our approach and our emphasis on certain aspects of the treatment. . . . The basic concept has not changed. . . . We have been guided by the [client's] reactions and in this way we have improved our knowledge . . . and have learned to test the value of a particular technique by the [client's] response to it" (B. Bobath & K. Bobath, 1980, p. 7). Over the years, with experience, knowledge, and insight, the Bobaths changed many of their clinical methods and underlying assumptions to provide better solutions to clients' problems of motor control. The clinical approach evolved as the Bobaths learned more about clients' responses to their methods. More recently, the changes in the movement sciences have caused clinicians to question the underlying theoretical model of NDT. Now, advances in understanding the nature of movement–how it develops and is produced–provide more accurate answers to Mrs. Bobath's ongoing challenge, "Why does this work?"

Although many of the concepts of NDT are accepted today as common knowledge in the therapeutic community, the belief that a therapist could have an impact on a client's functional movement by influencing the central nervous system (CNS) through carefully guiding the motor output (and the sensory feedback from the movement) was a revolutionary idea in the late 1940s and early 1950s. At that time, the dominant therapeutic approach focused on changing function at the muscle level by identifying isolated muscle weakness and tightness and designing specific exercises to strengthen, stretch, or support these muscles. This was an effective technique for treating poliomyelitis, and polio was the most frequent reason that children and adults with problems of neurologic origin were referred for therapy (Pearson & Williams, 1972). Mary Quinton (personal communication, 1999) recalled that when she went to Malta as a physiotherapist during World War II, she was sent because of a polio epidemic among children. She had very little experience with children, none with babies, and here was a hospital with hundreds of infants with paralysis, a typical caseload for a therapist who wanted to work with children. (The adults had a natural immunity due to earlier outbreaks of the disease, but babies and young children did not.) Orthopedists were the leading medical managers of clients with polio because once this lower motor neuron disease was diagnosed and the patient survived the acute viral impact, the remaining problems were of an orthopedic nature (i.e., how to support a weak spine and extremities, stretch tightened muscles, and strengthen or substitute for any muscles with partial paralysis).

With the advances in prevention of polio through the Salk and Sabin vaccines, polio disappeared as a major cause of disability, and resources–both manpower and finances–became available for other clients with neuropathology. This change led to two problems. First, therapists, who were now more likely to see children or adults with cerebral palsy (CP) or stroke, found that their methods for treating polio were ineffective in solving the problems of these new clients. Second, physicians, mainly orthopedists, who directed the medical and therapeutic management of individuals with neuropathology, were not trained to identify and treat patients who had complicated motor control problems related to damage of the higher centers of the nervous system. At that time, physicians and therapists treated disorders such as CP and hemiplegia following stroke primarily from an orthopedic perspective, with surgery, bracing, and muscle reeducation.

New ideas often develop because old ones don't work, and therapists and physicians looked for new ways to solve their clients' problems. Among others, Mrs. Bobath challenged the belief that changing muscle strength and length would lead to improved function in children with CP or adults with hemiplegia following stroke, as it had in clients with polio (B. Bobath, 1948). She recognized that these individuals had weakness and tightness, but, more importantly, had a disorder of coordination of posture and movement (B. Bobath, 1953). In her thesis (B. Bobath, 1954), for which she was awarded a fellowship in the Chartered Society of Physiotherapists in England, Mrs. Bobath reported on 305 clients of whom 160 received treatment for 6 years. She hypothesized that a lesion in the CNS led to impairment of the coordination of muscle action and prevented these clients from gaining functional skills. She concluded that examination of the neurophysiological problems was helpful in determining the severity of individual cases, in planning treatment, and in assessing improvement. Through her astute clinical observations, and, by her own admission, trial and error, she realized that more normal movement patterns were possible and that therapists could assist the individual in gaining these movements by treating the impaired coordination.

The original philosophy, basic assumptions, and clinical concepts can be attributed directly to the Bobaths. To support their approach, Dr. Bobath expanded on the then-dominant neurophysiological theory with its hierarchical organization and reflex base. Even as they were developing their ideas, their work was enhanced by the clinical practice of Mary Quinton, physiotherapist, and Dr. Elsbeth Köng, pediatrician, who had trained with them in England. Quinton and Köng applied the Bobath principles to their practice with infants in Berne, Switzerland. Köng's work (1992) emphasized methods for early detection, even when definitive diagnosis was not possible. Quinton developed a specific approach for the treatment of infants based on her insights into the development of infants with and without CNS dysfunction. Quinton's experience and skills allowed her to detect differences in development of typical and atypical movements, and intervene prior to the establishment of abnormal posture and movement (Quinton & Wilson, 1981; Quinton, 2002). She developed treatment strategies addressing this "competition" between normal and abnormal patterns. The contributions from Dr. Köng and Ms. Quinton to the examination and management of at-risk infants have become a fundamental part of the Bobath approach.

Since the early days of the development of the Bobath Approach, numerous clinicians and instructors trained in the NDT approach have added new ideas and expanded the concepts of this approach. In order to differentiate between the ideas contributed by the Bobaths and the current information that combines their efforts with contributions from many others, this book will use the term *Bobath Approach* to denote the Bobaths' original concepts. Chapter 5 describes the history and development of these ideas. The name *Bobath Approach* or *Bobath Concept* is still used in many countries today to identify this treatment. The term *Neuro-Developmental Treatment Approach,* or *NDT*, is the name used by the North American Neuro-Developmental Treatment Association (NDTA) and will be used in this publication to describe the theory, assumptions, and intervention strategies accepted by the NDTA membership and used today (DeGangi & Royeen, 1994).

The Bobaths believed that pathology in the neural system was the source of greatest impairment in clients with stroke or CP, so they changed the name from *Bobath Approach* to *Neuro-Developmental Treatment Approach* in the 1960s, to place a greater emphasis on the neuropathology. Mrs. Bobath wrote, "So far the emphasis in treatment has been placed . . . on the developmental side of the problem. Although most people are aware . . . of the many symptoms of the neurological disorder and the effect . . . on the cerebral-palsied child's motor development . . . this aspect has been neglected in treatment, which (up until now) has been planned only by advancing the child's activities along developmental lines" (B. Bobath, 1963, p. 242).

The Bobaths emphasized an interactive process within an interdisciplinary team composed of the client and family; physical, occupational, and speech therapists; and the physician. In order to ensure a cohesive approach for the benefit of the client, the Bobaths began training medical professionals in advanced clinical education courses that included hands-on experience with clients and their families. Currently, NDT courses are available around the world for physical, occupational, and speech therapists working with children and adults with neuropathology and resulting sensorimotor dysfunction. In some countries, these courses include physicians and teachers as well. The training of the different disciplines together gives each discipline an appreciation of the other professions' roles and contributions to the care of the whole person.

Because of the many changes in movement sciences and the impact on the practice of NDT, in 1990 the NDTA board of directors charged the NDT Instructors Group with the tasks of first, reassessing the NDT approach along with data from the neural science and motor behavior fields, reflecting a new paradigm for examination and intervention; and second, developing a position paper defining the theoretical base of NDT from this new perspective. Lois Bly served as chairperson of a small interdisciplinary group. This was to be a 5-year project. As the scope of this work took shape, members of the group changed and in 1997 the task force became a standing committee. Various consultants were engaged over the years and in 2000, under the direction of Lois Bly and Judith Bierman, the theory committee organized a very successful conference as a first step in introducing the changing aspects of the theory accepted by the North American NDTA. This conference highlighted the enormous task still ahead of preparing this material in a single publication for NDT members and the scientific and therapeutic community. They contracted with Janet Howle to write and edit, in collaboration with the committee, a comprehensive publication that clearly and explicitly describes the current theoretical basis, operational assumptions, and principles that guide NDT intervention.

This publication describes how these ideas have evolved from the original Bobath concepts and how they continue today to form a cohesive and well-defined set of principles that guide intervention strategies. Whenever possible, this book includes the clinical and scientific research that supports and promotes the standards of practice of NDT.

The NDT theory committee and the NDTA hope that the outcome of the task reflects the spirit of the Bobaths' legacy and will serve to guide clinical practice and form testable hypotheses that can validate the efficacy of this approach to improve the care of individuals with CNS pathology.

References

Bobath, B. (1948). The importance of the reduction of muscle tone and the control of mass reflex action in the treatment of spasticity. *Occupational Therapy and Rehabilitation, 27* (5), 371-383.

Bobath, B. (1953). Control of posture and movement in the treatment of CP. *Physiotherapy, 39* (5), 99-104.

Bobath, B. (1954, September/December). A study of abnormal postural reflex activities in patients with lesions of the central nervous system. *Physiotherapy, 40* (9), 10-11.

Bobath, B. (1963). A neuro-developmental treatment of CP. *Physiotherapy,* 242-245.

Bobath, K. (1980). *A neurophysiological basis for the treatment of cerebral palsy.* Philadelphia: J. B. Lippincott.

DeGangi, G., & Royeen, C. B. (1994). Current practice among Neuro-Developmental Treatment Association members. *American Journal of Occupational Therapy, 48* (1),803-809.

Köng, E. (1992). Early detection of cerebral motor disorders. In H. Forssberg & H. Hirschfeld (Eds.), *Movement disorders in children* (vol. 36, pp. 80-85). Basel, Switzerland: Medicine and Sport Science/Karger.

Pearson, P. H., & Williams, C. E. (1972). *Physical therapy services in the developmental disabilities.* Springfield, IL: Charles C Thomas.

Quinton, M., & Wilson, J. (1981). Competition of movement patterns applied to the development of infants. In D. Slaton & J. Wilson (Eds.), *Caring for special babies* (pp. 164-172).Chapel Hill: Division of Physical Therapy, University of North Carolina-Chapel Hill.

Quinton, M. (2002). *Making the difference with babies: Concepts and guidelines for baby treatment.* Albequerque. NM: Clinician's View.

Chapter 1

Current Theoretical Foundations

> "I would implore you to push . . . on. We've given you what we know. Whenever I teach, the first thing I say; look, learn, . . . look at other methods . . . we hand you the torch. We have achieved what we set out to achieve in one lifetime." (K. Bobath & B. Bobath, 1979, p. 6)

Development and Philosophy

In the United States, the Neuro-Developmental Treatment approach (NDT) is the most commonly used model for therapeutic management and treatment of children with cerebral palsy (CP) and a regularly used model for adults with hemiplegia following stroke (Cherry & Knutson, 1993; Hayes, McEwen, Lovett, Sheldon, & Smith, 1999; Sweeney, Heriza, & Mrakowitz, 1994). The basic philosophy underlying all the assumptions of this approach is that lesions in the central nervous system (CNS) produce problems in the coordination of posture and movement combined with atypical qualities of muscle tone that contribute directly to functional limitations (K. Bobath & B. Bobath, 1984). Like the Bobaths, NDT clinicians believe that these functional limitations are changeable when intervention strategies target specific system impairments in activities and contexts that are meaningful in the life of the person. From the beginning, the Bobaths believed, as NDT clinicians do today, that much of the disability that these individuals face is related, directly or indirectly, to their posture and movement dysfunction (Bierman, 1989; K. Bobath & B. Bobath, 1956).

NDT is a concept that focuses on the strengths and impairments of the individual client rather than a prescribed treatment of exercise. Clinicians systematically analyze impairments within a framework that includes the neurological and body systems and, in the case of CP, the developmental aspects of these systems. Therapists who use NDT observe and analyze each client's functional skills and limitations to determine the best choice of intervention strategies for that client. Clinicians believe that goal-directed examination and intervention leads to the best functional outcome that minimizes impairments and prevents secondary disability (Mayston 2001). Treatment is a problem-solving concept that allows for a wide variety of strategies flexible enough to be adapted to the impairments of the individual client (B. Bobath, 1990). In addition, NDT clinicians maintain that therapeutic handling is integral to the NDT approach. Facilitating movements with a hands-on approach is a natural part of interactions between two persons, and therapists use facilitation techniques in a carefully applied manner to establish or reestablish the postures and movements that will enhance the individual's capacity to carry out meaningful life roles. NDT clinicians believe that this approach will continue to grow and thrive as clinical experience and scientific inquiry supply new information.

Over the years, the Bobaths made many changes in their approach, and alterations continue today. The clinical practice of NDT evolved as the Bobaths questioned and challenged their own clinical concepts and scientific theory. Chapter 5 describes the development of the Bobaths' thinking, to give the student of NDT a feeling for the evolution of this approach and a point of reference from which to understand that NDT is still evolving. The Bobaths discarded the belief that voluntary movement was built on reflexive movement and that treatment must follow the normal developmental sequence. Currently NDT therapists accept that neural control is not a simple hierarchical function and that, along with the nervous system, multiple body systems participate in executing movement that is organized by the specific task and constrained by physical laws and the environment. There is recognition that both feed-forward and feedback sensory mechanisms are equally important in different types of movement control. Clinicians expect the client to participate actively in treatment, taking part in goal setting and initiating and completing movements directed toward function. Although the Bobaths always emphasized carryover into daily life activities, intervention is now overtly directed toward functional objectives in real-life settings.

These examples demonstrate how new knowledge has been working its way into this still-maturing method. Currently, clinicians are reexamining the concepts of clinical practice within the context of models of motor control, motor development, and motor learning to form testable hypotheses that can withstand the rigors of scientific inquiry. There is still a great deal to learn about the complicated issues of movement in individuals with and without neuropathology.

If so much has changed, what remains that defines NDT as a unique approach to the examination and treatment of individuals with CNS neuropathology? And what sets NDT apart from other approaches? The answer is that NDT continues to be a problem-solving approach to system impairments and provides clinicians with flexible guidelines for selecting treatment strategies integrated in their various fields of specialization to manage the individual functional problems of infants, children, and adults. These basic ideas began with the Bobaths, evolved with their increasing knowledge, and continue to expand with the emergence of contemporary models of motor control, motor development, and motor learning.

NDT Redefined

NDT is a problem-solving approach to the examination and treatment of the impairments and functional limitations of individuals with neuropathology, primarily children with CP and adults with stroke or traumatic brain injury (TBI). These individuals have dysfunction in posture and movement that lead to limitations in functional activity. NDT focuses on the analysis and treatment of sensorimotor impairments and functional limitations that physical, occupational, and speech therapies can address.

A thorough examination and evaluation is the basis for treatment. The examination begins with the identification of an individual's abilities and limitations. The NDT approach considers the individual as a whole and recognizes that every expression of the person–psychological, emotional, cognitive, perceptual, and physical–has value and contributes to the overall level of function. Examination focuses on identifying functions and their limitations. Evaluation analyzes and prioritizes the effectiveness of posture and movement and the body systems that affect function. Examination and evaluation lead to the establishment of treatment goals and the development of treatment strategies commensurate with the individual's current needs, while aiming for the long-term outcome of achieving the best possible inclusion in society across the life span through improving the client's perceptual-motor performance.

The NDT clinician's understanding of typical movement and how it changes across the life span provides a critical framework for problem solving and treatment planning. In addition, the clinician must anticipate the progression of atypical postures and movements and understand how they develop from limited neuronal repertoires, the individual's unique movement experiences and the attempt to compensate with stereotyped movement strategies. The clinician plans treatment in partnership with the client and meaningful persons in the individual's life. Implementation of treatment depends on the examination and evaluation outcomes, the client's competencies and integrity, and the limitations of the multiple internal systems and external resources. The clinician constantly guides and modifies treatment according to the individual's response to the selected strategies.

Therapeutic handling is integral to the NDT approach. It is an essential tool in both examination and treatment. Therapeutic handling allows the therapist to (a) feel the client's response to changes in posture or movement, (b) facilitate postural control and movement synergies that broaden the client's options for selecting successful actions, (c) provide boundaries for movements that distract from the goal, and (d) inhibit or constrain those motor patterns that, if practiced, lead to secondary deformities, further disability, or decreased participation in society.

The clinician selects the appropriate model of service and treatment intervention strategies that will fit the client's lifestyle, then helps to integrate the activities developed in treatment into the client's daily life to broaden the contexts for carryover. Active carryover, which is essential for motor learning, requires practice by the client throughout the day, independently or with caregivers.

As a result of NDT intervention, the individual will use the new or regained posture or movement strategies to carry out life skills more efficiently. These strategies will minimize secondary impairments that can create additional functional limitations or disability.

The NDT approach continues to be enriched with the new information, new theories, and new models that are emerging in the movement sciences. In addition, as the characteristics of the populations with CNS pathophysiology change, the approach will continue to evolve to meet their needs.

General Assumptions in the NDT Approach

The NDT approach continues to accept the following ten assumptions that originated with the work of the Bobaths:

1. **Impaired patterns of postural control and movement coordination are the primary problems in clients with CP or stroke.** This impaired coordination is somewhat predictable and is the direct or indirect result of neuropathology of the CNS, complicated by the intrinsic characteristics of the individual, including genetic makeup, morphology, motivation, prior perceptual-motor experiences, and environmental demands and the stage of neural recovery.

2. **These identifiable system impairments are changeable and overall function improves when the problems of motor coordination are treated by directly addressing neuromotor and postural control abnormalities in a task-specific context.** The NDT approach recognizes that continued maladaptive performance can result in increasing impairments, new impairments, and other pathophysiologies such as compromised cardiorespiratory function or joint and muscle contractures and deformities. This occurs because repeated practice strengthens the possibility of selecting maladaptive synergies and applying them to a wide variety of tasks.

3. **Sensorimotor impairments affect the whole individual–the person's function, place in the family and community, independence, and overall quality of life.** Atypical posture and movement are an expression of that individual and can affect the person's body image, adaptation to the environment, and sense of self in life roles. The perception of "disabled" can become so ingrained that even when more typical expressions are possible, they do not carry over into life roles.

4. **A working knowledge of typical adaptive motor development and how it changes across the life span provides the framework for assessing functions and planning intervention.** NDT therapists recognize that there are general patterns in the acquisition and timing of skills during development and maturation, and loss of some skills during aging. These consistencies provide a standard of reference for proficient human motor function and make it possible to identify the differences in individuals, both normal deviations and atypical, maladaptive motor development.

5. **NDT clinicians focus on changing movement strategies as a means to achieve the best energy-efficient performance for the individual within the context of age-appropriate tasks and in anticipation of future functional tasks.** Quality includes accuracy, quickness, adaptability, and fluency. In particular, the focus is on the musculoskeletal alignment of body parts relative to the base of support (BOS) and to other body parts prior to and during a movement sequence, as well as on the complex neural components of movement synergies. Normal movement is the ability to link a number of behaviors together, to do more than one thing at a time, and to perform tasks effectively under a variety of conditions. For this reason, NDT treatment includes practice with slightly different versions of the same task.

6. **Movement is linked to sensory processing in two distinct ways.** From the inception of NDT, the Bobaths identified sensory information as playing an important role in modifying motor responses. They believed that movement activates sensory receptors through a feedback control model. Feedback from muscles, movements,

and the environment also contributes to the detection of errors, comparing and correcting movement as it occurs to reach a goal. Currently, the NDT approach also includes the concept of feed-forward or anticipatory control, in which rapid complex movements and automatic postural reactions require anticipatory sensory information to prepare and initiate postural and movement requirements of the task in advance of the motor act (Keele & Summers, 1976; Kelso, 1976; Stelmach, 1976). In real-life situations, functional movement uses feedback and feed-forward systems simultaneously to respond to the dynamics of the physical world. NDT therapists recognize that it is not possible to teach sensory feed-forward, but they can structure the task and provide the best alignment prior to motor execution so that the client experiences an optimal anticipatory position and benefits from linking posture with the movement outcome (Bly, 1996).

7. **Intervention strategies involve the individual's active initiation and participation, often combined with the therapist's manual guidance and direct handling.** The clinician uses direct handling to facilitate postural alignment and movement synergies that enhance the individual's capacity to select and achieve successful motor outcomes. Direct handling also provides boundaries, inhibiting or controlling those movement components that interfere with efficient action, components that, if practiced, contribute to secondary deformities or further disability.

8. **NDT intervention utilizes movement analysis to identify missing or atypical elements that link functional limitations to system impairments.** Clinicians identify components of movement in the musculoskeletal system, observing movement in all three planes (for example, flexion/extension in the sagittal plane, lateral flexion and abduction/adduction in the frontal plane, and rotation in the transverse plane). In addition, the therapist identifies biomechanical components of a movement, including base of support (BOS), the center of gravity/center of mass (COM) alignment, weight shift, and range of motion (ROM) throughout a functional sequence. Clinicians then combine this information with analysis of neural components of movement and contributions from other body systems and contextual elements.

9. **Ongoing evaluation occurs throughout every treatment session.** This was a very important concept for the Bobaths. The therapist assesses the treatment strategies and outcomes according to the client's response to the various strategies used in the therapeutic setting. The clinician then modifies the treatment strategies based on the client's level of success in meeting the system and motor goals and functional outcomes set for the single session.

10. **The aim of NDT intervention is to optimize function.** Optimal outcomes are achieved when intervention occurs during periods of development and recovery, prior to the establishment of atypical postures and movement (K. Bobath & B. Bobath, 1984). NDT clinicians accept that plasticity and neural reorganization capacity occur throughout life and that recovery can take place at any period during the life span of an individual. There are periods of stable organization of movement, as well as transitions in the organization that result in the development of new or

compensatory movement strategies. During these periods of transition, the individual is more receptive to change through intervention or other influences (Thelen, 1994). The therapist assesses outcome by measuring changes in the success and efficiency the individual achieves in expanding his or her function that enhances participation in society and independence in life roles (K. Bobath & B. Bobath, 1984).

These ten assumptions are the characteristics that identify and separate NDT from other approaches. These ideas were set forth by the Bobaths and have been modified over the past 50 years to reflect changes in emphasis and terminology (see Chapter 5). The additional assumptions (11-19) that are part of NDT best practice standards have been incorporated more recently from the motor sciences to complete the current therapeutic model of NDT.

11. **NDT accepts that human motor behavior/function emerges from ongoing interactions among multiple internal systems of the individual, the characteristics of the task, and the specific environmental context, each contributing different aspects of motor control (Bernstein, 1967; Kelso, 1984; Thelen, Kelso, & Fogel, 1987).** The control of movement includes the individual's neuromuscular, sensory, musculoskeletal, regulatory, cognitive/perceptual, integumentary, cardiovascular, respiratory, and gastrointestinal systems. The importance of each system (and its subsystems) changes continuously before and during a movement, as determined by the goal of the movement, the strategy that the individual uses to accomplish the goal, and the environmental context in which the action takes place. The will of the individual, his or her motivation, the nature of the task, and the environment, all present powerful incentives (or disincentives) for movement.

12. **Movement is organized around behavioral goals.** In motor planning, multiple systems are organized according to the inherent requirements of the task being performed and the current status (postural, motivational, emotional, cognitive, and so forth) of the individual. NDT recognizes that, on the one hand, the *same function* can result from quite different movements while, on the other, the *same movement* might occur for a variety of reasons.

13. **All individuals have competencies and strengths in various systems.** In the NDT approach, examination and treatment identify these strengths, place the focus on the individual's capabilities, and utilize these strengths to build a framework for solving specific functional problems.

14. **A hallmark of efficient human motor function is the ability of the individual to select and match various global neuronal maps with a potentially infinite number of movement combinations that are attuned to the forces of gravity, forces generated by contracting muscles, and constraints posed by a variety of environmental conditions (Bernstein, 1967; Latash, 1998; Sporns, Tononi, & Edelman, 2000).** The individual must have a broad range of posture and movement experiences under a wide variety of environmental conditions to efficiently link the requirements of postural stability, movement strategies, sensory processing, cognition, and memory before and during an action. Varying the environmental constraints

and requirements of various body systems provides increased opportunity to teach individuals to organize and select their own strategies to solve motor problems.

15. **NDT uses the model of enablement/disablement based on the *International Classification of Function 2001* developed by the World Health Organization (2001) to categorize the individual's health and disability.** The NDT model organizes the information about the pathology of stroke (CVA) and CP and adds a dimension of motor function and dysfunction to the ICIDH-2 model that includes system integrity or impairments, function or activity limitations, and participation or restrictions in life. The use of this model allows the clinician to clarify the impact of pathology on various dimensions of the individual and also classifies the impact of intervention on the different dimensions, so that outcome measures can be more exact.

16. **Clinicians can best design intervention by establishing functional outcomes in partnership with the client and caregivers.** Treatment acknowledges that every person, with or without disability, changes during the progression from infancy through adulthood. Treatment planning and execution consider the client's age, capabilities, needs, and values within the constellation of family and community.

17. **Intervention programs are designed to serve clients throughout their lifetime**. With this longitudinal perspective, the therapist must establish goals, outcomes, and methods that are appropriate for the present, consider past experiences, and hypothesize future directions. NDT clinicians must provide clients and their families with the available evidence related to intervention, so that they can make informed decisions and take responsibility for directing the quality of their own lives (Campbell, 1997).

18. **Learning or relearning motor skills and improving performance requires both practice and experience.** Practice by the client, independently or with supervision, is essential for learning (Larin, 2000). Only through experimentation and practice will clients learn to solve their own motor problems. Therapeutic handling can help the client establish options for efficient function, but only by trial and error will the client make the posture and movement his own. NDT provides sufficient time to practice in real-life situations so that new movement becomes part of the individual's body scheme.

19. **Treatment is most effective during recovery or phase transitions.** These are periods before the person has experienced and used atypical posture and movement to the extent that these factors limit the variety of movement options, or during times of increased variability and instability of posture and movement due to growth, development, new experience or recovery from neural insult. NDT recognizes that plasticity of the neural system continues throughout the life span with phases of stability interspersed with phases of instability. These periods of transition are the times that intervention can promote and direct efficient motor patterns as the client is working out new ways to reinvent efficient movement in increasingly complex contexts.

20. **NDT clinicians assume the responsibility to provide clients with the available evidence related to all intervention methods, outcomes and service delivery systems.** This assures that each client can make informed decisions regarding optimal care that fit their lifestyle, priorities and personal goals.

NDT from a New Theoretical Perspective

The North American NDTA Theory Committee has worked to develop a theoretical model for NDT clinicians that organizes these basic assumptions and clinical methods to address changes in thinking about motor control, motor development, and motor learning. Some parts of this theory have been published in the *NDT Network* (Bierman, 1989; Birkmeier, 1997; Bly, 1996; Cupps, 1997; Rast, 2000). The theoretical model on which the clinical practice of NDT is currently based assimilates and synthesizes information from many areas of science to use the best available knowledge to support clinical decision making and clinical practice.

The acceptance of a revised theoretical base has resulted from the acknowledgment that the hierarchical/reflex model on which Dr. Bobath based the original Bobath Approach offered only limited explanation for the changes in the practice of NDT. By 1990, at which time the Bobaths were no longer contributing to the development of this approach, they had already made considerable changes in the treatment. This is a point not always acknowledged even in the current literature (Fowler, Ho, Nwigwe, & Dorey, 2001), due in part to the fact that, although they changed treatment, the Bobaths did not offer theoretical explanations that kept pace with the changes in clinical practice, and also because alternative neuroscientific explanations had not been widely published in the clinical literature.

The neurophysiological basis of the Bobath Approach used the work of others to provide insights into the neural processes thought to be responsible for movement. The accepted reflex/hierarchical model from Jackson (1932/1958) and Sherrington (1947) assumed that the CNS was "hard-wired," with clear separations of high-level voluntary control and low-level reflexive control. Change occurred only as the various levels of neural integration matured or recovered after damage to the CNS. (See Chapter 5 for discussion of the hierarchical model.) In spite of this popular theory, the Bobaths adopted a much more flexible view of the CNS that was still based on the hierarchical/reflex model, however, they also believed that it was possible to produce change in the CNS through intervention techniques. Nevertheless, this model did not provide the multidimensional distribution of neural control now accepted by NDT therapists. Other models, particularly systems models and neuronal selection models, seem to provide more accurate descriptions of the clinical concepts. The theoretical model of NDT described in this chapter represents a unification of models based on sound scientific and clinical research by neuroscientists and other investigators such as Bernstein (1967), Bradley (2000), Edelman (1987), Giuliani (1991), Horak (1991), Keele & Summers (1976), Kelso (1992), Schmidt & Lee (1999), Sporns & Edelman (1993), and Thelen, Kelso, & Fogel (1987) and applied in a therapeutic-intervention framework by Campbell (1994, 2000b), Carr & Shepherd (2000), Hadders-Algra (2000), Heriza (1991), Scholz (1990), Shumway-Cook & Woollacott (2001), and Tscharnuter (2002), among others.

NDT continues to be an evolving theoretical approach. Dr. Bobath frequently used the term "living concept" to convey the idea that these concepts are working hypotheses (K. Bobath & B. Bobath, 1979). The teaching and writings of the Bobaths in the late 1980s to 1990 already represented significant changes in the approach, incorporating many of the ideas expressed in systems theory, such as the importance of the task and the environment, the role of a feed-forward mechanism, and directing treatment to functional outcomes (B. Bobath, 1990). In the introduction to the third edition of *Adult Hemiplegia: Evaluation and Treatment* (1990), Mrs. Bobath wrote, "More than ever before, all treatment is done in real life situations with the use of furniture which the patient has in his own home. . . . In this way the patient learns the all important lesson that what he does in treatment is part of his daily routine" (p. x).

Over the past decade, the understanding of the mechanisms of movement execution has expanded immensely. Theories in motor control, motor learning, and motor development have added to the knowledge base of a very complex topic that Bernstein (1967) described as the "science of human movement" (Whiting, 1984). This next section examines the contributions of each of these areas and describes their relevance to changes in theoretical and clinical aspects of NDT.

Models of Interactive Systems

Systems perspectives and, even more recently, selectionist perspectives of motor control have gained acceptance as appropriate models with which to study human motor behavior. These models emphasize process (How does motor behavior occur?), rather than product (What is efficient motor behavior?). These models accept that in order to understand the neural control of movement, it is also necessary to understand the influence of other body systems, the specific task that organizes the motor components, and the environmental context within which the action occurs. In addition, control of movement depends on the interactions of variables within a single body system and between internal and external systems.

The model of systems interaction illustrated by Chiel and Beer (1997) is helpful in visualizing this concept (Figure 1.1).

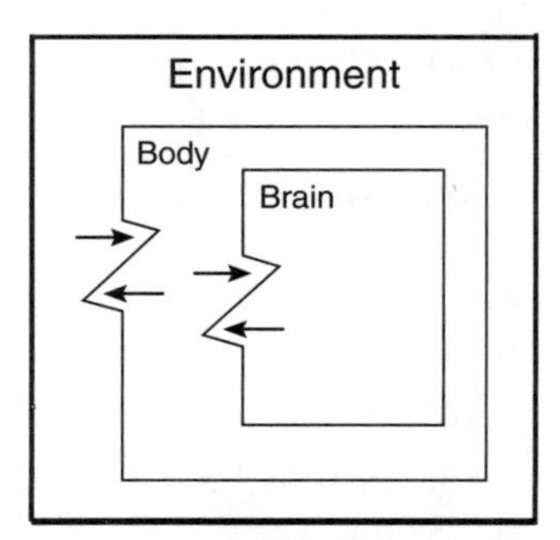

Figure 1.1. The nervous system is contained in the body that is contained in the environment. Each system is a rich, complicated, highly structured, dynamic system coupled to each other, producing constraints and opportunities for motor behavior. (Redrawn with permission from Chiel & Beer, 1997, p. 554.)

NDT Focus: NDT recognizes that the control of posture and movement relies on the interactions of many elements of various neural and body systems, the purpose of the task, the individual, and the context.

The following premises form a broad context in which to understand how the assumptions of NDT can be supported in a theoretical framework that includes selectionist and system perspective models. These premises can apply to movement of individuals with and without neuropathology. Later sections of this chapter cover additional premises related to motor development and motor learning.

NDT acknowledges that:

1. The ensemble of the brain and body systems is dynamically organized into interactive structures and functions that are determined by individual genetic characteristics, development, contextual learning, and environmental laws (Chiel & Beer, 1997). Self-generated exploration and the continuous processing of afferent information gradually results in selection and assembly of the most effective, variable, and adaptive motor behavior that meets the needs of the individual at a particular point in life (Thelen & Ulrich, 1991). For example, early reaching behavior includes swiping and batting with little directional or intentional outcome. As the infant explores and experiments over many months, this motor ensemble takes on timing and spatial characteristics of adult reaching. This mature ensemble includes not only muscles, joints, and neuronal components, but also vision, postural control, and object perception (Thelen et al., 1993; von Hofsten, Vishton, Spelke, Feng, & Fosander, 1998).

2. Multiple intrinsic and extrinsic variables establish a context for movement initiation and execution. Following Chiel and Beer's (1997) model, intrinsic variables of the nervous system, which depend on genetic constraints and developmental selection, include sensory, perceptual/cognitive, regulatory, and limbic (arousal, attention, and motivation) systems for stimulus identification, response selection, and patterns of neural activation to regulate and scale the force, onset, timing, direction, speed, sequence, and velocity of general action synergies of agonists, antagonists, and synergists.

   In addition to processing inputs and outputs from the nervous systems, intrinsic variables of the musculoskeletal system include muscle power and mass, extensibility, and tone; skeletal alignment; and joint ROM. Biomechanical characteristics include variables in body mass, size, structure and growth parameters, mechanical and compressive forces, weight bearing, and genetic makeup.

   Extrinsic variables (the environment) include the characteristics of the specific task, such as novelty or difficulty; relationship of the target to the body; need for speed, power, precision, and coordination for execution; the physical setting, including persons in it, and physical forces such as gravity, friction, and inertia. NDT assumes that, in individuals with neuropathology, identifiable changes in these variables affect the individual's ability to produce movement that is efficient, functional, and adaptive.

3. Intrinsic and extrinsic variables are involved in prior planning as well as shaping the features of a movement as it unfolds. These variables, which reside in the individual or within the environment, can constrain movement at one time and support it at another. They change throughout the life span and from moment to moment and can have significant influence on movement outcome during transition periods or little influence during nontransitional periods (Heriza, 1991). Intrinsic variables change with development, maturation, experience, practice, fatigue, therapeutic intervention, aging, disability, disease, or learning. Extrinsic variables change with the physical environment (home versus school, snow versus sand) or the persons in the environment (or missing from it) (e.g., new teacher, change in therapist, birth of a sibling, or addition of a step-parent). Loss by death, divorce, or moving also changes the external variables. Relationships with these persons (e.g., supportive, caring, competitive, or critical) constrain or contribute to changes in the external variables. NDT utilizes these variables to influence outcomes, adapting intervention to account for age and specific client characteristics, and provide a supportive environment and client-therapist relationship (Mayston, 1992).

4. The human motor system shows adaptability and flexibility in the presence of continually changing environmental tasks. The regulation (initiation and execution) and expression of movement possibilities does not lie in any one system or subsystem but is organized to effectively and efficiently utilize the elements of multiple systems that offer the best solution for the individual at that time, conserving power and energy (Kamm, Thelen, & Jenson, 1990; Morris, Summers, Matyas, & Lansek, 1994; Ryerson & Levit, 1997). Systems are assembled in the most efficient way within the contextual framework to accomplish a specific task or goal. The interactions of multiple systems are represented and strengthened in interconnected neuronal global maps based on use and purpose. For example, withdrawal from painful stimuli does not require precise coordination or independence of any one joint. This action requires only selection of a few neural groups that regulate activity of mass intralimb synergistic action at the musculoskeletal level. Contrast this mass action synergy with the precision and control needed to dance with the New York City Ballet. This skill requires regulation by multiple neural networks, quickly changing stability and mobility, precise postural control, strength and power, visual and spatial attention to self, use of sensory feed-forward and feedback as the dance is executed, and sensitivity to the forces of gravity, friction of the support surface, lighting, and other moving dancers in the environmental context. No wonder these performers are breathtaking! NDT recognizes this ongoing need to modify and adapt the organization of movement as one of the greatest problems confronting the individual with CNS impairment. The Bobaths wrote that the client with neuropathology is unable to modify, change, or use movement patterns in selective and varied ways with precision while adapting to the demands of the environment (K. Bobath & B. Bobath, 1956).

5. Any one or more of the various systems and subsystems can be rate-limiting or constraining to the performance of any specific behavior at a specific time. Subsystems develop at their own rate, but each is constrained or supported by physical and environmental factors, such as fitness, growth of various body segments over time, or the opportunity to practice (Edelman, 1989). Rate-limiting factors are present in the subsystems of the nervous system, the body, and the environment. For example, in children who are developing typically, the large mass of the infant's head in proportion to the body places constraints on the functions that are possible. Lifting the head and sustaining its upright position while the body is prone entails coordinating the neck, trunk, and extremities to create a stable base for head movements (Edelman, 1989). Another example demonstrates that strength and postural control do not develop at the same rate. A 4-month-old infant can support full body weight while standing **only if** external support is provided for balance. It will be many additional months before the rate of development of postural control in a standing position will catch up with the development of strength and these variables come together to allow independent standing and walking (Hadders-Algra, 2000; Sveistrup & Woollacott, 1997). In the adult, walking or running might be limited by muscle strength or cardiovascular endurance. This premise suggests that specific rate-limiting factors can be identified and manipulated therapeutically to produce change in motor abilities (Darrah & Bartlett, 1995), and that specific components of a task might have to be prepared before the task can be performed or practiced as a whole, an important aspect of NDT intervention.

6. Systems and their subsystems organize movement within a stable range of behaviors. Disruption of this steady state can result from normal growth and development, aging, or recovering from pathology such as joint replacement, muscle paralysis, and neuropathology. This disruption produces transient variability in movement strategies, followed by reorganization in which new or compensatory strategies develop and a new state of equilibrium is sought. An example is the child with hemiplegia who can walk with a flat-foot pattern but during periods of growth (when muscle length does not keep up with skeletal growth) walks up on the toes on the hemiplegic side. Normal periods of transition or instability are a part of systems in flux and are viewed as opportunities to manipulate the system toward a more favorable outcome (Byl et al., 1997). In NDT intervention, therapeutic handling takes advantage of situations in which patterns of movement are unstable, to assist the reorganization of the system. In addition to specific treatment strategies, other ways to take advantage of instability might include intensifying intervention following growth periods, after orthopedic surgery, during the emergence of new motor milestones, or during the spontaneous recovery process following stroke (Campbell, Vander Linden, & Palisano, 2000; Heriza, 1991). Optimizing outcomes for children with CP or adults with stroke by altering the intensity of treatment during periods of system instability is an important treatment principle of NDT (B. Bobath, 1990).

7. The internal components (such as; neural networks, sensory, and musculoskeletal systems) and external context of the task are equally important in determining the

outcome of behavior because behavior is task-specific. For example, cortical activity is necessary for the more discrete aspects of motor control of the hand (Muir & Lemon, 1983), but if the body is not sufficiently stable to support the reaching hand, or if the object does not spark interest, reaching still might not occur (Beauregard, Thomas, & Nelson, 1988). Motivation itself makes multiple contributions to the control of movement and meaningfulness of the task and can alter the strategy an individual uses to reach for an object (Van der Weel, van der Meer, & Lee, 1991; von Hofsten, 1991). The occupational therapy aspect of NDT in particular has contributed to recognizing the importance of structuring the environment with meaningful, age-appropriate tasks so that movement is initiated by the client or optimally facilitated by the therapist (Blanche & Hallway, 1998; Dunn, Brown, & McGuigan, 1994; Giuffrida, 1998).

8. New behaviors can emerge that are properties of interacting systems belonging to two separate individuals linked by a common environment (Mayston, 1992). Imagine the choice of evasive movements that are available to a hockey player. The unfolding behavior depends on the player's own skill in practiced maneuvers as well as the changing postures and movements of the other team members, resulting in a unique, spontaneous strategy of movement that emerges because the two individuals interact through a common environment (the ice rink and the moving puck). In another example, the NDT therapist has learned and practiced many handling skills utilizing various key points of control to facilitate movement, but the strategies and modifications the therapist makes during any one treatment session depend on how that client moves with respect to the specific goal. The therapist spontaneously alters assistance, leading or following the client, integrating skill and intuition. This spontaneous improvisation is an important factor in producing successful movement and is a key difference between experienced and novice therapists (Embry & Adams, 1996). (This inability to separate the changes of strongly linked yet independent systems is one of the reasons why research on the effectiveness of NDT is so difficult to document. The therapist influences the behavior and actions of the client just as the client influences the therapist.) Because this ability to improvise is so important, NDT courses include practical experience in applying movement strategies during practice with adults with stroke and children with CP, under the guidance of experienced clinical teachers.

9. The variables in any of the cooperating systems can be manipulated to produce significant changes in motor behavior. Changes in motor behavior or skill performance occur as a consequence of changes in one or more variables that add to or subtract from the expression of an action. For example, *adding* stability to the trunk by using an adapted chair with trunk supports, improves respiration in the child with CP (Alexander, Cupps, & Boehme, 1993). *Removing* stiffness by selective dorsal rhizotomy improves joint range and muscle length (Wilson, 1989 Ross, Engsberg, Wagner and Park 2002). *Removing* some of the body weight through a suspension system improves gait characteristics in adults with hemiplegia and children with CP

(Hesse, Bertelt, Schaffrin, Malezic, & Mauritz, 1994; Schindl, Forstner, Kern, & Hesse, 2000). *Adding* weight bearing through the upper extremities (UEs) improves performance in several reach and release components in children with CP (Barnes, 1986, 1989; Chakerian & Larson, 1991). This research supports the NDT assumption that guiding motor output through therapeutic handling can change the client's strategies, leading to more effective motor behavior. This hypothesis underlies the intervention strategy of therapist-facilitated movement in NDT. The Bobaths maintained that inhibiting unwanted patterns of movement and controlling the speed, timing, and direction of motor output helped to develop the most appropriate neural pathways to encourage maximal use of returning and developing functions. This concept has been a basis for the clinical methods since the inception of NDT in 1943 (K. Bobath & B. Bobath, 1979; Valvano & Long, 1991; M. Mayston, 2001).

10. Each movement is not entirely new because it is based on previous experiences and exploration, the strength of neuronal groups, learning, and practice. Neither is any movement exactly like any other, because all systems involved in producing any movement are affected simultaneously by what came before, the selection of interconnected neuronal groups, and the need to adapt to constraints imposed by the body systems and the environmental context of the task. This premise provides the context for two assumptions of NDT: (a) the need to understand previous adaptive or maladaptive experiences and their affect on currently occurring movement strategies, and (b) the impact of typical growth, aging, or neuropathology on the individual's body systems.

Can the practice of NDT be better understood within this context? Accepting these premises represents a change in orientation and emphasis in both theory and practice. They demonstrate that NDT has discarded the idea that the CNS is *the* most important aspect of motor control and singularly responsible for the appearance of abnormal posture and movement in clients with CNS damage. NDT intervention strategies take into account the movement, the purpose, the individual, and context. It is impossible for the clinician to understand purposeful movement without considering the current state of the body and its relationship to external context. There is much that we do not know about the control of movement in normal systems. We know less about the development and control of movement in children and adults with motor dysfunction. Exploring these areas from a new theoretical perspective hopefully will provide insights for new directions in therapeutic intervention strategies.

How Does NDT View the Organization of the CNS for Efficient Motor Control?

NDT Focus: Many variable neuronal networks are organized as interactive, functional units or maps, distributed widely throughout the brain.

Neuronal input for movement is distributed among many sites in the CNS, each contributing to the final motor outcome. In a distributed model, many levels of the nervous system cooperate in the production of movement behaviors, and no single site is responsible for any particular behavior (Kandel, Schwartz, & Jessell, 1991). These sites, which might be quite distant and distinct from one another, include not only the elements controlling posture and movement, but also elements of perception (somatosensory and exterosensory), cognition, and emotional aspects of movement (Thelen, Kelso, & Fogel, 1987). These functional circuits are formed from neuronal groups that have adaptive value for the individual and have been strengthened through the use and experience of moving (Edelman, 1987). This concept of motor control views the nervous system as an active agent capable of initiating, anticipating, comparing, and directing patterns of motor activation at every level. Various characteristics of a movement are represented in different parts of the nervous system that are widespread and overlapping. For example, directional control might take place in a different part of the nervous system than force production through the selective recruitment of motor units (Campbell, 1999a). Research shows that various aspects of vision–visual flow, color, pattern, and form–are represented in as many as 30 different and distinct neuronal maps and are organized into a global map of the image (Treisman, 1988). In order to create a functional movement that achieves the task goal while maintaining the stability of the body as a whole, selection from various regions of the brain and from the entire nervous system must occur.

Additionally, any resulting motor behavior is subject to input from several different sites, and communication among sites takes place in ascending, descending, or lateral fashion (Keshner, 1991; Schotland, 1992; Thelen, 1995). Because each site is capable of analyzing and processing information, the transmitted message is never the same as the message received, and the final response is controlled neither from peripheral nor central origins but through a distribution among all levels of the nervous system. In a distributed model, there is no "controller." Any site in the CNS can assume a command or subordinate role; consequently, the sites that are selected and strengthened are those sites that can most efficiently respond to the demands of the external circumstances. As the experience of moving occurs, the sites that receive input become more strongly interconnected into neuronal maps. Less frequently selected neuronal circuits continue to exist and can be called upon to enhance movement performance if certain contextual elements are present to trigger them, such as the need for increased strength or speed. Increasingly, theorists are modeling the CNS as a flexible complex of systems and subsystems of neuronal maps that share information in the process of influencing the final motor behavior (Connolly & Montgomery, 1987). This is not to suggest that any area of the nervous system can substitute for any other, but it might explain, to some extent, why a client's MRI can look so abnormal and yet the individual shows little functional limitations or vice versa.

There is evidence that these overlapping networks, or neuronal maps, do exist in the CNS (Brooks, 1983). For example, electrophysiological recordings have shown the existence of circular pathways between the cerebellum and the motor cortex (Allen & Tsukahara, 1974; Delong, Gerogopoulos, & Crutcher, 1983). Every neuron in the CNS receives convergent inputs from a variety of intervening synapses that derive from both peripheral and central origins. Neurons that have received input from many sources transmit to many other neurons that then transmit along their respective pathways (divergence) (Keshner, 1991). The final output of the network reflects a response selected and calculated to achieve the overall goal of the system, determined through the dynamic interactions of distributed neuronal populations (Carson & Riek, 2001; Schotland, 1992, Sporns et al., 2000). This convergence and divergence of information over various levels of output shifts the responsibility for control for the final response among various sites in the CNS. Theorists view patterns of coordination as being temporally or "softly" assembled for a particular purpose specifically in response to the total task context (Massion, 1992). This distributed model of neural organization proposes a much richer and more complex functional system than a model based on the assumption that purposeful movement relies on sensory inputs and that the CNS simply matches the incoming sensory stimuli with appropriate motor patterns of stability and movement matched to the task.

Although the Bobaths explained motor control with a hierarchical/reflex model in which "lower" levels produced and controlled simple reflexes and "higher" levels produced highly coordinated balance reactions and self-directed movements (Walshe, 1961), Dr. Bobath stated that the hierarchical/reflex model "should be thought of as a gross simplification of a very complex interplay of functional . . . levels" (K. Bobath, 1980, p. 79; see Chapter 5). A multilevel hierarchical model of function described by Bernstein (Latash, 1998) proposed significant differences in understanding the hierarchical model of organization and its role in control of movement. Bernstein's explanation separated the structures from functions and describes a system in which "higher" levels of the brain are those levels concerned with abstract components of movement, including decision-making, information processing, and the selection of motor strategies needed to accomplish a particular task. "Lower" levels control many finely coordinated movements and are concerned with detailed monitoring and regulation of the response to make it appropriate for the context (Bradley, 2000; Schmidt & Lee, 1999). Viewed in this way, the hierarchical processing model is not necessarily incompatible with a distributed processing model. Although the hierarchical model assigns functions to various levels, communication among all levels is recognized as a *requirement* for the final adaptive motor response. Although there is a structural hierarchy and unique functions of specific structures do exist, the functions of these structural units occur with circular, overlapping networks in which each level can influence those above and below or in parallel (Shumway-Cook & Woollacott, 2001). Therefore, any specific site (brain stem, basal ganglia, cerebellum, etc.) is part of a process, rather than an independent structure contributing to a motor function (or dysfunction) with the task characteristics organizing the response. The control level for a given movement varies, depending on task requirements and previous experience with similar tasks. This multilevel hierarchical processing model acknowledges the importance of being able to shift away from the decision-making level for repetitive or well-learned tasks, freeing the attentional mechanisms for use on higher-order aspects of the task or when doing simultaneous tasks. This ability to allocate attention, when engaged in multiple activities, is one of the major events that occurs when people learn (Schmidt & Lee 1999; Shumway-Cook & Woollacott, 2000). A distributed organization of the CNS implies almost unlimited possibilities for movement combinations and raises another question: How does the CNS work in conjunction with the musculoskeletal system to produce movement that is precise in timing, direction, force, and selectivity of muscles and joints, and efficient for the intended goal?

How Does Efficient Movement Occur?

NDT assumes that it is possible to identify variables in both typical and atypical posture and movement and that it is necessary to understand not only the neural elements, but also the characteristics of the body systems that are moving, the forces acting on the body systems, and the context in which the body moves in order to understand movement variations.

> ***NDT Focus: The structures of the musculoskeletal system (muscles, joints, ligaments, etc.) form functional groups or coordinative structures, constraining the number of independent parts in flexible yet stable relationships. These coordinative structures can be instantaneously selected to reduce the complexity of motor control.***

Systems Theory in NDT

The evidence that body systems reduce the complexity of motor control and remove the control from the CNS comes from ideas developed by the physiologist Nicoli Bernstein. In a departure from other neurophysiologists of his time, Bernstein (1967) applied the principles of dynamic systems to the understanding of human motor behavior. He contended that biological organisms, like other physical systems, are complex, multidimensional, cooperative systems in which no one subsystem has priority for organizing the behavior of the system. He maintained that when two or more independent parts (muscles or joints) combine to perform as one functional unit or synergy, they act as a unit, which he termed a "coordinative structure" (Zernicke & Schneider, 1993).

The following example of breathing (Tuller, Turvey, & Fitch, 1976) demonstrates the functional linkage among biomechanical properties and musculoskeletal structures and functions. When a person inhales and exhales, the mechanical properties of the muscles and joints in the thorax and spine push and pull the spine backward and forward, linking the timing of the muscle action to the respiratory functions (Massery, 1996). The biokinematic linkage of head and spine dictates that the head should move with the spine; but instead, the head is stable throughout the cycle of spinal movements. This stability occurs because, with inhalation, rather than responding to the biokinematic link, the pelvic girdle and the cervical region move forward to the same degree that the thoracic region is pushed backward, thereby maintaining head stability. There appears also to be a functional linkage among the muscles of the cervical-thoracic-pelvic groups. The muscles relevant to inhalation are anatomically separate from those muscle groups involved in the movement of the pelvic girdle and also separate from those muscles involved in the movement of the upper part of the spine, yet they are linked to produce efficient movement of the chest with stability of the head. This is an example of functional linkage, indicating that muscles are not controlled individually but are linked with other muscles to form coordinative structures as dictated by the functional task. Establishment of functional linkages between groups of muscles simplifies motor control. Following this example, therapists can appreciate the impact that contractures at the hips and pelvis or immobility of the scapula and thoracic spine might have on head control or efficient respiration. It is also possible to hypothesize how intervention strategies designed to promote efficient coupling among spinal posture, head control, and respiration enhance any one of these functions. How often Mrs. Bobath told us, "If you want better head control, gain control of the pelvis!"

Although many muscle groups exhibit a predisposition toward coordinative structures, the most flexible solution of task requires modification and flexible coupling. As described above, normally there is efficient, *complementary coupling* of the anatomical structures, muscles, and tendons needed for head stability and respiration. This coupling is also important for efficient transitional movements that utilize the shared musculoskeletal resources that link rotational trunk movements and respiration. Mutual isotonic patterns of inspiration and expiration enhance trunk rotation to solve the task of producing energy-efficient rolling over, twisting around in sitting, and even walking (Massery & Moerchen, 1996). However, the use of the muscles of the external chest wall in situations that demand excessive postural stability, result in breath holding. In this situation, the muscles of ventilation (intercostals) function as trunk stabilizers and are linked in a *competitive coupling*, interfering with the ability to rotate the trunk, placing stability in competition with mobility. In still another situation, muscles of ventilation can be linked in *augmentative coupling*, to increase the stability of the head and eyes. For example, if an individual looks through binoculars at a distant marker while standing on a moving boat, breath holding augments the stability of the trunk, head, eyes and even the hands to effectively solve a different task.

In the three situations described here, the muscles used in respiration and trunk movements are coupled in typical or atypical (but not necessarily abnormal) relationships that complement or compete with the desired movement or postural pattern, depending on the task requirements (Carson & Riek, 2001).

Bernstein (1967) theorized that effective control of the musculature results from reduction in the number of elements or "degrees of freedom" that are assembled into functional patterns, not by direction given by the nervous system, but by the organization of the body systems alone. In this theory, motor behavior is the end-product of a process of self-organization among the many elements, or subsystems, comprising a system, including but not limited to, the CNS. The "controller" is the motor behavior as it is produced. In this framework, the context for the behavior and the task are equally important parts of the system. These concepts placed a new emphasis on the body systems (muscle power, biomechanical properties, body mass, and skeletal configuration), the task requirements (meaningfulness, predictability, and the array of movement conditions), and the laws that govern the environment (forces opposing gravity, friction, and the support surface). These ideas are the basis of various systems models and, although the importance of the task and the environment has been included in NDT treatment strategies for a long time, the importance of the biomechanical properties of the body systems and the specific context for the actions necessary to complete a task are now given more specific focus in NDT treatment strategies. For example, Finnie (1997) described one way to develop the functional patterns that involve combining posture with arm and hand strategies and age-appropriate play in sitting (Figure 1.2). The parent, sitting in a chair, seats the child on the floor between the adult's legs, leaving the child free to use his or her hands and develop various ways to explore pots and pans, lids, and measuring cups and spoons to figure out how things "work" by stacking, nesting, and combining various items. With this positioning, the parent can encourage appropriate alignment and stability and guide shoulder protraction (by limiting the degrees of scapular retraction) for reach and play with the hands while providing boundaries for the BOS and promoting weight shift with reaching.

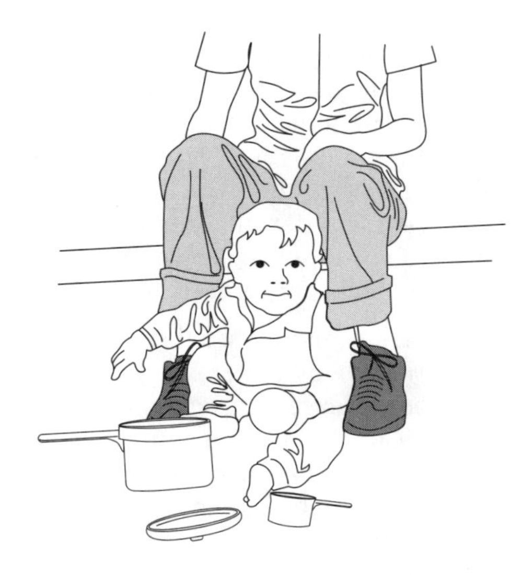

Figure 1.2. The parent structures the environment through the placement of her own body, positions the child (between her legs) to limit ineffective shoulder and arm movements, and increases the opportunity for the child to select useful combinations linking posture and movement as the child experiments with various problem-solving strategies while playing. (Illustration by Claire Wenstrom.)

Bernstein (1967) also suggested that there is a change in the flexibility of coordinative structures as learning takes place. When first learning a movement sequence, the learner attempts to control the degrees of freedom by "fixing" or limiting the freedom of the number of muscles and joints to an excessive degree, a familiar concept in NDT that contributes to increased stiffness in many clients. This initial coupling takes advantage of normal biomechanical constraints and controls many more sets of movement combinations than necessary, resulting in movements that are rigid and energy- and attention-consuming. As learning takes place, the mechanical constraints on the degrees of freedom give way to flexible functional mechanisms of neural and musculoskeletal constraints that allow for greater motion, more variability, and a higher level of success when skill is required because more movement options are accessible to adapt to subtle changes in task requirements.

For example, most individuals can recall a skill gained as an adult–such as skiing, ice skating, typing, archery, needlepoint, fly fishing, tap dancing, etc. –that might have required unlearning a motor pattern the person learned as an child. After the first few attempts, every muscle is sore and fatigued, including those very distant from the muscles necessary for the task completion (even jaw muscles). There is a general sense of exhaustion and a desire to retreat to previously learned patterns that require little attention or effort, even when these patterns do not solve the problem efficiently. If the individual perseveres at the task, not only do the movements show greater spatial and temporal stability, they become more rapid, fluid, coordinated, reliable, and accurate. The individual finds that he or she can grade the posture and movements appropriately to the changing requirements of the task. This same situation exists in clients with CNS dysfunction, and the therapist must permit the client to use previously learned patterns when the individual needs to retreat to a "comfort zone," recognizing that the new movement patterns will not be easy, smooth, or efficient. However, the therapist must identify which patterns can develop into smoother and more flexible ones and which might limit further functional skills. NDT does not always allow the client's own solution to a motor task because this might be limiting to overall function in the long run (K. Bobath, 1980; Davies, 1985).

It is not difficult to take this one step further to see that *if* individuals are driven to control the degrees of freedom of the various body systems in the attempt to acquire posture and motor skills, and *if* strategies involving excessive coupling of biomechanical combinations are functionally preferred early in learning, *and if* the presence of CNS pathology limits the possibilities for development of flexible coordinative structures, *then* constrained movement combinations can become increasingly stable and prevent the effectiveness of more effective flexible couplings of the neurolgic and musculoskeletal systems. The client will appear stiff and restricted in motion, further restricting the ability to form new movement strategies to solve novel motor problems. This is the explanation that NDT uses the appearance of abnormal stiffness and limited movement synergies in clients with neuropathology.

Dynamic Systems Approach

Several theorists have expanded systems theory, incorporating ideas of how complex systems work together within the physical world. The contribution to motor control and development by dynamic systems theory (DST) is placing greater value on body systems and the importance of considering movement in a context-specific perspective (Heriza, 1991; Kelso, 1984; Kugler, Kelso, & Turvey, 1980; Thelen, 1985). Dynamic systems theorists propose that movement and changes in movement patterns generated by various systems are organized by the interactions of multiple component parts of cooperating systems, such as body weight, muscle strength, joint configuration, postural support, mood, attention, specific environmental conditions (such as inertia and gravity), and patterns of neural firing. Due to the properties of dynamic pattern formation, these components spontaneously adopt a specific organization (Ulrich, 1997). This theory de-emphasizes instructions or neural commands to achieve coordinated action and instead looks at explanations based on physical parameters (Perry, 1998, Tscharnater, 2002). Change occurs because one control parameter, or variable, reaches a critical value, which causes a change in the entire system. For example, change in velocity regulates a change from walking to running (Thelen, 1992).

There are three key principles that define dynamic systems theory (Darrah & Bartlett, 1995).

1. **Self-organization.** The concept of self-organization implies that interacting systems, through repetition and practice, can organize themselves and create motor patterns out of this continual activity (Perry, 1998). Self-organization is contingent on prior events as well as current experimentation. Heriza's (1991) studies on preferred kicking behavior in preterm infants support this premise. She proposed that the differences in amplitude and velocity of kicking among low-risk preterm infants result from multiple causes: differences in arousal level, body build, and passive muscle tone among the infants. Self-organization supports the assumption that movement cannot be isolated from the context of the functional task and that spontaneous exploration of movement possibilities is necessary for accomplishing efficient, goal-directed activity (Darrah & Bartlett, 1995). For example, studies by van Vliet, Sheridan, Kerwin, and Fentem (1995) and Wu, Trombly, Lin, & Tickle-Degnen (2000) reported that persons with stroke showed nearly normal reaching kinematics (velocity patterns and decreased movement time) when the goal of reaching and grasping was placed in a task context that offered real objects (such as reaching for and drinking from a cup or picking up coins).

2. **Rate-limiting factors.** Each subsystem develops at its own rate, but is constrained (or supported) by physical and environmental factors. Any component that prevents success at a functional task can be rate-limiting. This suggests that clinicians can identify constraints that limit functional change and develop intervention strategies that directly target these rate-limiters. For example, in early infancy, the mass of the child's head relative to the size of the rest of the body places constraints on, or limits the rate at which, head lifting and visual following can occur (Campbell, 2000a). In adults with CP, moderate weakness or markedly increased muscle tone are independently responsible for limitations in independent activities of daily living (ADL), as evaluated by the Barthel Index (Maruishi et al., 2001). Jorgensen, Nakayama, Raaschou, and Olsen (1995) found that they could predict the timing and degree of walking function recovery in stroke patients based on the initial impairment of walking and leg weakness. These examples support the NDT assumption that impairments to function can be identified and that treatment must be directed toward reducing these rate-limiting factors and at the same time explain why changes in the rate of development are not a stated outcome in NDT programs.

3. **Transitions.** Motor behavior is made up of a series of states of stability, instability, and phase shifts, in which new states become stable aspects of behavior (Thelen, 1998). Even stable aspects of behavior are "softly" assembled so that different aspects of motor behavior (i.e., need for greater stability or variability of movement against the force of gravity) vary in response to changes in adaptive value as the infant develops. During development, as the subsystems of developing systems change, motor behaviors can either become more stable or destabilize. It is during these periods of destabilization, referred to as *transition states,* that new forms of movement are most likely to occur. These transitions are characterized either by an

> increased latency in time to return to a stable state after perturbation, or by increased variability in behavior (Thelen, 1998). Wimmers, Savelsbergh, Beek, and Hopkins (1998) demonstrated that just prior to transitioning from reaching without grasping to reaching with grasping, infants demonstrated instability and increased variability in reaching patterns during a single session of reaching opportunities. Both Fetters (1991) and Heriza (1991) proposed that transitional phases, during which time behavior is less stable, are the optimal times to effect changes in movement by providing experiences directed toward functional goals or tasks, structuring the environment, and manipulating control parameters that constrain the movement.

Although DST has helped to broaden the assumptions of NDT (particularly placing more emphasis on the role of the environment and body systems as strategies for intervention), this theory, with its emphasis on self-organization, does not seem to support manual guiding or facilitating movement as a strategy for gaining the best movement possible for individuals with motor dysfunction. However, it is possible to deduce support for this intervention strategy within a dynamic systems approach. Self-organization implies that the spontaneous motor strategies will emerge from the contribution of many subsystems in the most efficient way, given the present constraints on the motor abilities of the individual. Frequent repetition of these movement patterns causes them to become more stable (Thelen, 1992). Although this is not a problem for persons with intact sensory and motor systems who can develop their individualized, efficient movement by selecting from many movement options, this increased stability of tightly coupled patterns might cause individuals with fewer options for variability to become "stuck" by constrained and repetitive postures and movements that could lead to further disability. Cusick (1990) offered the following example. The W-sitting posture is a frequently used postural pattern for children with spastic diplegic CP who have persistent antetorsion of the femurs after age 2. W-sitting provides a wide, stable BOS with the pelvis stabilized in an anterior tilt by the position of the femurs, aiding symmetrical trunk extension (see Figure 1.3). The child then has the necessary (if inefficient) proximal stability for arm and hand functions. However, as this position becomes more stable from constant use, it inhibits variability in transitions between sitting, quadruped, side-sit, and kneel-stand. In this case, the transitions to kneel-stand and quadruped positions with the hips medially rotated, activate hip flexors and adductors, quadriceps, and lumbar extensors, while forces of hip extension and lateral rotation are absent (Cusick, 1990).

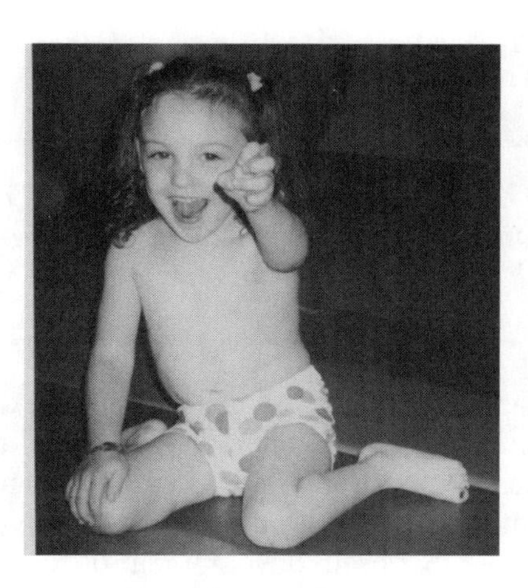

Figure 1.3. W-sitting is a functional sitting posture for children with either spastic diplegic CP or generalized hypotonia and joint hyperextensibility that represents their "best solution" to the problem of gaining stability in sitting. Repetitive selection of this posture, however, prevents more adaptive patterns from being assembled.

It is not hard to see how the W-sitting position contributes to the posture of hyperlordosis with flexion and adduction of the hips, when these children assume standing, leading to the typical skeletal deformities and muscle hypoextensibility in the lower extremities (LEs) that children with diplegic CP exhibit. NDT considers manual facilitation to be an effective way to uncouple these tight constraints on movement. Through facilitation, the therapist guides the active movements needed to destabilize the W-sitting synergy and provides experience with multiple sitting postures and transition options. These variations provide more movement combinations (and new sensory-perceptual feedback), which in turn builds flexibly assembled synergies of the musculoskeletal structures of the trunk, pelvis, and hip joints needed to accomplish these common tasks.

Dynamic systems theory directly supports the NDT treatment strategy of reducing impairments that result in a change in the biomechanics of the musculoskeletal system and alter the emergent movement strategy. For example, asymmetry in alignment of the trunk and unequal weight-bearing in a sitting position is a common problem for adults with hemiplegia. These changes in the trunk posture create an abnormal starting alignment for movement in the sitting position, interfere with efficient muscle activation and weight transfer, and limit the movement patterns that can safely be executed (Ryerson & Levit, 1997). Restrictions in muscle tissue length and joint mobility can develop as secondary impairments due to the abnormal biomechanics of asymmetrical sitting. The NDT therapist uses movements of the trunk to increase mobility in the spine and ribcage and lengthen tight muscles. This allows a more symmetrical postural alignment, equalizes the weight bearing, and increases the possibility that the client will be able to select more efficient movement patterns.

Neuronal Group Selection Theory

NDT Focus: NDT acknowledges that the emergence of coordinated movements and the ability to solve problems require an adaptive nervous system simultaneous with growth and change in the body systems.

Recent work by Edelman (1987) and Sporns (1994) has extended dynamic theory by offering a balance between maturation and interactive physical systems. Selection acts to match possible motor commands to constraints posed by neural and body structures and the physical laws of the environment (Sporns & Edelman, 1993). Neuronal Group Selection Theory incorporates the knowledge that brain development or recovery from brain damage is aided when the individual engages in activities that occur in functionally or developmentally appropriate environmental contexts and when the individual generates movement to meet specific task requirements. NGST describes how selection produces the species-specific yet uniquely individual human brain, as well as how experience strengthens certain patterns of responses and solves the problem of managing movement in an organism with multiple degrees of freedom (Sporns & Edelman). According to NGST, the brain's ensemble of cortical and subcortical systems is dynamically organized into variable networks, the structure and function of which are selected by development and behavior. The units of selection are collections of strongly interconnected neurons, called neuronal groups, that act as functional units. Gray and Singer (1989) have identified the presence of neuronal groups in several cerebral cortical regions. Each neuronal group receives overlapping inputs from a wide variety of afferent sources. The neuronal group consists of hundreds to thousands of strongly interconnected neurons and, according to NGST, serves as the basic functional unit of the nervous system. Neuronal groups are arranged in neural maps in segregated areas of the brain; however, there are long-range reciprocal connections between groups that integrate activities of multiple sensory and motor areas of the brain. Edelman's theory is based on findings from biologic research, but is also consistent with behavioral observations.

NGST has three basic tenets that describe how the anatomy of the brain arises and takes shape during development, how experience selects for strengthening certain patterns of responses, and how the resulting maps of the brain give rise to uniquely individual behavioral functions (Edelman, 1992).

The first tenet of NGST describes the developmental selection by which the characteristic neuroanatomy of brain formation occurs. Edelman (1987) proposed that a genetic code forms the neuroanatomy but not specific neural structures of a species. This genetic code and the local behavior of specific molecules establish the borders of different neuronal areas in the brain whose connections are not preprogrammed. The neural cells compete to make connections. Because of this competition and the interaction of neural elements, diversity develops as a result of the dynamic way in which the brain is formed. Consequently, each individual has a unique brain yet one that is characteristic of its species.This uniqueness is expressed by Woodruff (2000, p. 105) in *Someone Else's Child*: ". . . any mother knows the differences in her babies, could identify any one of them by the weight of their hands, the way their mouths moved in sleep, the feel of their hair, anywhere, anytime, no matter how many years passed." This neural development, along with the development of a sensory system capable of detecting and recognizing movements that have value to the infant to accommodate and adapt to the environment, and with the somatic development of muscles and joints, result in a primary repertoire of species-specific yet unique behaviors.

The primary repertoires include (a) orienting the head and eyes toward light, (b) bringing the mouth to the hand, (c) sucking and rooting on the fist or nipple, (d) coordinating suck-swallow and respiration, (e) following moving objects with the eyes, (f) visual preference for the human face, (g) projecting the arm toward moving objects, (h) reciprocal kicking, and (i) orienting the head toward the vertical and toward sounds (Alexander et al., 1993; Campbell 2000b). The formation of the primary repertoires does not rely on experience from the environment but on genetically endowed movement structures. For example, Ronnqvist and Hopkins (2000) found that newborns' preference for turning and maintaining the head to one side (most often a right-sided preference) reflected active neural processes related to the infant's state regulation, but was not dependent on either biomechanical or postural constraints imposed by gravity.

The second tenet of NGST proposes that the experience of moving (which activates sensory receptors and the ability to perceive the effects of various movements in the environment) eventually strengthens or weakens selective activation by adaptive value (Sporns & Edelman, 1993). A secondary repertoire of functional circuits thereby develops from the neuronal groups that are part of the primary repertoire of behaviors and which have proven to have value for the individual by experience in the environment. Moving activates the sensory receptors and the ability to perceive the effects of various actions in specific contexts. This secondary repertoire consists of the functional synergies underlying skilled motor activities and includes memory and success in accomplishing the task. As the experience of moving in the environment occurs, the neuronal groups that receive more input become more strongly interconnected through the enhancement of pre- and postsynaptic efficacy. The movements experienced in the context of given tasks and appropriate environments, and utilizing the biomechanical characteristics of the musculoskeletal system competitively, select neuronal groups that meet motor requirements efficiently. Because infants demonstrate very poor postural responses, part of the formation of a secondary repertoire must include the strengthening of synaptic connections that organize posture for anticipating the forces created by the activation of muscles, as well as anticipating the need to link posture with movement and sensations and to create efficient actions while maintaining stability of the body in space (Campbell, 1999b). NGST hypothesizes that anticipatory postural control is part of a synergy that includes a self-directed component as well as the component that meets the demands of posture within a particular context. The selection process creates favored functional synergies or strategies for performing the movements associated with desired actions from among the many combinations that could be effective. This differs from Bernstein's systems theory solution, in which the control of degrees of freedom is solely dependent on the body systems and the environment. NGST proposes that the development of synergies is the means by which the nervous system solves the problem of redundant degrees of freedom in the motor ensemble; thus synergies are the fundamental units of movement.

Those neural circuits that are less frequently selected continue to exist with the probability that they might be called upon to enhance movement performance if certain contextual elements are present to trigger them (such as the need for increased force or speed). The precise editing or biasing of secondary repertoires continues throughout an individual's life, maintaining plasticity within the nervous system in response to the adaptive value of a movement experience, changing spontaneously with requirements consistent with growth, maturation, or aging. NGST emphasizes plasticity of the nervous system whose purpose it is to create individuality in movement in response to sensory input. As a result of lifelong plasticity, many synaptic connections or neural circuits are available for immediate selection in the event of a brain lesion that renders the primary synergy nonfunctional (Sporns & Edelman, 1993).

The third tenet of NGST describes how the selection process forms neural maps. These global maps are connections of neuronal groups distributed among vast areas of the nervous system and are organized so that very distinct and sometimes distant areas of perception, cognition, emotion, posture, and movement are spontaneously activated in response to the task conditions and the environment. Because of the parallel and reciprocal connections among many areas, the combination of neuronal groups from selected multiple maps of an area's function allows the production of a movement that is precisely adapted to the contextual demands for performance yet unique to the individual's nervous system capacity for receiving sensory inputs and selecting neuronal groups from individual regional maps. Each neuronal group has a combination of excitatory and inhibitory connections, allowing the final motor output to be assembled selectively based on current demands and past experience with the task that has either strengthened or weakened the tendencies to select particular groups from particular maps (Edelman, 1992). Selection from various maps occurs throughout a particular region of the brain and the nervous system as a whole, linking various systems in movement synergies. For example, a reach-and-grasp action might combine selections from the hand motor areas of a primary cerebral motor-sensory cortex, from maps that receive visual and tactile information, and from areas concerned with the postural function of the neck and shoulder (Campbell, 1999b).

Because each person has variations in his or her neural maps based on individual experience, individuals show unique yet similar strategies for accomplishing common tasks. That human movements share common patterns is a central concept in the Bobaths' explanation of movement control and movement dysfunction (K. Bobath, 1980). Studies of adults (Keshner, Campbell, Katz, & Peterson, 1989) and infants (Thelen et al., 1993) demonstrated that infants and adults use similar but unique combinations of synergistic muscle activation when performing the same task. As children and adults solve motor problems daily, they blend the discovery of the most stable trajectory, joint coordination and patterns of muscle activation, preferred posture, and energy level with memory and prior experience to create their own personal maps (Thelen et al., 1993). Essential to the development of global maps is sufficient experience with slightly different tasks to permit the neuronal groups to respond differently to various objects and events in the environment and still produce a movement synergy that solves the problem (Sporns, 1994).

How are Dynamic Systems and Selectionist Theories Applicable in NDT?

These systems and selectionist models of motor development and motor control support many of the current assumptions in NDT described earlier in this chapter and in Chapter 4's discussion of the principles of intervention. NDT considers the development of broad sensorimotor experiences to be important in producing effective, reliable movement that the individual can then select to achieve multiple functional outcomes. To help students in NDT training courses gain a better understanding of the differences in movement strategies, student therapists perform motor tasks, such as getting up from crossed-leg sitting, while others observe the many variations on the general features. Another exercise is to ask one student to imitate precisely the way a colleague performs an ADL function, to appreciate how difficult it is to imitate exactly another adult with typical skills. These experiences help the students understand their clients' postures and movements and the variety of ways in which individuals solve similar problems. These exercises also help to identify intervention strategies that respect the individual's motor solutions while at the same time directing the client toward efficient motor solutions.

In NDT intervention, repeated experience in movement ensures that a particular synergy is readily accessible for motor performance–the more one does it, the easier it becomes to do. The synergies that NDT intervention strives to obtain are those that are economical for the client and link requirements of postural stability, sensory processing, and movement patterns in response to a broad range of tasks in a specific context. NDT sees movement as a means of activating sensory receptors, thereby linking neuronal maps that contain both movement and sensory components. NDT intervention uses active movement, requiring the client to attend to the aim of the task to improve the ability to generalize on the link between movement and function. NDT recognizes that clients with brain damage have a limited repertoire of movement synergies, and finding a treatment strategy that increases movement generally and develops functional actions is the basis of the NDT problem-solving approach to clients. In the absence of such a treatment strategy, the client most likely will develop a limited set of movement synergies that the individual applies to virtually all tasks. The repeated use of these limited synergies will hinder progress in functional positions.

NDT uses guided or facilitated movement as a treatment strategy to ensure correlation of input from tactile, vestibular, and somatosensory receptors and to expand global maps of useful movement synergies in a task context. NDT also recognizes that self-generated movements that require the client to solve motor problems that reflect the individual's neuronal maps is essential to motor learning and producing permanent changes in motor skills. NDT recognizes that motor behavior emerges from ongoing interactions among multiple internal systems of the individual and that systems theory models provide many ways to approach and alter the client's movement.

The following example of opening a cabinet door to remove a box of woodworking tools (Figure 1.4) demonstrates this new paradigm in the context of designing an NDT strategy to develop movement synergies for simple functions of the hand. The therapist selects a real-life setting in the client's home or in a simulated kitchen (this client's hobby is woodworking) and gives the client the aim of the task–"Get your toolbox from the cabinet below the sink"–so that he can prepare his posture in anticipation of the action to carry out the task. This includes positioning himself at the correct distance from the cabinet door and adjusting his posture anticipating the perturbation that will be caused by the resistance from the door, keeping in mind that he needs to bend down and see into the cabinet and yet stand so that he is out of the way of the opening door. The therapist might first use verbal directions to help the client focus on the motor elements of the task, such as distributing his weight equally on both feet to ensure a stable standing posture with hips and knees slightly bent, anticipating bending down as the task proceeds. She then might add handling to inhibit his habit of shifting his weight to the less-involved side even when this does not aid his posture or support his movement. The client spontaneously places his left hand on the counter to reduce his fear of losing his balance while reaching with his right hand during the task. If the client's attempt is unsuccessful, the therapist might move her right hand onto the client's right arm to assist in isolating shoulder protraction and grade the variability of elbow extension as he directs his attention and energy to the movements of his hand as the task proceeds. The therapist correlates cognitive and memory maps with the motor synergy by asking at the appropriate time, "How did you do this at the end of our last session?" "Do you feel more secure when you stabilize with your left hand on the counter?" "Were you able to get your toolbox out of the cabinet in your workshop at home?" "Do you think this (strategy) will work as well or better than the last attempt you made?" These correlations of inputs from tactile and somatosensory systems, cognition, and memory can be helpful in linking global maps and strengthening the postural and movement components of the motor synergies in a meaningful task context and yet respect the client's ability to solve problems.

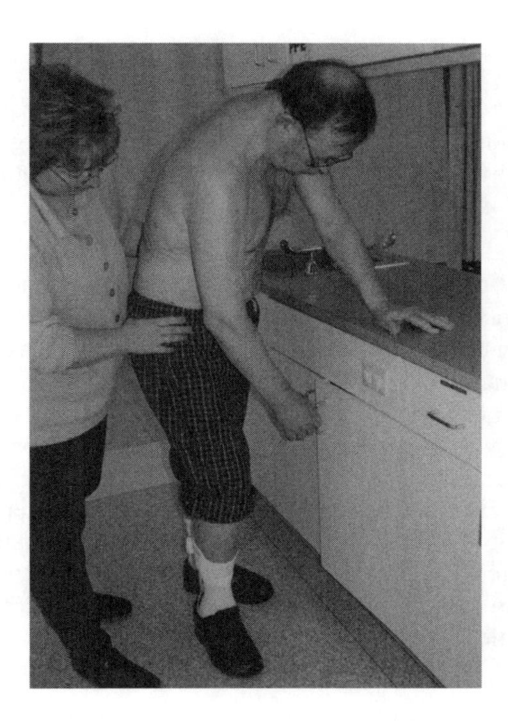

Figure 1.4. The therapist selects a real-life setting in the client's home or in a simulated space and presents the task goal: "Get your toolbox from the cabinet below the sink." The client prepares his posture in anticipation of the action, then plans and carries out the task with input from the therapist only as needed.

Whenever possible, the therapist should follow (rather than lead) the self-generated movements and promote practice with movement options (reaching into different shelves, with different time constraints, obtaining items of different sizes and weights, and sequencing additional steps in the task) to build on the possibilities of multiple systems to self-organize into a global plan that works best for the individual. Finally, combining systems theory and NGST, the therapist allows the client to try and fail, so that the client can sense the effect of his or her movements on the resulting actions, allowing selective activation of neuronal groups to be strengthened (or weakened) by adaptive value. Viewing treatment in this way requires the therapist to be extremely astute to all the elements that make up function, so as not to impose distractions or values of the "right way" that will limit the client's systems to organize for the best success at that time.

Generalized Motor Programs–An Alternative Theory

Generalized motor program theory (GMPT) is not compatible with systems or selectionist models that hypothesize that movements and postures are continually organized to task-specific sensory signals derived by the need for action. Generalized motor program theory assumes the existence of a motor program and provides an alternative to this concept of self-organization.

Current models of generalized motor programs (GMP) provide evidence that the nervous system stores abstract representations of movement, codes classes of action, retrieves, and produces movement plans with considerable flexibility and variability based on prior experience and learning that are context-specific and highly individualistic, without the need for sensory feedback (Keele & Summers, 1976). These neuronal networks generate complex activation patterns of muscles without the influence of peripheral sensory signals (Keele & Summers; Stelmach, 1976). Motor programs, first described by Keele and Summers and more recently by Schmidt (1976; Schmidt & Lee, 1999), have considerable experimental support (Bouisset, 1987; Klapp, Anderson, & Berrian, 1973; Rosenbaum, 1977; Taub & Berman, 1968). These programs are activated by a variety of effector systems, including peripheral sensory stimuli and central processes (Carson & Riek, 2001). This concept expands the flexibility of the role of the nervous system to include its ability to create movement without feedback.

A GMP model acknowledges that sensory information is important in providing information about accuracy of a movement, body posture, and equilibrium and environmental demands when learning or changing a movement. This model considers sensory feedback to be an important component in error detection. Comparing incoming information to prior movement experience enables the CNS system to determine the appropriate course of muscle sequencing to activate muscles subserving postural control or movement in a specific context (see Figure 1.5). This means that movement accuracy and coordination are dependent on guidance from the periphery (Schmidt & Lee, 1999).

GMP contain both invariant and variant features and consist of components or subprograms that can be recruited separately in a task-specific manner (Bradley, 2000). Invariant features are those characteristics of movement that are difficult to change, such as the sequence and relative timing of muscle activation. The invariant features of motor programs account for the commonality of many human movement patterns, such as the general movement synergies for rolling over, getting up, walking, or grasping (in contrast to NGST, which states that common features are based on common experiences). The "personal signature" of one's own movements, such as the way one walks or writes, might be more dependent on individual genetically programmed body characteristics and the way one prefers to execute a posture or movement than the GMP.

Duration, force, amplitude, and muscle selection are variant features and are activated and combined depending on the specific motor plan, strategy, and goal direction (Schmidt & Lee, 1999). The particular combination of variables determines how the motor program is expressed and executed in a given environmental context. Changing the combination of variant features of a GMP permits production of a wide variety of movements that have not been performed previously, because only the general action pattern has to be learned. For example, according to this model, once the general program for crossing one's legs while sitting is stored in the CNS, the specific way in which an individual crosses legs when sitting on the floor in jeans, or when seated on an elevated stage in front of an audience while wearing a tight skirt, depends on the context and does not require the individual to learn a new pattern. This supports the idea that, once learned, much of an individual's movement and posture is more or less "automatic" and does not require attention for the individual to perform the movement effectively and efficiently. These programmed movements act as the supporting system for the intentional elements of a particular self-initiated movement (Keele, Cohen, & Ivry, 1990).

GMPT can account for control of anticipatory postural adjustments. Various researchers have documented the finding that postural muscles of the trunk, pelvic girdle, and scapula contract before a person lifts an arm in standing; however, postural support starts from the BOS or perceived BOS, not the trunk muscles (Aruin & Latash, 1995; Hodges, Cresswell, & Thorstensson, 2001; Hodges & Richardson, 1997). These adjustments occur prior to the voluntarily initiated tasks, are predictable, and allow the CNS to initiate a specific pattern of muscle activation and trunk movements that are independent of sensory feedback. (DST and NGST describe these postural adjustments as one element of a self-organized system.) The Bobaths described postural adjustments as part of the postural control mechanism that they believed occurred automatically as a basis for skilled movement. They used the term *postural set* to describe the anticipatory adaptive movements that maintain equilibrium during all activities involving changes of parts of the body in relation to each other (K. Bobath & B. Bobath, 1984).

GMP models can also support rapid movements, which include well-learned and repetitive movements. Rhythmical movements that would be controlled by GMP include respiration, locomotion, sucking, and mastication (which NGST identifies as primary repertoires). Studies on perturbations to rapid movement and reaction time indicate that these movements proceed faster than the nervous system can process and use the sensory information (Morris et al., 1994). Try this: Place your hands as though you are going to type on your computer keyboard. (This exercise assumes that you type with all fingers!) Now, look at your fingers and move your fingers to strike the "b" key. Did you know which finger to use and what direction to move? Now, without looking at your fingers, type the word *cab*. The ease with which you found "b" is probably apparent to you. Once a pattern is learned in context, it becomes very difficult to initiate the same motion with the same speed and skill if you try to take it out of context. This concept might also explain why, once learned, a pattern of movement, whether adaptive or maladaptive, is likely to remain part of an individual's movement repertoire and is difficult to change without excessive attention and energy. However, well-learned movement might occur not because a GMP exists, but because the selection of a specific synergy has become so frequent that the specific synapses are activated more economically (automatically) than others in a neuronal pathway. This supports the idea that it is important to practice the whole task and not just the components of the task.

The concept of motor programs supports the idea that changes are possible when intervention begins before maladaptive motor synergies become well established and "programmed" and limit an individual's movement patterns. Acknowledging motor programs does not mean that movement cannot change, but it does suggest that there are elements to every posture and movement that are invariant and difficult to influence.

How Do the Sensory Systems Contribute to Motor Control?

NDT Focus: NDT recognizes two different types of sensory systems that complement each other to produce well-coordinated movements. Feed-forward, a proactive system, anticipates and initiates movement; feedback, a reactive system, regulates and adapts movement execution to produce an optimal response within a context.

Sensory processing is the ability to receive, register, and organize sensory input for use in the individual's adaptive responses to interactions with people and objects in the surrounding environment. It includes awareness, orientation, and ability to benefit from combinations of sensory input that support action.

Movement uses sensory information in two systems of control–feedback and feed-forward. Theorists have long considered sensory feedback to have a major role in the acquisition of complex, intentional, coordinated movement requiring accuracy (Horak, 1991). Sensory feedback contributes to the planning and execution of purposeful, goal-directed movement. Feedback control is important when an individual is learning movement and adjusting to unexpected perturbations as movement occurs (Schmidt & Lee, 1999). In a feedback model, external disturbances destabilize the state of the individual and activate peripheral sensory receptors. The sensory afferents report and update the information about the destabilized state of the individual and the environment, to allow the motor neurons to increase movement precision and timing accuracy to regain a stable state (Stelmach, 1976). Exteroceptors report about the environment, and somatosensors (tactile and proprioceptors) report about the individual's own movements. With this information, the individual is operating in a *closed-loop* or *feedback* system that is capable of detecting errors and correcting for them.

A third group of sensory receptors, interoceptors, describes the internal state (e.g., hunger pains, a "lump in the throat," or "butterflies in the stomach") and are associated with regulatory, emotional, and autonomic states (Greenspan, 1997). In the past, these receptors have been considered relatively insignificant in contributing to motor control, but in an NGST, interoceptors, which are associated with motivation, interest, attention and arousal, and autonomic nervous system regulation, have a higher level of importance than once thought because they contribute to the emotional qualities or "value" of a particular sensation. Theorists consider the regulation of arousal and physiological state to be essential for successful adaptation to a complex environment. Researchers have linked irregularities in such regulation to the problems that occur in children with autism, learning disabilities, and pervasive developmental disabilities. Infants with regulatory disorders have difficulty regulating the autonomic nervous system to support the behavioral state required for attention, social responses, sensory reactivity, and information processing (DeGangi, DiPietro, Greenspan, & Porges, 1991). These differences are evident at birth (Weiner, Long, DeGangi, & Bataile, 1996).

A closed-loop, feedback system depends heavily on the involvement of particular types of sensory information as the system executes its function. The visual system is generally considered the most critical exteroceptor for supplying focal information about *what* is in the environment and therefore makes important contributions to movement ("I want to reach for, hold, walk to what I see around me"). More recently, studies have credited the visual system with a proprioceptive or ambient function, providing information about *where* things are in the environment and how these objects are moving (exocentric motion) or how the person is moving (egocentric motion) in relation to them (Gibson, 1966). This is considered a proprioceptive function of the visual system because it requires movement of the eyes, head, and body to detect placement. The consideration of a proprioceptive visual system is particularly relevant to motor control because it contributes to orientation of position in space, provides general information about the accuracy of movement and postural control and error detection, matching information with the somatosensory and vestibular systems (Padula & Argyris, 1996). According to Schmidt and Lee (1999), the exteroceptive visual system contributes to the individual's consciousness of the environment, whereas the proprioceptive visual system participates in the control of actions.

A number of published studies suggest that the auditory system also plays a role in the perception of movement requiring temporal regulation (Jenison, 1997; Schmidt & Lee, 1999). The auditory system, like the visual system, needs to be thought of as a proprioceptive as well as an exteroceptive system because, as the individual moves the head and body, the auditory system provides information about where objects are in the environment (e.g., the sound is coming from the left side) as well as providing accuracy by orienting to the feedback from the individual's own movement (Butterworth & Castillo, 1976). For example, in a popular water game, children move around a pool and call out to "Marco Polo" to the person seeking them. The child who is Marco Polo must, with eyes closed, rely on auditory and tactile (the movement of the water on skin) systems to explore, locate, and tag the other players. This game relies on hearing the voices, the sounds, and movement of the water as the children move in the pool, determining direction and distance of the voices, and finally orienting, moving, and changing direction toward the sound.

The vestibular system and the somatosensory system (including muscle, joint, and cutaneous receptors) are fundamental in their importance for closed-loop control (Abbs, Gracco, & Cole, 1984; Abbs & Winstein, 1990). Many sources describe the structure and function of these systems (Kandel et al., 1991; Schmidt & Lee, 1999; Shumway-Cook & Woollacott, 2001), and PTs, OTs, and SLPs are quite familiar with them. The question is, how do the various receptors of the exteroceptive and somatosensory systems contribute to motor control?

In a closed-loop, feedback system, the sensory systems contribute to motor control in two different ways–regulatory and adaptive–depending on the nature of the motor behavior (Gordon, 2000). The regulatory role occurs during ongoing movements to shape the movement characteristics (speed, direction, force, timing, and error detection) to meet the demands of the task in the environment. Regulatory roles are generated primarily by the way that either the exteroceptive or somatosensory systems see, hear, or feel the need to make adjustments in the environment. The adaptive role relates to the subsequent actions that follow an initial action and allow the individual to update either the decision-making process or effector selection based on information about how well the performance matches the goal (see Figure 1.5). A reference of correctness or "goal to be achieved" is part of a closed-loop system. The reference of correctness represents a comparison of the state of the feedback associated with execution of the desired movement. Once a movement begins, muscle contractions cause the limb and body to move, producing changes in the environment. Each of these effects generates information from the various somatosensors and exteroceptors. The system compares the feedback it receives with the desired goal. If the two sources are the same, the implication is that the movement is correct and no adjustments are necessary. If a difference exists between the reference and the feedback received, then an error is signaled and correction is required. In these ways, sensory information contributes to motor control in a closed-loop system (see Figure 1.5).

Recently, along with the development of motor programming theory, an *open-loop* or *feed-forward* system has evolved to explain the organization of a movement that does not rely on feedback from the body or environment (Bly, 1996; Schmidt & Lee, 1999). Although theorists have most often described the open-loop system along with GMP, it is not inconsistent to consider this a dimension of a motor synergy that develops by selection. Feed-forward occurs when the client anticipates and initiates the postural and movement requirements of a task proactively, in advance of the motor act. These might be relatively simple postural adjustments or rapid complex movements. Bly (1996) provided the following example (updated here) to distinguish these two mechanisms. If I am a passenger in a moving car and I am talking on my cell phone, writing down a message, and not noticing or anticipating a upcoming turn, my body will be displaced in the direction of the turn when the car goes around a corner. Even as my body is moving, I sense the movement via feedback from my somatoceptors (and, if I look up, from my visual exteroceptors, as well) and respond by making the proper postural adjustments to prevent falling and regain stability. However, if I am looking out the window as I talk on the phone and notice the upcoming corner, I can anticipate the speed and effect of cornering from prior experience. I use my visual exteroceptors and vestibular and somatosensory receptors in a feed-forward manner, preparing the postural adjustments prior to the movement, tensing those muscles to counter the disturbance in equilibrium. Anticipation of the postural requirements of a task results in a rapid and automatic execution of the necessary movement responses. Feed-forward occurs as a result of learning through experience and means that in NDT intervention, the therapist must structure the environment and the task, setting up a variety of similar experiences, providing the best alignment prior to the task, permitting repetition and practice, and allowing the client to learn through experiences of self-initiated movement. Beginning with the optimal anticipatory position, the client will experience the benefits of this posture on the movement outcome. The therapist must assess the client's current feed-forward system, that is, the way the client currently anticipates, organizes, and plans a task, in order to address this in treatment.

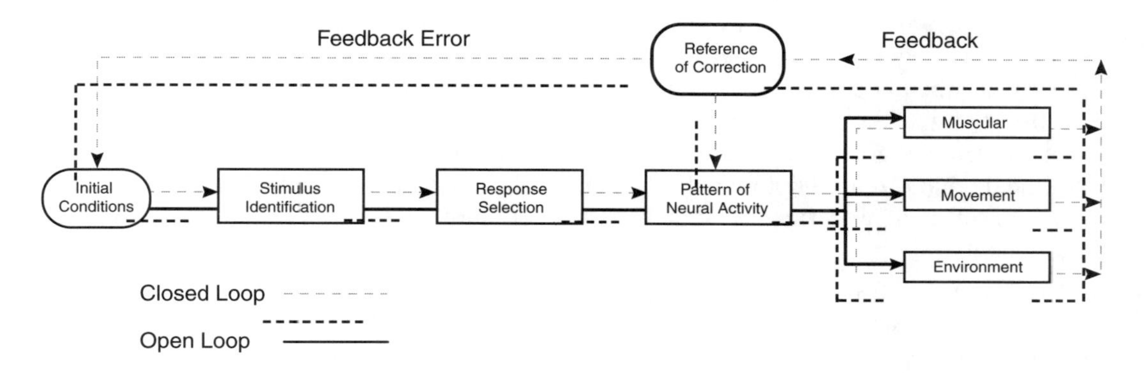

Figure 1.5. The feed-forward (open-loop) and feedback (closed-loop) systems complement each other as necessary to anticipate, regulate, and adapt actions to the dynamics of the physical world.
(Illustration by Claire Wenstrom.)

The open-loop (feed-forward) system proposes that information either from peripheral sources or from an internal self-directed command is distributed throughout the spinal cord and brain stem, as well as the motor and premotor cortex that predicts constraints associated with the physical laws governing the biomechanical aspects of the musculoskeletal systems and the environment (Horak, 1991; Massion, 1992). The sensory information from peripheral sources is assimilated in the CNS, matched with memory of similar experiences, selected and prepared in advance, and executed as part of a tightly linked sensorimotor synergy, without additional feedback and without reference to the consequence the movement or action has on the context. The final sensorimotor outcomes are relatively fixed under stable conditions, but are adapted in less stable situations by flexibility in selection and learning from past movement experiences, not from sensory feedback. Horak (1991) presented the following example: At the end of swing phase in gait, the gastrocnemius-soleus muscles contract in advance, in anticipation of their stretch on heel-strike and weight bearing. This anticipatory muscle activation accounts for "missteps" when stair height unexpectedly changes, because slow feedback systems must substitute for the appropriately timed anticipatory activation. The efferent command is sufficient to initiate certain types of coordinated movements that do not rely on afferent input. In movements controlled in an open-loop fashion, the parameters of the movements are carried out to completion without alteration, even if, as the example illustrates, the result does not produce appropriately adapted movements. Fortunately, movements are organized with spontaneously adaptive synergies that solve immediate functional problems so that new movement responses emerge to correct the error. As mentioned earlier, the scientific evidence suggests that three types of movement are produced as a result of an open-loop system: rapid movement sequences (such as those found in Jean-Pierre Rampal's flute fingering or Gregory Hines's tap-dance sequences), anticipatory postural strategies, and well-learned movement sequences (Massion, 1992).

The need for rich prior motor experiences and opportunities to practice a large variety of movement strategies to solve various motor problems is important in an open-loop model. The broader the experience an individual has in movement exploration, the more flexible options exist and the more precise the resulting movements will be in accomplishing a given movement goal. Individuals with CNS pathology will demonstrate maladaptive movements that often do not meet the demands of the task because these individuals have limited movement experiences with which to attempt to support new and varied task requirements.

In functional situations, control of movement fluctuates between feedback and feed-forward modes of control (Bly, 1996; Cupps, 1997; Giuliani, 1991). Bly gave the following example: When I want to reach for an object slightly out of my range, I select components of posture prior to the onset of the postural disturbance that occurs due to the movement of my arm and hand. By doing this, I reduce the possibility of falling as I reach. This feed-forward occurs as a result of learning posture and balance in sitting from prior experience and the ability to select from those neuronal maps that meet these requirements. As I reach, I use visual feedback to determine the characteristics of the object I am reaching for and the direction and distance I need to move. I use proprioceptive feedback to obtain information about my arm's position in space and during movement, as well as the relative position of each joint. But because I have reached many times for objects outside my range, much of this is "well-learned" and does not need sensory feedback for completion. However, because this object is unique and I have never seen anything quite like it, I will depend on sensory feedback to estimate its weight and size in order to match the tension I need in the muscles of my arm and hand to pick it up. Each of us has experienced the strange sensation (and inaccurate movement) that results when we have incorrectly guessed the weight of an object!

Motor control is the ability to regulate the mechanisms essential to movement, producing the optimal response in a context involving external and internal constraints organized around a task-specific goal. The systems and selectionist models require understanding the contributions of the CNS, the body systems, and the sensory systems. However, this is not the whole picture. Understanding movement requires a systematic consideration of the physical dynamics of the environment as well.

How Does the Environment Contribute to Motor Control?

NDT Focus: NDT recognizes the importance of the environment and the persons in it as a powerful incentive for movement

In systems theories, the characteristics of the task and the specific environmental context are as important as the contributions from the nervous system and the body systems. The environment, including the people in it, is a powerful incentive or disincentive for movement in individuals with and without neuropathology (Ada, Canning, & Westwood, 1990; Fetters, 1991; Gibson, 1988; Howle, 1999). For example, infants who sleep in the supine position, as recommended by the American Academy of Pediatrics task force on SIDS, were less likely to have rolled over at 4 months of age and had lower developmental scores at 6 months of age than infants who slept in prone (Jantz, Blosser, & Fruechting, 1997). Changing the infants' relationship to the environment and therefore the ability to practice the movements of rolling to prone from supine appears to have affected the timing of motor development. (This does not mean, however, that therapists and parents should oppose the "Back to Sleep" movement, because the differences in developmental scores at 6 months were undetectable at 18 months of age.) Belanger, Bolduc, and Noel (1998) evaluated the importance of the environment on the social integration of persons with stroke and found that environmental characteristics, including a regular supportive presence of children or other relatives at home, had a positive correlation with retention of motor skills gained after stroke. Studies of the relationship of the home environment and infant motor development found that more supportive and stimulating home environments correlate with higher infant motor development scores (Abbott & Bartlett, 1999; Abbott, Bartlett, Fanning, & Kramer, 2000). In another study, siblings who were educated about CP and included in home programs had a positive effect on the functional independence of the sibling with CP (Craft, Lakin, Oppliger, Clancy, & Vander Linden, 1990). Bass-Haugen, Mathiowetz, and Flinn (2002) described the importance of an active learning environment in an OT task-oriented approach that includes creating an environment that encompasses the common challenges of everyday life and an organization of the environment that matches the level of performance of the client.

Researchers have documented changes in posture or function in children or adults with modifications in the environments, such as using adaptive equipment. Several studies have credited proper seating as an important factor contributing to motor function and voluntary control of the UEs in children with CP (Reed, 1996; Sochaniwskyj, Koheil, Bablich, Milner, & Lotto, 1991). Other studies on the impact of walker design on the mobility of children with CP found that the use of posterior walker designs produced a more upright posture during walking, more "normal" alignment when standing, and improved gait characteristics, including stride length, step length, and speed, than did anterior walker designs (Greiner, Czerniecki, & Deitz, 1993; Logan, Byers, Hinley, & Ciccone, 1990).

The effects of providing a positive, supportive learning environment are not new to NDT therapists (Embry & Adams, 1996; Larin, 2000). Larin described the following characteristics of the environmental context in which tasks take place as variables in developing strategies to improve performance:

1. **Abstract aspects of the environment:** a context that is appropriately motivating, stimulating, and challenging for the age, cognitive level, emotional stability, attentional, sensoriperceptual processing, and motor abilities of the client; organized to match the level of performance of the client; considers the cultural and social aspects of the context

2. **Physical aspects of the environment:** size and physical layout of the room; placement of furniture and persons; level of noise, light, color, temperature, and safety and comfort factors; encompasses the common challenges of everyday life that can directly or indirectly affect movement

3. **Interactive context:** supportive, confident instructor-learner interaction; promotion of initiations by the learner; creation of problem-solving situations; effective guidance with shared control of decision-making and incorporation of risk-taking; mental and motor challenges; timely, responsive feedback that focuses on modifying, recommending, or expanding motor behavior rather than on corrective feedback

4. **Multicontext situations:** application of newly learned skills to multiple situations and in real contexts, such as home, school, and community, for varied practice leading to motor learning under a variety of conditions, aimed at decreasing dependence on the instructor or any one particular context

5. **Task characteristics specific to the environmental context:** characteristics that drive motor behavior; purposeful, meaningful tasks that are initiated by the learner; specific tasks with which the learner has some prior knowledge and experience; tasks containing components that can be generalized in other settings and to other tasks; tasks that provide both an action goal ("Can you put on your jacket?") and a movement goal ("Can you make a fist, straighten your elbow, and push your arm through that sleeve?"); tasks that are specific, consistent, and attainable; tasks that are basic for solving a variety of motor problems in the client's home; tasks that capitalize on the individual learner's strategies

Gentile (2000) proposed a taxonomy of tasks moving systematically through 16 levels of environmental conditions, from level 1 (Closed Context/Body Stable) to level 16 (Open Context/Body Transport with Manipulation), which describe the kinds of requirements the environments impose on the learner. This taxonomy is extremely helpful for the systematic evaluation of environmental contexts, task complexity, and their influence on motor behavior.

Gentile's (2000) taxonomy described "closed" environmental conditions in which the critical features of the environment (including objects, other people, and the support surface) are stationary. Movements are controlled by the spatial features of the environment (such as the length and width of the room and placement of doors, lighting, furniture, and persons). The learner is free to perform at his or her own pace, to decide when to start, and how long the movement will take. These conditions, while predictable and safe, with few environmental variables, lack stimulation, challenge, and problem-solving possibilities. This is often an appropriate environmental context for learning new tasks because it reduces the need to adapt to a variety of variables and allows the individual to attend to the task; but at the same time, such predictability reduces the opportunity for transfer of the skill to functional settings. At the lowest end of the taxonomy, the individual is stable, sitting or standing, and is not engaged in manipulation–for example, sitting on a bench, listening to a story, watching television, or the activity in the room.

In the "open" environment, the spatial and temporal conditions are variable. The motions of people and objects in the environment determine the learner's movements, and conditions change with successive attempts. This environment helps the client to develop flexibility in motor performance and actively search for critical environmental cues to determine successful task completion. This is a much more demanding context for movement, because the learner must become adept at developing and controlling movement patterns that fit environmental variations. An example of an open environment is shopping in the mall, coping with a constant but perhaps irregular change in the individual's own position, and interpreting changing visual and auditory stimuli while adapting to changing velocities of other shoppers.

Physical laws governing the environment enhance or constrain motor control. The support surface characteristics and the forces of gravity, friction, and inertia are variables that affect the individual's COM relative to the BOS. All movement involves changing the body's relationship to the support surface. Efficient contact with the support surface is necessary as a foundation for movement from that surface (Tscharnuter, 1993, 2002). Increasing the friction of the surface decreases the ease in moving away from that surface, but increases the stability of maintaining posture in contact with the surface. For example, sometimes something as simple as placing a nonskid material such as Dycem™ on the seat, or changing the seat depth and back height, increases the amount of body in contact with the surface, which increases stability and body alignment. If the goal, however, is to move in a sitting position to dress, then a low-friction seat without a back and with a surface such as varnished wood enhances weight shift and movement within a seated position.

The effects of gravity are so fundamental to motor control and motor development, that it is difficult even to think of this in a separate context. It is the one consistency among highly interactive, interdependent brain, body, and environmental systems. Throughout life, individuals (with or without neuropathology) must adjust and adapt to the invariant effects of gravity. The job of the newborn is to organize movement against the forces of gravity. This is a particularly difficult job for small, premature infants, and neonatal nurseries have made many efforts to structure the environment to support behavioral organization and stimulate the flexed midline position, based on positioning against the force of gravity (Campbell, 1999b; Girolami & Campbell, 1994; Kahn-D'Angelo & Unanue, 2000). Gravitational forces, along with various mechanical and genetic coding, affect bone structure, growth, and resultant shape of the skeleton in developing children (Gajdosik & Gajdosik, 2000). The body segments change rapidly in mass and size in the first year, and the infant must constantly cope with the interactive effects of gravity and these dynamic physical changes. In addition, gravity affects posture, skeletal alignment, and strength in aging adults. Bones develop and change in response to external forces, such as gravity and dynamic biomechanical changes throughout life. In the examination of the adult, NDT is particularly concerned with compromises in alignment and posture of the spine and extremities, based on age-related changes in joint mobility, muscle extensibility, and joint mechanics that secondarily affect movement patterns (Davies, 1990; Ryerson & Levit, 1997).

Concepts in Motor Development in NDT

> ***NDT Focus: NDT recognizes that many of the differences in movements in infants and adults result from anthropometric changes and movement experiences rather than neurological influence.***

NDT has always had a strong foundation in motor development, especially in working with children with CNS dysfunction. Almost since the inception of the Bobath Approach, the Bobaths wrote and taught that understanding the development of movement supplied the means for recognizing differences in normal movement and movement pathology and provided a framework for timing various intervention strategies for children. Over the years, they developed, expanded, and discarded many of these original concepts. Based on the maturationist point of view described by Gessell (1928) and McGraw (1945/1963), and their observations of normal development at that time, the Bobaths initially wrote that it was important to teach control of movement by closely following the developmental sequence of motor behavior of the normal child (B. Bobath, 1953; K. Bobath & B. Bobath, 1979, 1984). The Bobaths discarded this concept as they explored why children move and recognized that many movements develop simultaneously for the purpose of expanding the means of interacting purposefully in the environment (Atwater, 1991). The Bobaths believed that understanding the interaction and coordination of various posture and movement combinations that compose a skill, including, but not limited to, the components of the neuromuscular and musculoskeletal systems and the purpose of the skill, emphasizes the importance of treating in many positions at the same time. The Bobaths stated, "Treatment should not attempt to follow the sequence of development described, regardless of the age and physical condition of the individual child. Rather it should be decided what each child needs most urgently at any one stage or age, and what is absolutely necessary for him to participate for future functional skills, or for improving the skills he has but performs abnormally" (K. Bobath & B. Bobath, 1984, p. 11). They believed that the sequence of development was less important than developing the components for age-appropriate skills. For example, in NDT treatment, a method of developing trunk and hip extension and orientation to the vertical position is to treat while standing even before earlier "milestones" are in place. However, it is equally important, when using this treatment strategy, for the clinician to pay close attention to the client's alignment and BOS when the person is in a standing position.

As Dr. Elsbeth Köng and Mary Quinton had the opportunity to observe and treat babies and infants and communicate their findings with the Bobaths, and as younger children and infants were referred to the Bobaths, it became clear that using motor milestones as a frame of reference was not enough. By the time the Bobaths wrote the book *Development of Movement in Different types of Cerebral Palsy* in 1975, their concepts of normal development were well-defined and included the idea that movements develop in overlapping patterns that make possible the complex functional skills referred to as "motor milestones." The Bobaths acknowledged that development does not proceed in a linear fashion. Rather, a child develops many different motor skills simultaneously, practicing a large variety of combinations of movement patterns in different positions against the force of gravity, eventually preferring some over others to solve motor tasks (K. Bobath & B. Bobath, 1984; Hadders-Algra, 2000). As the child becomes more active, these motor abilities find expression in a number of related activities and not only in one particular milestone.

The Bobaths strongly maintained that observing and describing the quality of posture and movement, rather than changes in the achievement of motor milestones, differentiated the normally developing infant from the infant with motor dysfunction and gave the therapist a means to intervene before atypical patterns of coordination became established and habitual. The Bobaths focused on the progressive development of postural control as a foundation for skilled movement via supporting directed movements of the UEs, as well as control of the body moving in and through space. Their attention to the righting reactions (which support transitions) and equilibrium responses (which support alignment and balance) was a critical contribution to the understanding of movement in children and adults.

The Bobaths found that experience was a driving force. Every new activity built on previous sensorimotor experiences (typical or atypical), which could be expanded and modified for new purposes. They realized that in individuals with neuropathology, it was not necessary, in fact in some situations was harmful, to perfect one motor milestone before continuing to another. They found that it was more useful to identify basic motor patterns that the child could then use in a whole group of new activities. They viewed gravity as a major constraint on posture and movement. The Bobaths wrote that the full force of motor dysfunction would not be manifested until the individual developed upright posture and movement, confronting all the physical forces of the environment (B. Bobath & K. Bobath, 1975; K. Bobath & B. Bobath, 1984).

Two other important contributions expanded the developmental framework in NDT treatment. Milani-Comparetti (1967) analyzed the development of movement patterns by their adaptive value, and the Bobaths applied this concept in NDT. Mary Quinton (Quinton & Wilson, 1981; Quinton, 2002) developed and described the "competition of motor patterns" that she observed in young infants who were at risk for motor dysfunction and taught this as an essential part of NDT Baby Courses. This concept was particularly useful for observing and analyzing premature or very young infants who had not developed classic signs of CP. She divided patterns of competition into three subdivisions:

1. **Competition between normal patterns of movement,** which compose the repertoire of movement patterns in the typically developing infant. The competition of normal patterns has three characteristics.

First, one pattern never dominates the baby's movement to the exclusion of any other pattern. For example, at 2 months, the baby might turn the head to sound or moving sights and find him- or herself with the head turned and the face arm extended, so that the infant is now able to regard his or her hand. This asymmetry links vision (or hearing) and hand movements. At another moment, the infant can select to put both hands simultaneously in the mouth and suck them. The competition between symmetry and asymmetry is obvious as one observes the baby, but both are functional patterns and have value for the infant as he or she learns about him- or herself.

Second, competing patterns develop simultaneously. For example, at 4-5 months, while in the supine position, the infant reaches out to knees and feet, showing strong flexor control of the neck, shoulders, and hips. At the same stage, while in the prone position, the infant practices patterns of neck, shoulder, and trunk extension as the baby bears weight on the arms and reaches.

Third, each new pattern can use the experience of previous patterns and, in turn, is necessary for the emergence of later patterns. Development is contingent and dynamic. As a new pattern emerges, it can temporarily overpower the structure of the old pattern, destabilize the organization of movement, and then reorganize the baby's movements into broader functions. For example, an infant in prone might use a strategy for head lifting with little trunk or pelvic stability, marked cervical spine hyperextension, and weight on the chest, and arms. By 4-5 months, the infant lifts the head, producing a second pattern that shifts the weight caudally, so that the pelvis is against the support surface, hips are extended, and weight is on the lower rib cage, elbows, and forearms. Head lifting now includes head and upper trunk extension combined with forward shoulder flexion. This stability makes it possible for the infant to lift and turn the head freely and easily. As this new pattern emerges, it competes with the earlier pattern and, during this period of transition, the baby might demonstrate either pattern. With repeated experience, the typically developing infant prefers and repeats those posture and movement patterns that fit the child's morphology and the need to solve motor problems that can be produced most easily.

2. **Competition between normal and atypical patterns** occurs in infants that have brain injury. These infants begin with a smaller repertoire of movements and a nervous system that is less capable of managing competing motor patterns. This means that as this infant practices with the limited movements he or she does have, particular patterns become more tightly linked and constrain the expansion of additional movement repertoires. For example, in the baby's effort to turn the head to sound or visual stimuli, the infant spends more time in an asymmetric posture. The more time the child spends in an asymmetrical posture, the easier it becomes, and the infant requires greater effort to maintain the head in midline and in bringing the hands to the mouth. Subsequently, rather than symmetry and asymmetry competing equally, asymmetry dominates over symmetry.

3. **Competition of atypical with abnormal patterns** occurs as the infant with neuropathology continues to practice and experience movement. The movement patterns

become more strongly linked and stereotypic. In the desire to solve problems with the movements that are available, the child will compensate for these early abnormal synergies with more atypical movements. The outcome will be persistent patterns of posture and movement that are poorly adapted for the task. For example, it will be harder for the infant to gain symmetry when he or she is dominated by asymmetry and uses this pattern repeatedly. Placed in sitting, the child will find it increasingly difficult to use both hands together. The child might try to compensate for the loss of bilateral hand use by persisting with orientation to one hand at the increasing disuse of the other. Subsequently the child's use of one hand perpetuates and increases what is now a maladaptive asymmetry.

This analysis of the competition of patterns gives physicians and therapists a tool to recognize a growing dominance of atypical patterns in babies. This process also alerts professionals to begin intervention before the ineffective patterns become so well practiced and dominant that they prevent the development of a broad range of movement patterns.

The third contribution to the understanding of motor development came from Lois Bly (1983), who identified and described the components of normal movement based on the contributions of the musculoskeletal systems. She identified the components of the musculoskeletal system (weight shift, control of antigravity extension, flexion, and rotation) and proposed that these elements develop in a systematic way to support the appearance of motor milestones. She maintained that it is important for therapists to identify these musculoskeletal components in order to evaluate typical or atypical development. She described these components in various positions (supine, prone, sitting, and standing) and focused on movements in the sagittal, frontal, and transverse planes and on transitions from one position to another. Babies typically activate and elongate their muscles by moving on all three planes of movement. They play with flexion and extension in supine; extension and flexion in prone; lateral weight shifts to each side in supine, prone, sitting, and standing; and rotation around the body axis in all positions. Flexion and extension occur on the sagittal plane; lateral movements, abduction, and adduction occur on the frontal plane; and rotation occurs on the transverse plane.

Bly's detailed analysis of these components allows therapists to identify atypical or missing elements in children with motor dysfunction. Bly's analysis (1983, 1994, 1999) reinforced the Bobaths' concept that the developmental sequence is not a continuous process in which one milestone is the foundation for the next milestone, but that milestones are the expression of age-appropriate behavioral characteristics.

The Bobaths originally thought that therapists needed to guide adults through the developmental sequence, so that they could relearn control of the neural and kinesiological components of movement (neuromuscular and musculoskeletal) in the same way that children did (Bly, 1991). Later, the Bobaths changed the way they looked at the use of the developmental sequence and began to consider the critical components that were developed within the various positions. For example, infants develop scapular and glenohumeral stability in prone-on-elbows or hands-knees positions. This stability of the shoulders needs to develop in adults, but does not necessarily have to be developed in the prone-on-elbow position. More age-appropriate positions and activities could be used. For example, the therapist can encourage an adult with hemiplegia to take weight on elbows and forearms by leaning forward onto a low table as the client rises from a chair, or to sit with forearms on a desk and lean into the elbows and forearms (Ryerson & Levit, 1997).

These key contributions made the NDT approach extremely strong in analyzing both the neuromuscular and musculoskeletal components of movement. In addition, the increased understanding of the role of the sensory systems in learning to move and in moving has enhanced this analysis. More recently, as NDT has embraced contemporary systems and selectionist theories, NDT has focused attention beyond the neurological and muscular systems in motor development to recognize that the motor system provides a means of interacting, and that motor development must include the value the task has for the individual, the context of the development, and the physical laws of the environment. The consistencies described in normal development provide a standard of reference for proficient human motor function and make it possible to identify the differences in individuals, both normal deviations and atypical, maladaptive motor behavior.

The physical laws of the environment influence the biomechanical, kinesiological, and anthropometric changes in the musculoskeletal system. Alignment, gravity, and the BOS affect the activation and elongation of muscles and muscle groups. These effects, along with growth and development, subsequently effect changes in body configuration (anthropometric changes). NDT currently views the processes by which functional postures and movements develop in a framework consistent with the systems and selectionist theories described earlier in this chapter. Assumptions in motor development have been expanded to take advantage of this recent information.

NDT Assumptions in Motor Development

1. Motor development is an ongoing process that occurs throughout the life span. Experience and learning within specific environmental contexts strengthens certain motor patterns, giving rise to uniquely individual characteristics while retaining the same general form across all human motor behavior in typical individuals.
2. Motor development emerges from the cooperation of many subsystems in a task-specific context. Development of specific motor synergies depends on a combination of mechanical, neurological, cognitive, and perceptual factors; the individual genetic code; and environmental contributions that provide a context for experience and learning. Neural maturation is only one process in an interactive model of multiple systems that drive motor development.
3. Neural and body systems and their subsystems develop at different rates to share in the control of motor behavior, enhancing or constraining the development of particular motor patterns at different times. Rate-limiting variables include muscle strength and length, postural control, perceptual capabilities, and body morphology.
4. Motor development is a series of states of stability and instability of motor synergies, reorganizing with new combinations of posture and movement better suited to

accomplishing tasks commensurate with emerging physical capabilities and adaptive values. Different phases of the human life span are characterized by different motor behaviors designed for efficient functions at those times.

5. Newborns have primary repertoires of movement that are both unique and species-specific, including visual orientation to moving objects, sucking and rooting, mouth to hands, reciprocal kicking, projecting the arm toward objects, and orientation to sounds.
6. The hallmark of normally developing movement is variability. Within this variability exist multiple synergies (producing functional combinations of flexion, extension, and rotation in symmetrical and asymmetrical patterns) that combine to serve postural control and mobility.
7. Infants discover preferred motor patterns that are flexible yet stable, selected in response to the sensory feedback from generalizing about specific tasks experienced in a particular context. Variability in motor synergies develops through individual experiences and alterations in the body subsystems of the infant, with respect to the physical laws affecting the environment, such as gravity, inertia, and friction.
8. Motor milestones appear as discontinuous, discrete, new behaviors with a definable onset. They arise from the continuous development of cooperating neural and body systems that, in and of themselves, do not contain the pattern of behavior.
9. Understanding typical and atypical motor patterns underlying motor function is useful in analyzing components of movement in adults with CNS pathology.

The following two examples illustrate these assumptions.

Development of Postural Control

Postural control involves controlling the body's position in space for the purposes of stability and orientation and emerges from the interaction of multiple systems that are organized around a task and constrained by the environment (Shumway-Cook & Woollacott, 2001). The gradual development of postural control constrains developmental milestones that require the body to be controlled against the force of gravity and enhances skills that entail orienting the body segments to each other and to the effects of gravity in task-specific relationships. For example, an infant can take full body weight on the legs at 4 months, but cannot stand unsupported until 11 months, when postural stability develops. The same 4-month-old infant changes from rolling as a unit to rolling with rotation between the pelvis and shoulder girdle as orientation between body segments develops.

Postural control requires the integration of sensory information to assess the position and motion of the body in space and the motor ability to generate forces for controlling body position and to prepare for the reactive forces of movement. In a general way, the development of postural control in the infant and child follows a cephalocaudal progression, control of the head and neck preceding that of the trunk, which precedes the hips and LEs. This progression results from the interaction of multiple neural systems and the biomechanical aspects of the musculoskeletal system to meet the goals of postural orientation and equilibrium. The relative importance of each system (and subsystems) appears to vary with age and contextual demands. Experimental studies suggest that the following components contribute to the emergence of postural control for independent stance and locomotion: (a) sensory subsystems, which include visual, vestibular, and somatosensory systems for detecting imminent (or threatened) loss of balance, (b) motor mechanisms, including postural tone and muscle synergies for controlling balance, (c) adaptive systems for modifying sensory and motor systems to changes in task or environment, and (d) biomechanical and kinesiological forces and body morphology for alignment and weight bearing (Shumway-Cook & Woollacott, 2001).

In infants and young children, vision is the most powerful sensory system in regulating posture, both in feedback correction and in feed-forward anticipatory postural strategies (Bradley, 2000; Forssberg et al., 1992). In several different studies, babies as young as 60 hours were able to orient by righting their heads toward a source of visual stimulation if their heads and trunks were supported (Bullinger, 1981). However, the lack of strength due to an immature musculoskeletal system and mass and weight of the head constrained the postural response so that babies were unable to maintain head stability and alignment. Several researchers have investigated the effects of vision on postural control in sitting and standing (Butterworth & Hicks, 1997; Lee & Lishman, 1975). Although results have varied somewhat, most researchers agree that newly sitting infants rely heavily on visual inputs to control body sway. This dependency on the visual system decreases with experience and with the formation and control of postural muscle synergies. As children mature, they become less dependent on vision and rely on the faster vestibular and body proprioceptors to control postural action. By the time an infant can sit independently, postural responses are controlled primarily by somatosensory inputs at the hip joints, not by vestibular or visual stimulation. When confronted with conflicting sensory information, children are able to ignore misleading visual information and utilize somatosensory information to control equilibrium shortly after they begin to walk (Foster, Sveistrup, & Woollacott, 1996). Adult-like responses with minimal sway, however, are not apparent until after age 6 (Foudriat, 1993). These adaptive capabilities indicate that the child is able to modify sensory information and form new motor strategies in accordance to changing task and environmental conditions even though this capacity is not refined until the child is approximately 7 years old.

Postural control requires generation and coordination of forces that effectively control the position of the body in space. The activation of muscle synergies that control spontaneous sway to remain upright develops over time (Hartbourne, Giuliani, & MacNeela, 1993). Infants without prior experience are unable to control the degrees of freedom sufficiently and do not show consistent, directionally appropriate responses to perturbations (Forssberg & Nashner, 1982; Hartbourne et al., 1993; Woollacott & Sveistrup, 1992). As neuromuscular responses become better organized, the infants demonstrate a decrease in sway velocity, decrease in onset latency, improvement in timing and amplitude of muscle responses, and decrease in variability of muscle responses. For example, the emergence of independent sitting is characterized by the infant's ability to control spontaneous sway of the head and trunk with anterior/posterior and side-to-side perturbations. By the time the infant can sit independently, postural muscle synergies relating the head and trunk segments for postural control activate spontaneously and the infant is stable (Hadders-Algra, Brogren, & Forssberg, 1996a).

Stable posture is affected not only by the development of sensory and neuromuscular elements, but also by the alignment of body segments that contribute to stability in the upright position. *Alignment* refers to the arrangement of body segments with respect to one another, as well as the position of the body with reference to the force of gravity and the BOS. In ideal alignment, the various parts of the body are maintained in a state of equilibrium with the least expenditure of energy. Musculoskeletal changes progress rapidly in the first few years of life and are influenced by internal muscle and skeletal development and external mechanical and gravitational forces (Zernecki & Schneider, 1993; Gajdosik & Gajdosik, 2000). Periods of instability in postural control can result from changes in skeletal growth and the child's attempt to adapt body alignment to new skeletal length and morphological relationships among body segments.

Anticipatory components of posture establish a stabilizing framework that supports intentional movement. Infants as young as 9 months show activation of the postural muscles of the trunk in advance of most reaching movements (von Hofsten & Woollacott, 1989). This same activation relationship occurs in children in standing at a later age. These feed-forward, anticipatory components of posture take place before the child is able to sit or stand unsupported, suggesting that the ability to activate postural muscles in patterns of feedback and feed-forward develop simultaneously (Forssberg & Nashner, 1982). The feed-forward components of posture are necessary for the child to initiate skills in postures against gravity (Bly, 1996).

Additionally, biomechanical variables constrain the development of mature patterns of postural control in children under age 4 (Bradley, 2000). Particularly in the first year, the COM is proportionally higher than at any other age because of the large head and short limbs, requiring large force generation and regulation by neck and upper trunk musculature. Woollacott and Shumway-Cook (1990) suggested that these differences in body morphology affect the selection of appropriate motor strategies. As children grow and body proportions change, the emergence of adult-like postural responses is no longer constrained by these biomechanical variables. Children are not just small adults; rather, young children use strategies adapted to the task that are appropriate for their body size and proportions.

Finally, practice and experience influence the activation and organization of postural muscle responses. Two different studies, one with pre-sitting infants (Hadders-Algra, Brogren, & Forssberg, 1996b) and the other with pre-standing infants (Sveistrup & Woollacott, 1997), demonstrated that experience with balance training produced postural muscle responses that were more organized than in infants who did not receive this practice. In both cases, latency in the onset of postural responses did not change, suggesting that neural maturation might be a rate-limiting factor associated with myelination of the nervous system, whereas organization of the response is affected by practice (Shumway-Cook & Woollacott, 2001).

Postural control continues to change over the life span. Many factors contribute to declining balance in older adults. Various studies have documented impairments in the sensory systems (including changes in visual, somatosensory, and vestibular senses), impairments in the neuromuscular system (including changes in muscle strategies and anticipatory control), impairments in the musculoskeletal system (including changes in ROM and loss of spinal and extremity joint flexibility, muscle strength, and endurance), and impairments in cognitive-emotional systems (including fear of falling), all of which can contribute to decline in balance control (Butchner & DeLateur, 1991; Shumway-Cook, Baldwin, Pollisar, & Aruber, 1997; Wade, Linquest, Taylor, & Treat-Jacobson, 1995). No one predictable pattern is characteristic of changes in postural control in the aging population, but NDT views such changes in clients with CNS dysfunction as a result of the interaction of normal aging and specific disease processes (Shumway-Cook & Woollacott, 2001; Woollacott & Shumway-Cook, 1989).

In summary, postural control, the ability to control the body's position in space, is fundamental to everything we do. Every task requires a stability component (to maintain the COM over the BOS) and an orientation component (to maintain appropriate relationships between body segments in specific contexts) to support skilled behavior. Changes in postural control that occur in clients with CNS dysfunction might be normal variations that develop with various experiences in movement during the developmental and aging process, or might result from the type, location, and extent of neural lesions and the primary or secondary impairments resulting from this pathology. In short, postural control is a multidimensional issue, and the specific relationship of postural control and functional limitations is difficult for clinicians to determine.

Development of Reach and Grasp

The capacity to reach for and grasp an object is a complex and important motor milestone. This skill involves the development of many systems, culminating in the ability of the infant to move the hand and arm through space and contact a target that the infant perceives by vision. Reaching for and grasping an object begins as one of the newborn's primary repertoires described by Edelman (1992).

Reaching and grasping has its origin in the developing fetus. Without the aid of vision, the fetus is able to reach out, explore the uterine wall, the umbilical cord, and the legs, chest, and arms, suggesting that reaching is either an inherent motor program (Humphrey, 1978), or a spontaneous generation forming part of a primary movement repertoire (Prechtl, 1997). von Hofsten and Ronnqvist (1993) presented evidence that neonates' spontaneous arm movements demonstrate distinct patterns of spatiotemporal organization that have one acceleration and one deceleration phase similar to those that occur in the reaching patterns of 5-month-old infants. However, in the neonate, the movements of the two arms are strongly coupled in all three planes, moving together along the body's longitudinal axis, abducting and adducting together, and extending together in the forward direction. The differences in postnatal reaching and manipulation involve, at the very least, postural control; development of control of arm movements (kinematics) against the force of gravity; development of a flexible coupling in eye-head and hand coordination and between the two hands; shaping and molding of the hand as a terminal device; interpreting exteroceptive and proprioceptive visual information; developing control of strength, velocity, timing for initiation, and braking; as well as experience, learning, and desire. Yet by 5 months, an infant can reach out with accuracy and grasp objects of different sizes and shapes.

Researchers generally accept that reaching in the newborn is visually triggered and that hand trajectories are directed actions. The role of exteroceptive and proprioceptive vision changes with development. In the newborn, visual location of the target initiates movement; however, visually guided reaching, which requires the ability to attend to the hand as it moves toward the target, is not part of early reaching. (Proprioceptive vision is available to newborns as they are able to reach toward their mouths without vision in a goal-directed way; von Hofsten, 1982). Vision is used in a feed-forward way with no correction for incorrect timing or direction. Visual attention to the reaching hand does not develop until the fourth or fifth month of life (Clifton, Muir, Asmead, & Clarkson, 1993; von Hofsten & Ronnqvist, 1993). Eye movements to track a moving object also occur in the neonate, but are most likely reflexive and must develop further during the first 5 months (McCarty, Clifton, Asmead, Lee, & Gojubet, 2001; von Hofsten, 1982). Coupling eye movement with head movement does not develop substantially until 5 months, at which time head control includes stability and mobility independent from the trunk and arm. This means that exteroceptive vision is not a rate-limiting factor in the infant's initial attempts at reaching. It is available for initiating movement, but the lack of visual feedback for correction of movement and visual proprioception for perceiving the position of the arm and hand in relation to the target is a constraint on precise, smooth trajectory for reaching.

A study by Thelen et al. (1993) concluded that the inability to control the arm to contact an object is a major constraint on coordinated reach and grasp. This study suggested that infants begin with preferred (innate) movement patterns and progressively restructure reaching strategies until the hand path trajectory straightens to a nearly adult pattern by 9 months. Changes in trajectory of the arm during the first year suggest the development of new, flexibly linked coordinative structures.

The arm and hand are strongly coupled in patterns of flexion or extension synergies, limiting the patterns for reaching in the neonate. Appropriately coordinated reach and grasp require that the arm extend and the hand flex around an object, a combination that is not available to the neonate. von Hofsten and Woollacott (1989) demonstrated that neonates do have a large variety of differentiated finger-thumb movements, yet neonates do not use these movements for manual skills. In this study, the neonates used finger movements for social gesturing to maintain contact with the mother. Until 2 months of age, the coupling between the arm and the hand requires that whenever the infant extends the arm, the hand opens in extension at the same time, so grasping rarely occurs. At 2 months, this strong synergy uncouples, allowing a more flexible arm-hand coordination. Now the fingers begin to flex as the arm extends. At 4 months, reaching changes again; the hand path trajectory consists of several steps, which causes the trajectory to appear less coordinated, and the hand begins to close just before contact with the object. This occurs with a change from dependence on feed-forward to a feedback control mechanism. It is interesting to note that the pattern of reach with grasp does not appear to change between 5 and 9 months, suggesting that other control parameters limit the development of this skill during this period of time.

Postural stability undergoes change with development of postural control in the trunk. As described in the preceding section on postural control, there can be an uncoupling of the head, arm, and hand synergies and development of flexible coordinative structures as the trunk muscles assume the role of controlling postural stability, leaving the biomechanical structures of the arm and hand available for mobility functions, for which they are better suited. This is also the point at which the infant begins to use proprioceptive visual information at the end of the reach, as the child sees the hand approach the target and corrects for errors in hand path trajectory and hand shape. This attention to visual feedback and desire to mold the hand for grasp, as well as changes in postural control, might account for the development of new strategies. This is an example of variable rates of development in multiple systems acting as constraints on the emergence of specific motor skills.

Reaching and grasping are intimately related in a functional sense, but control of grasp differs from control of reaching in several ways. Reaching and grasping are most likely dependent on two different groups of descending neural pathways that control the shoulder and hand and that mature together, but at different rates (Kuypers, 1981; Pehoski, 1995). Additionally, the anatomical and biomechanical structures differ as well. Successful reaching depends on the structures and kinematics of the shoulder girdle, one of the human body's most complicated kinesiological systems, which also includes the arm, forearm, wrist, and hand (Boehme, 1987).

The scapula, humerus, forearm, and hand are coupled in a flexible synergy during reach. Boehme (1987) described the biomechanical processes of the UE and hand during reach and grasp. Specifically, the job of the humerus and its muscles is to project the hand in a wide and varied range of space and to direct the hand to an object. The kinematics, including linear and angular displacement, velocity, and acceleration, allow the upper arm to reach, hold the posture in midspace, and correct or change the direction based on task-specific feedback during the movement. Large muscles move the humerus, and smaller rotator cuff muscles that hold the humeral head in the glenohumeral joint also function to alter the rotational component of the humerus during reach. The elbow brings the hand to and from the body. The dynamic control of the elbow permits the elbow to move through its range of motion slowly or quickly, stop and hold a midrange position, and produce the force to make the arm longer or shorter when loaded. The development of elbow control depends on both glenohumeral control and wrist and hand placement. This complicated relationship, which further allows the forearm and wrist to orient and adapt the hand relative to the object, is not available to the infant. Preparatory adjustments of hand orientation begin to occur at 4-5 months, when the infant first begins to grasp objects. To reach smoothly, the infant must time the grasp appropriately in relation to the object.

Grasping depends on the correct hand orientation and the ability to switch between power and precision grips. Generally, the hand shape depends on specific objects in the environmental context. The hand shapes itself around an object and accommodates its own shape to the shape of the object. In order to do this, the hand must be expandable and malleable enough to shape around both large and small objects. At times, the hand needs to be powerful and at other times delicate in its approach to grasp and manipulation. The ability of the hand to be functional in all these situations depends on the balance between the long finger flexors and extensors, the capability for alignment between wrist and hand, mobility of the carpal and metacarpal bones, and the activity of the intrinsic muscles of the hand. These biomechanical contributions, including the kinetics and kinematics of the UE, play an important role in the development of reach and grasp. Compromise of any of these anatomical structures or intrinsic movement dynamics will constrain hand trajectory, joint coordination, and muscle activation patterns as well.

Finally, combining visual-perceptual processes with motor synergies is important in developing reach with grasp. The ability to judge weight and texture is dependent on the emergence and integration of these systems.

In summary, reach, grasp, and manipulation emerge gradually during development and are characterized by changes in the neural, sensory and musculoskeletal systems, experience with external forces and adaptation to increasing complexity of task demands. With the maturation of each of these systems, there are changes in timing, coordination, and modulation of forces the infant uses for reach, grasp, and manipulation.

The development of locomotion is another motor skill that researchers have investigated using a systems approach. Heriza (1988) and Thelen (1985, 1986) have described these changes in extensive publications; consequently, this text will not address development of locomotion.

Theories and Strategies of Motor Learning in NDT

Motor learning is a set of processes directly related to practice or experience leading to relatively permanent changes in the capability for movement (Schmidt & Lee, 1999). These concepts are particularly pertinent to NDT because strategies for improving motor learning are used in NDT training courses and in client treatment. Many changes have taken place in the application of motor learning principles in NDT, moving from an early time when the therapist determined the patient's problems and directed treatment to recognizing the importance of self-determination in goal setting and in the motor learning process to ensure functional changes in everyday life (K. Bobath & B. Bobath, 1984). Early in the development of the Bobath Approach, the therapist controlled all aspects of the client's movement experiences. The extensive use of "reflex-inhibiting postures" (see Chapter 5) required the therapist to physically control the position and movements of the client. Bobath treatment was recognized by the physical contact and control the therapist maintained throughout the session. The therapist led the treatment and determined when the client would be allowed to move, how much, and in what direction. The therapist was also responsible for determining the success of the outcome. The client was the recipient of highly structured, well-controlled treatment that stressed changes in performance rather than motor learning.

Over time, the Bobaths discovered the importance of allowing clients to control their own movements, directing and actively participating with only guidance by the therapists while learning or relearning functional movement. The amount of physical handling has decreased, and verbal and nonverbal coaching and cognitive strategies have increased with practice variability. The Bobaths also discovered that practice conducted in meaningful, natural contexts reduces the gap between treatment and function and provides a clear link between "therapy" and daily living (K. Bobath, 1980).

In the past, NDT has received criticism for its lack of attention to the principles of motor learning (Goodgold-Edwards, 1993; Van Sant, 1991). However, three fundamental aspects of motor learning theory that Schmidt (1991) described–developing strategies for solving motor problems, structuring the instructions, and use of feedback–have been a part of the NDT approach from its early stages.

1. **A problem-solving approach.** NDT clinical practice has always involved planning and developing strategies and experimenting with solutions for motor problems. NDT treatment planning is not a prescriptive set of methods or techniques. The process, used in both examination and treatment, of observing functional limitations, analyzing the task and the movements needed for performance, hypothesizing underlying impairments, and assessing the success of application of treatment strategies toward overcoming these limitations is in keeping with concepts of motor learning. In addition, the feedback from the client allows the therapist to either retain treatment strategies or modify them based on the client's responses during the intervention. At the same time, the client experiences success in solving the movement problems.
2. **Structuring instruction.** Therapists trained in NDT learn to pay close attention to all aspects of the instructional process, including the influence of their own physical relationship with the client during a treatment session, the decision to use manual facilitation, verbal or nonverbal instruction, the use of feedback during or after practice, the active participation of the client during treatment, and the ability to assess the client's reaction to the selected strategy. Although certainly guilty of overstructuring in the past, the NDT approach has evolved to selectively apply various strategies, letting the client progress as he or she demonstrates the ability to produce the optimal movements for task performance in various positions and with the speed, force, and ROM appropriate for the function. Larin (2000) pointed out that appropriate instruction can enhance the client's ability to distinguish task-relevant information from task-irrelevant information and attend to the appropriate components for learning.
3. **Use of feedback.** Mrs. Bobath taught and wrote that success of any strategy used in NDT required the therapist to assess the capability of the client to respond to the selected strategy, interweaving assessment and treatment and using the knowledge of results (KR) to modify the treatment approach. This has always been important in NDT because therapists consider treatment techniques as tools and do not hold any specific technique responsible for the outcomes and results (K. Bobath & B. Bobath, 1984). During treatment, therapists regularly augment the inherent feedback provided by the outcome with knowledge of performance (KP). The clinician gives feedback to the client via physical or verbal guidance to provide information about performance errors and by suggesting modifications to correct the movement.

NDT Assumptions in Motor Learning

The following assumptions have developed from motor learning concepts and are currently part of the NDT framework.

1. Motor learning results as the individual gains experience and practice in specific environments in the pursuit of new or different motor behaviors. It is important that the environment and the task be conducive to the client's or student's learning capability (i.e., appropriately motivating, stimulating, achievable, and meaningful).
2. NDT intervention structures motor learning experiences to evoke active responses from the client. Active movement does not necessarily mean voluntary movement; postural reactions performed automatically during skilled activities require a great amount of coordination, strength, and endurance.
3. Goals and outcomes that the learner selects and that are specific, meaningful, attainable, and of moderate difficulty have a greater effect on the motor learning than goals or outcomes that the clinician sets.
4. During NDT intervention, the therapist helps the client plan and develop strategies for solving motor problems, recognizing that each person works out ways to perform various tasks in ways that are most functional for them. Individuals form their own specific strategies based on their musculoskeletal and neuromuscular competencies and limitations as well as motivation, priority, value, and necessity of the task. Individuals alter their plans as the solution for a motor problem evolves from the specific task and environmental constraints at the moment, taking into consideration the structure and capabilities of their body systems.
5. NDT intervention uses specific instructional strategies in a task-oriented approach that recognizes that functional tasks help organize motor behavior. The selection of instructional strategies reflects the stage of learning of the client. Therapists present these strategies in such a way that clients gradually select and then optimize the strategy that best matches their needs and desires with the task and the environment.
6. Practice is a prerequisite for motor learning. Repetition through random practice is an important component in motor learning. Motor activities that are task-specific and that the client repeats, throughout an NDT therapeutic session and in functional ways in other settings, have a better chance of becoming part of the client's movement repertoire than infrequently practiced skills. Changes in motor skills occur under conditions that most closely resemble the conditions the client will normally encounter during the performance of that skill.
7. Training courses and client treatment utilize physical, cognitive, verbal, and nonverbal guidance along with verbal and nonverbal feedback.
8. Hands-on guidance is a naturally occurring, motor-teaching strategy that influences motor learning and is particularly useful when eliciting specific behavior in the early stages of motor learning or during the refinement of skills at any stage. NDT

recognizes that parents' normal daily handling of their infants influences motor development, as well as effecting positive parent-infant relationships. Physical guidance, as a therapeutic strategy, strives to duplicate this natural relationship between two individuals, whether adults or children.

9. An optimal state of readiness, including attentional, physical, emotional, cognitive, and sensorimotor systems, prepares the individual for the consequence of the motor action. NDT focuses on preparing the client for movement through a supportive therapist-client relationship, an appropriately comfortable environment, motivational activities, physical preparation through alignment and position, and "just-right" challenges (Fisher, Murray, & Bundy, 1991).
10. Experience, experimentation, memory, and recall are additional elements that bring about improvement in motor learning.
11. NDT recognizes that improved performance (the ability to perform better immediately following practice) does not automatically equal motor learning (the degree of long-term retention of performance capability). NDT recognizes the importance of transfer of skills to the daily life setting.

These principles of motor learning are directly applicable to NDT treatment planning and execution. This section discusses these concepts as they relate to NDT theory in a therapeutic environment. Chapter 4 on the principles and process of NDT intervention covers applications of motor learning principles to treatment in specific client contexts.

Motor Learning and Motor Performance

It is important to distinguish between motor learning and performance. *Motor learning* occurs as the direct result of practice or experience that influences the individual's ability to process information and leads to relatively permanent changes in the capability for producing skilled actions (Higgins, 1991). Skill is the consistent attainment of an action-goal with some economy of effort and is the result of organizing movement as an individual solution to a motor problem. Motor learning is the set of underlying events, occurrences, or changes that happen when practice enables a person to become skilled at some task. Motor learning can be measured by the degree of long-term retention of performance capability or the amount of transfer to other tasks or different settings (Larin, 2000; Schmidt & Lee, 1999). *Performance* is the change in motor behavior that comes from a variety of temporary factors following practice. Initially, NDT focused on changes in performance following treatment, rather than changes in motor learning. The lack of carryover into life settings became obvious, and the Bobaths made changes in the intervention strategies to establish a more direct link between treatment and the performance of functional skills at home (K. Bobath & B. Bobath, 1984). Research has shown that the more closely the demands in the practice environment resemble those in the actual environment, the better will be the transfer of skill (Winstein, 1991). Improved performance, observed immediately following practice, does not necessarily imply that learning has occurred. It is important to make the distinction between improved performance and increased motor learning. In fact, research has shown that practice conditions that promote long-term retention might be different from the practice conditions that produce immediate improvement in performance. Setting up conditions for long-term retention for motor learning may actually decrease the quality of immediate motor performance (Schmidt & Lee, 1999). Errors during practice can facilitate learning.

Preparation for Motor Learning

Preparation for a motor learning experience involves addressing the overall context that is conducive to the individual's learning ability and style. (See this chapter's section entitled How Does the Environment Contribute to Motor Control.) In summary, children and adults respond positively to a multicontext approach that requires the individual to apply the newly learned skill to multiple situations (Toglia, 1991). Providing real contexts for varied practice leads to motor learning under a variety of conditions. For example, children with CP demonstrated differences in quality of movement when reaching for a doll while playing a game, compared to reaching with limited purpose (Beauregard et al., 1988). The narrower the context, the narrower the solution and the more consistent, or stereotyped, the movement (Higgins & Spaeth, 1972).

Movement is the means by which individuals solve motor problems and includes awareness of the kinematics of the movement as well as the external and internal forces needed to exactly match the features of the movement with the task (Higgins, 1991). In addition, the structure of the movement can be consistent (stereotypic) or variable (nonstereotypical), depending on the problem and the context. For example, to place a key in a lock, the body must be stable so that the arm can elongate the right distance and direction to reach the lock. The individual must control velocity, decelerating at the end of the motion so that precise placement in a small target is possible. Mobility must combine with stability to then hold the arm in space, while the hand shapes to the configuration of the key. Grasp must be precise with fingers and thumb and include changing the force applied against the surface of the key to place it successfully in the lock and then turn it against the stiffness of the lock mechanism. However, because every learner has a different set of physical characteristics (variations in height, weight, limb length, strength, and flexibility), no single pattern can be used to place a key in the lock. In addition, all keys and locks are different, so the final motor skill must vary with the individual and the environment's constraints. In this example, the critical features of the environment (size, shape, and weight of the key; dimensions and location of the lock) shape the spatial characteristics of the movement, and the task shapes the movement's temporal and kinetic characteristics (velocity, acceleration and deceleration, power, and force). Understanding these movement characteristics can increase effectiveness in planning motor learning tasks. Changing movement characteristics enhances learning, affecting such factors as fluency, flexibility, originality, and elaboration on movement patterns that can lead to an increased problem-solving capacity (Larin, 2000). The individual who solves similar movement problems using a number of different organizational strategies is more likely to develop permanent changes in motor skills.

These concepts are basic to designing motor learning experiences in NDT training courses. The practicum sessions include modeling, demonstration, independent movement experiences, and practice with a wide range of peers and treatment settings that involve a variety of children or adults with motor dysfunction.

Goal setting and instructions before practice are part of motor learning preparation. The pre-task period is important for information processing, decision-making, and response programming (Clark, 1982). Various investigators found positive effects on performance and learning when the learner selected specific movement goals of moderate difficulty, contrasted with the results when the instructor selected vaguely stated movement goals (Lewthwaite, 1990; Lin, Wu, & Trombly, 1998; Kyllo & Landers, 1995). In addition, the learner must be motivated to learn a motor task for intentional learning to occur. Larin (2000) described three factors in motivated learning:

1. The learner must perceive that the skill is meaningful, useful, desirable and has personal value and implications. For example, a woman who has had a stroke might find cooking tedious and difficult if she never liked to cook prior to her stroke, while a man who jogged regularly before his stroke might enjoy learning various swimming strokes as part of his rehabilitation program.
2. The learner must experience satisfaction from executing a movement. Movements that are self-initiated and self-controlled are most satisfying and therefore of great importance for motor learning. Children often engage in movements that seem purposeless to adults. This is particularly true of newly learned movement in which the child engages in the activity over and over "for no apparent reason." Adults usually refer to this as play or practice, but these activities are functional behaviors representing important components of motor learning and motor behavior. Repetition might serve a variety of useful functions such as muscle strengthening, trial of various organizational strategies, tests of postural control and balance, or learning about the reactive forces produced elsewhere in the body by muscle contraction of prime movers (Howle, 1999).
3. Third, the learner must find encouragement toward higher, achievable goals after task execution by feedback from significant persons, from self-monitoring, or from the pleasure of the experience. Children are wonderful at the "watch me" game, setting up their own program of feedback, which invariably leads the "watcher" to suggest, "Can you climb higher, run faster, or jump or swim further?" If the watcher's attention fades, the child will attempt to achieve more to reingage the watcher. Adults use more subtle means for encouragement from external sources and more often set up their own rewards: "I will swim four laps this week, run 2 miles on the treadmill, or walk every night after dinner."

Instructions for Motor Learning

Instructions prior to the motor task are important for motivational purposes and also as feedforward input to convey information about the task requirements. This information includes a description of the task based on the learner's competencies in movement and processing information. Appropriate instruction can enhance the individual's selective attention and foster the ability to separate task-regulatory information from nonregulatory information

(Gentile, 2000). Regulatory conditions are those environmental features to which the movement must accommodate to successfully reach the goal, in contrast to the background information that is irrelevant for movement organization. In the example of placing the key in the lock, the size and weight of the key and the shape and placement of the lock (in the door or car) are regulatory conditions that directly affect the organization of the movement. The presence of other persons in the environment, sounds in the background, or color of the key are irrelevant to the movement features and therefore are nonregulatory.

Instructions (a) can be verbal or nonverbal (demonstration or modeling), (b) include information about the general action ("See if you can do this," then demonstrate and model touching toes) and the movement goal ("Keep your knees straight, bend over, reach your arms down toward the floor, and touch your toes"), and (c) include a way to recognize goal attainment ("Once you have touched your toes, see if your knees are straight"). The description of functional, relevant goals elicits faster and smoother movements than nonfunctional goals (Lin et al., 1998). Boyd and Winstein (2001) found that when explicit factual knowledge about the task and sequence was provided prior to practice, participants with stroke were able to demonstrate motor sequences. Instructions to children sometimes need to be more concrete, depending on the child's age and abilities. Van der Weel et al. (1991) found that children with CP responded with greater movement excursions when they received concrete instructions rather than abstract instructions.

Physical or verbal guidance during the task is an effective method for limiting movement errors during the performance of a task. Guidance can assist the learner through the proper movements needed for task completion. Guidance has a considerable positive effect on performance during the trials of the practiced task, but not on learning. In particular, continuous physical guidance can modify the feel of the task, reducing its specificity and transfer potential (Salmoni, Schmidt, & Walter, 1984). Trial-and-error or "discovery" procedures result in effective retention and transfer performance. If the therapist includes guidance as a method of instruction, more effective learning will occur, if there is an alternation between trial and error, independent movements, and guided movements.

The current view in NDT treatment is that physical guidance or handling, used judiciously, is an appropriate strategy for enhancing both performance and motor learning (see Chapter 3 for further discussion). Goodgold-Edwards (1993) expressed concern that physical guidance or handling in NDT treatment might direct attention away from the appropriate sensory cues, encourage dependence on the therapist's cues, and possibly interfere with the client's ability to perform actions independently. However, in two separate studies with typically developing infants and their mothers, the mothers' handling enhanced motor skills. Stack and Arnold (1998) showed differences in gaze and affect when the mothers included touch and hand gestures during face-to-face interchanges with their 5-month-old infants. Hopkins and Westra (1989, 1990) found that mothers who included "formal handling" (including stretching movements, massage, and interventions to provoke active movement) were able to influence the timing of their infants' motor abilities. NDT views physical guidance as a way to permit clients to allocate their attention to the component of performance that will lead to motor learning when they are engaged in multiple activities.

NDT Focus: Physical guidance or handling is used during the early stage of practice and is gradually withdrawn as the client indicates readiness for independent movement. Combined with periods of trial and error and self-initiated movements, therapeutic handling remains an important contemporary NDT treatment strategy.

Practice in Motor Learning

Practice is the most important condition for motor learning. However, practice has different effects depending on the stage of learning (Gentile, 2000; Giuffrida, 1998). Practice during *early learning* allows the learner to discover a reasonable, effective approach to goal attainment. Practice during *later learning* allows the learner to concentrate on achieving skilled performance that includes expedient solutions characterized by economy of effort and successful action (Gentile). During the early-learning phase of a novel task, the learner establishes an organizational framework for the behavior, learns which environmental conditions are regulatory, plans the initial movement patterns, and attends to feedback for organizing subsequent attempts. Verbal guidance appears to be very important for adults in this phase of learning. Fitts (1962) referred to this phase of motor learning as "cognitive" because the learner uses active problem-solving with a high level of attention to the task goal. In later learning, practice changes the processing of information and organization of movement. The learner becomes more proficient in coping with task constraints. Movements become more efficient with refinement of control processes, so that movement is consistent and smooth. Fitts referred to this stage in motor learning as "automatic" because there appeared to be minimal attention cost, freeing the learner to engage in planning strategies such as form and style of movement sequences.

These differences in early and late learning might not be applicable in young children. Adolph (1997) showed that the first movement strategies selected for a risky task, such as descending a steep slope, are goal-directed, but can be highly inefficient and do not take into account environmental cues. Children must "relearn" control in each position, and experience with the environmental conditions does not help. Children who had practiced descending slopes as crawlers tried to descend upright when they had learned to stand, even when it was not safe. They were no more proficient at the task than those children who had no previous experience with the slope. They did not recognize which conditions of the environment were regulatory or did not understand their own motor abilities. During development, children appear to try out a variety of movement strategies that happen to occur to them, perhaps accidentally, before selecting the most safe and economical one for the task at hand (Campbell, 2000a).

Practice can take place in blocked or random sequences. Blocked sequencing refers to practice in a drill-type repetition, during which the individual completes all trials of a given task before undertaking another task. Random sequencing refers to a mixed repetition of various tasks. In the early-learning stage, blocked practice is slightly more effective than random practice in acquisition of performance. Random practice has proven more beneficial than blocked sequence when measured on retention tests. Random sequencing requires a greater number of trials, and performance can actually deteriorate during the practice session.

Physical practice is essential to motor learning; however, mental practice is also a useful strategy of motor learning. Individuals can use this strategy pre-task, post-task, or between physical trials to enhance performance. Gabriele, Hall, and Lee (1989) found that learners benefited from mental practice in correcting errors in execution when they used random imagery practice. Alternating actual practice and imagery practice also facilitates motor learning (Kohl, Ellis, & Roenker, 1992). Rast (1986) described the benefits of visual imagery and imaginative play in children with CP and reported that mental imagery sparks interest and motivation, but also leads to spontaneous repetition of movement sequences. Other investigators examined the positive effects of mental practice on speed, balance, accuracy, and efficiency and found that mental practice can be particularly effective in the early-learning stage (Schmidt & Lee, 1999).

Scheduling of Practice

Scheduling practice trials is an aspect of motor learning that improves both performance and learning. Gentile (2000) determined that "distributed" practice, in which the amount of rest between trials equals or exceeds the amount of time of the trial, improves performance. Larin (2000) found that pediatric therapists used a distributed model of practice with intermittent breaks, implementing most of the recognized strategies for motor learning and teaching. In "massed" practice, the amount of practice time is greater than the amount of rest between trials. Distributed practice facilitates both performance and learning. Massed practice works best for discrete tasks in which the goal of practice is to increase peak performance on a well-learned task. This method of practice is useful in developing a high level of skill for a specific sport, gymnastics, or dance performance. Distributed practice has a positive effect on continuous or complex tasks, because tasks of this nature require greater energy expenditures and rest periods become increasingly important. Continuous practice can cause muscular fatigue. In children with CP, increased fatigue resulting from repetition of activities correlated with a lower rate of progress toward certain motor activities (Bower & McLellan, 1992). Schmidt (1991) suggested that to be effective, practice must be somewhat difficult and effortful; however, he cautioned that massed-practice designs for individuals with neuromotor impairment might increase the risk for injury because fatigue could put the learner at risk. Davies (1990) cautioned about the need to move without overexertion when using an NDT treatment approach for individuals following stroke. The NDT therapist always attempts to achieve the "just-right challenge," motivating and providing tasks that are somewhat difficult yet achievable.

Another factor that affects learning is the amount of variability within a practice sequence. There are two main purposes for including variability in motor learning. The first is to enhance generalizability and transfer or adaptability when the practice of one task contributes to the performance of another task in the same category. The second purpose is to establish competence throughout a movement sequence while maintaining the same fundamental pattern. Overall, low-variable practice translates into greater performance on the practiced task (Heitman, Erdmann, Gurchiek, Kovaleski, & Gilley, 1997). High-variable practice yields high performance on transfer to a task with a similar movement (Shea & Kohl, 1990) and better retention of learning when skill variations are from different classes of movement (Hall & Magill, 1995). In a study to evaluate long-term effects of intervention, Horn, Warren, and Jones (1995) found that children with CP were able to generalize movement components to unrelated skills from skills they had gained during NDT treatment sessions.

Many tasks are inherently variable and are called "open skills." Walking and maintaining balance in a moving metro or bus, or pedaling while steering a bike across a school playground, are examples of open skills. Tasks of this nature contain unpredictable perturbations. An important part of learning such tasks is acquiring the capability to cope with these novel situations. Achieving success in open skills requires the learner to constantly monitor the environmental context, identify advance cues, and process this information in a feed-forward manner. Movements become more diversified with flexible, adaptive coupling of coordinated structures. Random scheduling with variable practice generally leads to greater retention and error detection, at least for spatial performance (Sherwood, 1996). These types of activities are particularly difficult for children with CP or adults with sensory-perceptual problems following stroke (Toglia, 1990).

When the client is learning "closed skills," in which the environmental conditions are always quite similar, practice (certainly in the early stages of learning) should be consistent, enabling the learner to refine the movement pattern. Prior experience plays an important role. For example, every time a person stands up from a chair, the individual must bring the body forward over the feet to place the COM over the BOS. Changing the environmental context (such as chair height or seat configuration) or the kinematic demands (such as speed) does not change the movement synergy. The demands on information processing decrease with practice because conditions do not change. Movement combinations become more stable with fixed movement parameters that match the unchanging environment. Closed skills become "automatic," which reduces the need to monitor the surroundings continuously. Many real-life skills are made up of open- and closed-skill components. For example, learning to stabilize the body in relation to the support surface is a closed skill, whereas standing and reading as the bus moves, accommodating to the lurching motion and changing directions, is an open skill. Experienced therapists are able to make procedural changes in harmony with the learner's needs to process the necessary information successfully to solve various motor problems (Embry & Adams, 1996).

Feedback

Other than practice, feedback is the single most important variable for motor learning (Bilodeau, 1966). Feedback can occur before the task (in the form of initial instructions), during the task (as verbal or physical guidance), immediately after the task, or after and delayed in relation to task execution. The form of this information, the amount of it, and the time at which it is presented can affect performance and learning.

Feedback consists of two types, intrinsic and extrinsic. Intrinsic feedback occurs as a natural consequence of motor behavior and relates to the learner's various sensory channels involved when practicing a task. There are two categories of intrinsic feedback. The first provides information about the components of the movement, sensing speed, direction, accuracy, joint angles, muscle strength, and other factors. This feedback often involves the vestibular or somatosensory receptors. The second type of intrinsic feedback provides information about outcome and gives indications concerning the degree of goal attainment through vision, hearing, or feeling the success. Depending on the duration of the movement, intrinsic feedback often allows the learner to evaluate the success of a movement prior to completion. Because the body does not retain specific sensory consequences, feedback about outcomes is organized with reference to the goal. Theorists propose that intrinsic feedback is compared to a learned reference of correctness in a closed-loop motor control framework (see Figure 1.5). This reference acts in conjunction with the feedback in an error-detection process (Schmidt & Lee, 1999).

Extrinsic feedback is external information about the task that is supplemental to intrinsic feedback, such as a buzzer in the client's shoe that sounds each time heel-strike occurs. Extrinsic feedback can occur as a movement takes place (as in the example of the shoe buzzer), or after the movement. Extrinsic feedback about the nature of the movement pattern is called *knowledge of performance* (KP). Two types of KP feedback relevant to clients with motor control problems are kinematic feedback and kinetic feedback. Kinematic feedback consists of verbal observations that refer to aspects of movement such as position, time, velocity, acceleration, and patterns of coordination ("You were able to hold your weight on your right leg without hyperextending your knee," or "You will need to slow down in order to step down safely from the curb."). An important component of kinematic feedback is that it informs the learner about some aspect of the movement pattern that the individual might not otherwise perceive, such as information about the relative timing differences in two joints, or subtle changes in velocity. Most of the research suggests that the effectiveness of kinematic feedback depends on the nature of the task goal (Newell, Carlton, & Antoniou, 1990). Researchers assessed the effectiveness of kinematic feedback in tasks in which the feedback was identical to the goal of the task. For example, if the goal of the task is to improve weight shift forward over the feet, a pattern necessary to rise from a chair, then kinematic feedback that describes what went wrong ("You need to bend your body more forward to help bring your weight over your feet before rising.") will be an effective way to improve this movement pattern.

Kinetic feedback gives information about the forces that produce the variables, including the muscular forces that organize movement and their durations ("Keep your hand lightly on the paper cup while you drink," or "Keep a tight grip on the jump rope handle."). Although researchers have done less work in this area, it appears that feedback about the force needed for successful task completion affects both performance and learning (Howell, 1956; Newell & Carlton, 1985). KP appears to have the greatest effect on learning when it precisely specifies information that is critical for movement efficiency. This information is most useful when it promotes active, problem-solving activities in the learner (Brisson & Alain, 1996a).

For example, Thorpe and Valvano (2002) examined the effects of KP during practice of a novel motor skill in 13 children with CP. The researchers found that, with or without KP, all children benefited from practice; but when KP was used and enhanced with cognitive strategies, children were able to make greater gains in the learning of the motor skill.

Extrinsic feedback that provides information about the outcome of the movement in the environment is called *knowledge of results* (KR). Very little learning occurs in the absence of KR. This type of extrinsic feedback provides information about how the outcome of a task compares with the level of success in attaining the goal (Brisson & Alain, 1996a). In many real-life learning situations, the goal of the task is not connected to a specific movement pattern; rather, the individual can achieve that same outcome through various movement patterns. In the example of rising from a chair, the client might push down on the chair arms or seat with his or her hands, or not use the hands at all and still successfully rise from the chair. The goal in this example is not to shift the weight, but to get up to standing from the chair in the most energy-conserving or quickest way. KR is particularly useful when the goal is for the individual to achieve the best possible result by taking into account his or her unique physical attributes. Feedback on the inaccuracy and direction of errors provides information about the ways in which the person must modify the movement the next time and prescribes means to improve performance. Brisson and Alain (1996b) found that subjects who received KR as a reference were able to discover and reproduce the most efficient generalized motor program. Schmidt and Lee (1999) found that the frequency of KR and the time between task completion and KR were variables in enhancing learning. More immediate feedback during practice facilitated performance but was detrimental to learning, producing dependence. Finally, both KP and KR make the task appear more interesting, keep the learner alert, and cause the learner to set higher performance goals.

In summary, applying the best available knowledge and research on motor learning contributes to a systematic approach promoting skill acquisition in individuals with or without neuropathology. This information is particularly applicable in NDT, where motor learning concepts shape the training courses as well as provide a framework for planning and assessing the outcome of patient care.

Chapter Summary

1. Since its inception by the Bobaths, NDT has undergone many changes while preserving the basic philosophy and approach toward the treatment of individuals with neuropathology. NDT considers impaired patterns of postural control and movement coordination to be the primary impairments in clients with CP or stroke resulting from CNS pathology.

2. NDT practice currently uses a theoretical framework that is compatible with systems and selectionist models of motor control and motor development. New information in motor learning has expanded ideas for structuring a positive environment for examination and intervention. Clinical experience and scientific understanding have produced the changes in the theoretical basis of NDT as therapists strive to answer questions and better meet the needs of their clients.

3. NDT is a problem-solving approach, providing examination and treatment of the system impairments, motor dysfunction, and functional limitations of individuals with neuropathology.

4. NDT considers the individual as a whole and recognizes that neural and body systems, as well as contextual factors, contribute to the overall level of function.

5. NDT accepts that movement control in the nervous system is achieved through the selection of multiple neuronal networks connecting global maps that are distributed widely throughout the brain.

6. NDT recognizes that movement emerges from ongoing interactions among internal systems of the individual, the characteristics of the task, and the specific environmental context as the individual attempts to solve motor problems.

7. The advantage of adopting current models of motor control in NDT is that these theories account for the variability and adaptability of motor behavior in a variety of environmental conditions during development and during recovery from neuropathology.

8. NDT recognizes that there are two different types of sensory signals that complement each other. An individual uses feed-forward in anticipation and initiation of movement, and feedback to regulate and adapt movement to environmental constraints. Together, these sensory systems contribute to well-coordinated posture and movement.

9. Understanding typical posture and movement, how they link functions and systems, and how they change across the life span provides a critical framework for examination, analysis of sensorimotor problems, and treatment planning.

10. Therapeutic handling remains an integral part of an NDT approach to direct active movement toward the best possible solution for the individual client. However, NDT clinicians have enormous flexibility in choosing treatment methods, manipulating the individual, the task, or the environment in order to positively influence function.

11. NDT believes that intervention strategies, aimed at the underlying system impairments, are currently the best way to positively influence function.

12. NDT therapists accept that motor milestones appear as discrete, age-appropriate behaviors with definable onset. They arise from the continuous development of cooperating systems, giving rise to uniquely individual characteristics that define the person.

13. Different phases of the human life span are characterized by different motor behaviors designed for efficient functions at those times. A working knowledge of typical adaptive motor development and how it changes across the life span provides the framework for examining functions, evaluating limitations, and planning interventions.

14. In this new framework, therapists must be clear about the functional outcomes and make certain that demands on the various systems are compatible and appropriate for accomplishing the task in both realtime and developmental time.

15. The goal of NDT intervention is to optimize function. Applying principles of motor learning to learn or relearn motor skills involves a process associated with both practice and experience designed to fit the individual's lifestyle and goals.

One word of caution: Although new theoretical models are appealing, the data in support of these theories have *not,* for the most part, resulted from research with individuals with neuromotor disabilities. NDT believes that it would be inappropriate to expect that clients with sensorimotor impairments could gain normal motor skills simply by setting a goal, manipulating the environment, and waiting for optimal movement to occur. Many unanswered questions remain, both about movement in typically developing children and aging adults, and about movement in individuals with neuropathology. We can use this current thinking to add new concepts and hypotheses to existing clinical practice. In this way, we can broaden our approach to the examination and treatment of clients and merge theories of clinical practice with theories of motor control.

References

Abbott, A. L., & Bartlett, D. (1999). The relationship between the home environment and early motor development. *Physical and Occupational Therapy in Pediatrics, 19* (1), 43-57.

Abbott, A. L., Bartlett, D. J., Fanning, J. E., & Kramer, J. (2000). Infant motor development and aspects of the home environment. *Pediatric Physical Therapy, 12,* 62-67.

Abbs, J. H., Gracco, V. L., & Cole, K. J. (1984). Control of multi-movement coordination: Sensorimotor mechanisms in speech motor programming. *Journal of Motor Behavior, 16,* 195-232.

Abbs, J. H., & Winstein, C. J. (1990). Functional contributions of rapid and automatic sensory-based adjustments to motor output. In M. Jeannerod (Ed.), *Attention and performance XIII* (pp. 627-652). Hillsdale, NJ: Erlbaum.

Ada, L., Canning, C., & Westwood, P. (1990). The patient as active learner. In L. Ada and C. Canning (Eds.), *Key issues in neurological physiotherapy* (pp. 99-124). Boston: Butterworth Heinemann.

Adolph, K. E. (1997). Learning in the development of infant locomotion. *Monographs of the Society for Research in Child Development, 62* (3), 1-140.

Alexander, R., Cupps, B., & Boehme, R. (1993). *Normal development of functional skills.* Tucson, AZ: Therapy Skill Builders.

Allen, G. I., & Tsukahara, N. (1974). Cerebrocerebellar communications systems. *Physiological Reviews, 54,* 957-1006.

Aruin, A. S., & Latash, M. L. (1995). Directional specificity of postural muscles in feed-forward postural reactions during fast voluntary arm movements. *Experimental Brain Research, 103* (2), 323-332.

Atwater, S. W. (1991). Should the normal motor developmental sequence be used as a theoretical model in pediatric physical therapy? In M. Lister (Ed.), *Contemporary management of motor control problems. Proceedings from II Step Conference. Foundation for Physical Therapy* (pp. 89-93). Alexandria, VA: American Physical Therapy Association.

Barnes, K. (1986). Improving prehension skills of children with CP. A clinical study. *Occupational Therapy Journal of Research, 6,* 227-239.

Barnes, K. (1989). Relationship of upper extremity weight-bearing to hand skills of boys with CP. *Occupational Therapy Journal of Research 9,* 143-154.

Bass-Haugen, J., Mathiowetz, V., & Flinn, N. (2002). Optimizing motor behavior using occupational therapy task-oriented approach. In C. A. Trombly & W. Radomski (Eds.), *Occupational therapy for physical dysfunction* (5th ed., pp. 481-499). Philadelphia: Lippincott, Williams and Wilkins.

Beauregard, R., Thomas, J. J., & Nelson, D. L. (1988). Quality of reach during a game and during a rote movement in children with CP. *Physical and Occupational Therapy in Pediatrics, 18* (3/4), 67-84.

Belanger, L., Bolduc, M., & Noel, M. (1998). Relative importance of after-effects, environment and socio-economic factors on the social integration of stroke victims. *International Journal of Rehabilitation Research, 11* (3), 251-260.

Bernstein, N. A. (1967). *The co-ordination and regulation of movements.* Oxford, England: Pergamon Press.

Bierman, J. (1989, September/October). Theoretically speaking. *NDT Network,* 4-5.

Bilodeau, I. M. (1966). Information feedback. In E. A. Bilodeau (Ed.), *Acquisition of skill* (pp. 255-296). New York: Academic Press.

Birkmeier, K. (1997, July/August). Curriculum and theoretical base committee update. *NDT Network,* 1, 3, 6.

Blanche, E. I., & Hallway, M. (1998). Historical perspective: Neurodevelopmental Treatment in OT. *Developmental Disabilities Special Interest Section Quarterly, 21* (3), 1-3.

Bly, L. (1983). *The components of normal movement during the first year of life.* Laguna Beach, CA: Neuro-Developmental Treatment Association.

Bly, L. (1991). A historical and current view of the basis of NDT. *Pediatric Physical Therapy, 3* (3), 131-135.

Bly, L. (1994). *Motor skills acquisition in the first year. An illustrated guide to normal development.* San Antonio, TX: Therapy Skill Builders.

Bly, L. (1996, September/October). What if the role of sensation in motor learning? What is the role of feedback and feedforward? *NDT Network,* 1-7.

Bly, L. (1999). *Baby treatment based on NDT principles.* Tucson, AZ: Therapy Skill Builders.

Bobath, B. (1953). Control of postures and movements in the treatment of cerebral palsy. *Physiotherapy, 39* (5), 99-104.

Bobath, B. (1990). *Adult hemiplegia. Evaluation and treatment* (3rd ed.). Boston: Butterworth Heinemann.

Bobath, B., & Bobath, K. (1975). *Motor development in the different types of cerebral palsy.* London: Wm. Heinemann.

Bobath, K. (1980). *A neurophysiological basis for the treatment of cerebral palsy.* Philadelphia: J. B. Lippincott.

Bobath, K., & Bobath, B. (1956). Control of motor function in the treatment of cerebral palsy. *Australian Journal of Physiotherapy, 2* (2), 75-85.

Bobath, K., & Bobath, B. (1979). Acceptance Speech (audiotape), First Currative Foundation Awards Dinner, Milwaukee, WI.

Bobath, K., & Bobath, B. (1984). The Neuro-Developmental Treatment. In D. Scrutton (Ed.), *Management of the motor disorders of children with cerebral palsy. Clinics in Developmental Medicine* (90, pp. 6-18). Philadelphia: P. B. Lippincott.

Boehme, R. (1987). Developing hand function. In B. H. Connolly & P. C. Montgomery (Eds.), *Therapeutic exercise in developmental disabilities* (pp. 155-166). Chattanooga, TN: Chattanooga Corp.

Bouisset, Z. M. (1987). Biomechanical study of the programming of anticipatory postural adjustments associated with voluntary movement. *Journal of Biomechanics, 20* (8), 735-742.

Bower, E., & McLellan, D. L. (1992). Effect of increased exposure to physiotherapy on skill acquisition of children with cerebral palsy. *Developmental Medicine and Child Neurology, 34,* 25-39.

Boyd, L. A., & Winstein, C. J. (2001). Implicit motor-sequence learning in humans following unilateral stroke: the impact of practice and explicit knowledge. *Neuroscience Letters, 298* (1), 65-69.

Bradley, N. (2000). Motor control: Developmental aspects of motor control in skill acquisition. In S. K. Campbell, D. W. Vander Linden, & R. J. Palisano (Eds.), *Physical therapy for children* (2nd ed., pp. 45-87). Philadelphia: W. B. Saunders.

Brisson, T. A., & Alain, C. (1996a). Should common optimal movement patterns be identified as the criterion to be achieved? *Journal of Motor Behavior, 28,* 211-223.

Brisson, T. A., & Alain, C. (1996b). Optimal movement pattern characteristics are not required as a reference for knowledge of performance. *Research Quarterly for Exercise and Sport, 67,* 458-464.

Brooks, V. B. (1983). Motor control. How posture and movements are governed. *Physical Therapy, 63* (5), 664-674.

Bullinger, A. (1981). Cognitive elaboration of sensorimotor behavior. In G. Butterworth (Ed.), *Infancy and epistemology: An evaluation of Piaget's theory* (pp. 173-199). London: Harvester.

Butchner, D. M., & DeLateur, B. J. (1991). The importance of skeletal muscle strength to physical function in older adults. *Annals of Behavioral Medicine 13,* 1-12.

Butterworth, G., & Castillo, M. (1976). Coordination of auditory and visual space in newborn human infants. *Perception, 5* (2), 155-160.

Butterworth, G., & Hicks, L. (1997). Visual proprioception and postural stability in infancy. *Perception, 6,* 255-262.

Byl, H. N., Merzenich, M. M., Cheung, S., Bedenbaugh, P., Nagarajan, S. S., & Jinkins, W. M. (1997). A primate model for studying focal dystonia and repetitive strain injury. Effects on the primary somatosensory cortex. *Physical Therapy, 77,* 269-284.

Campbell, S. K. (1994). *Physical therapy for children.* Philadelphia: W. B. Saunders.

Campbell, S. K. (1997). Programs to last a lifetime. *Physical and Occupational Therapy in Pediatrics, 17* (1), 1-15.

Campbell, S. K. (1999a). *Decision making in pediatric neurologic physical therapy.* New York: Churchill Livingstone.

Campbell, S. K. (1999b). The infant at risk for developmental disability. In S. K. Campbell (Ed.), *Decision making in pediatric neurologic physical therapy* (pp. 260-332). New York: Churchill Livingstone.

Campbell, S. K. (2000a). The child's development of functional movement. In S. K. Campbell, D. W. Vander Linden, & R. J. Palisano (Eds.), *Physical therapy for children* (2nd ed., pp. 3-44). Philadelphia: W. B. Saunders.

Campbell, S. K. (2000b). Reevaluation in progress: A conceptual framework for examination and intervention. Part II. *Neurology Report, 24* (2), 42-46.

Campbell, S. K., Vander Linden, D. W., & Palisano, R. J. (Eds.). (2000). *Physical therapy for children* (2nd ed.). Philadelphia: W. B. Saunders.

Carr, J., & Shepherd, R. (2000). *Movement science: Foundation for physical therapy in rehabilitation* (2nd ed.). Gaithersburg, MD: Aspen Publishers.

Carson, R. G., & Riek, S. (2001). Changes in muscle recruitment patterns during skill acquisition. *Experimental Brain Research, 138* (1), 71-87.

Chakerian, D. L., & Larson, M. (1991, September). The effects of upper extremity weight-bearing on hand function in children with CP. *NDT Newsletter,* 1, 4-5, 19.

Cherry, D., & Knutson, L. (1993). Curriculum structure and content in pediatric PT: Results of a survey of entry-level PT programs. *Pediatric Physical Therapy, 5,* 109-113.

Chiel, H. J., & Beer, R. D. (1997). The brain has a body: Adaptive behavior emerges from interactions of nervous system, body and environment. *Trends in Neurosciences, 20* (12), 553-557.

Clark, J. E. (1982). Developmental differences in response processing. *Journal of Motor Behavior, 14,* 247-254.

Clifton, R. K., Muir, D. W., Asmead, D. H., & Clarkson, M. G. (1993). Is visually guided reaching in early infancy a myth? *Child Development, 64* (4), 1099-1110.

Connolly, B. H., & Montgomery, P. C. (1987). *Therapeutic exercise in developmental disabilities.* Chattanooga, TN: Chattanooga Corp.

Craft, M. J., Lakin, J. A., Oppliger, R. A., Clancy, G. M., & Vander Linden, D. W. (1990). Siblings as change agents for promoting the functional status of children with cerebral palsy. *Developmental Medicine and Child Neurology, 32* (12), 1049-1057.

Cupps, B. (1997, January/February). Postural control: A current view. *NDT Network,* 1, 3, 5, 7.

Cusick, B. (1990). *Progressive casting and splinting for lower extremity deformities in children with neuromotor dysfunction.* Tucson, AZ: Skill Builders.

Darrah, J., & Bartlett, D. (1995). Dynamic systems theory and management of children with CP: Unresolved issues. *Infants and Children, 8* (1), 52-59.

Davies, P. M. (1985). *Steps to follow. A guide to the treatment of adult hemiplegia.* New York: Springer Verlag.

Davies, P. M. (1990). *Right in the middle. Selective trunk activities in the treatment of adult hemiplegia.* New York: Springer-Verlag.

DeGangi, G., DiPietro, J., Greenspan, S., & Porges, S. (1991). Psychophysiological characteristics of the regulatory disordered infant. *Infant Behavior and Development, 14,* 37-50.

Delong, M. R., Gerogopoulos, A. P., & Crutcher, M. D. (1983). Cortico-basal ganglia relations and coding of motor performance. In J. Massion & J. Palliard (Eds.), *Neural coding of motor performance* (pp. 30-40). New York: Springer-Verlag.

Dunn, W., Brown, C., & McGuigan, A. (1994). The ecology of human performance: a framework for considering the effect of context. *American Journal of Occupational Therapy, 48* (7), 595-607.

Edelman, G. M. (1987). *Neural Darwinism. The theory of neuronal group selection.* New York: Basic Books.

Edelman, G. M. (1989). *Bright air, brilliant fire.* New York: Basic Books.

Edelman, G. M. (1992). *Bright air, brilliant fire: On the matter of the mind.* New York: Basic Books.

Embry, D. G., & Adams, L. S. (1996). Clinical applications of procedural changes by experienced and novice pediatric physical therapists. *Pediatric Physical Therapy, 8,* 122-132.

Fetters, L. (1991). Cerebral palsy: Contemporary treatment concepts. In M. Lister (Ed.), *Contemporary management of motor control problems. Proceedings from II Step Conference. Foundation for Physical Therapy* (pp. 219-224). Alexandria, VA: American Physical Therapy Association.

Finnie, N. R. (1997). *Handling the young child with cerebral palsy at home* (3rd ed.). Boston: Butterworth and Heineman.

Fisher, A. G., Murray, E., & Bundy, A. C. (1991). *Sensory integration: Theory and practice* Philadelphia: Davis.

Fitts, P. M. (1962). Factors in complex skill learning. In R. Blasser (Ed.), *Training, research and education* (pp. 177-197). Pittsburgh, PA: University of Pittsburgh Press.

Forssberg, H., Kinoshita, H., Eliasson, A. C., Johansson, R. S., Westling, G., & Gordan, A. M. (1992). Development of human precision grip II. Anticipatory control of isometric forces targeted for object's weight. *Experimental Brain Research, 90,* 393-398.

Forssberg, H., & Nashner, L. M. (1982). Ontogenetic development of postural control in man: Adaptation to altered support and visual conditions during stance. *Journal of Neuroscience 2* (5), 545-522.

Foster, E., Sveistrup, H., & Woollacott, M. H. (1996). Transitions in visual proprioception: A cross-sectional development study of the effect of visual flow on postural control. *Journal of Motor Behavior, 28,* 101-112.

Foudriat, B. A. (1993). Sensory organization of balance responses in children 3-6 years of age. A normative study with diagnostic implications. *International Journal of Pediatric Otorhinolaryngology, 27* (3), 255-271.

Fowler, E. G., Ho, T. W., Nwigwe, A. I., & Dorey, F. J. (2001). The effect of quadriceps femoris muscle strengthening exercises on spasticity in children with CP. *Physical Therapy, 81* (6) 1215-1223.

Gabriele, T. E., Hall, C. R., & Lee, T. D. (1989). Cognition in motor learning: Imagery effects on contextual interference. *Human Movement Science, 8,* 227-245.

Gajdosik, C. G., & Gajdosik, R. L. (2000). Musculoskeletal development and adaptation. In S. K. Campbell (Ed.), *Physical therapy for children* (pp. 117-140). Philadelphia: Churchill Livingstone.

Gentile, A. M. (2000). Skill acquisition: Action, movement, and neuromotor processes. In J. Carr & R. Shepherd (Eds.), *Movement science. Foundations for physical therapy in rehabilitation* (2nd ed., pp. 111-187). Gaithersburg, MD: Aspen.

Gesell, A. (1928). *Infancy and human growth.* New York: McMillan

Gibson, E. J. (1988). Exploratory behavior in the development of perceiving, acting and the acquiring of knowledge. *Annual Review of Psychology, 39,* 1-41.

Gibson, J. J. (1966). *The senses considered as perceptual systems.* Boston: Houghton Mifflin.

Girolami, G., & Campbell, S. K. (1994). The efficacy of a neuro-developmental treatment program for improving motor control in preterm infants. *Pediatric Physical Therapy, 6,* 175-183.

Giuffrida, C. (1998). Motor learning: An emerging frame of reference for occupational performance. In M. E. Neistadt & E. B. Crepear (Eds.), *Willard and Spackman's Occupational Therapy* (9th ed., pp. 560-567). Philadelphia: J. B. Lippincott.

Giuliani, C. A. (1991). Theories of motor control: New concepts for physical therapy. In M. Lister (Ed.), *Contemporary management of motor control problems. Proceedings from II Step Conference. Foundation for Physical Therapy* (pp. 29-36). Alexandria, VA: American Physical Therapy Association.

Goodgold-Edwards, S. (1993). Principles for guiding action during motor learning. *Physical Therapy Practice, 2* (4), 30-39.

Gordon, J. (2000). Assumptions underlying physical therapy intervention: Theoretical and historical perspectives. In J. Carr & R. Shepherd (Eds.), *Movement science: Foundations for physical therapy in rehabilitation* (2nd ed., pp. 1-32). Gaithersburg, MD: Aspen Pub.

Gray, C. M., & Singer, W. (1989). Stimulus-specific neuronal oscillations in orientation columns of cat visual cortex. *Proceedings of the National Academy of Sciences, 86,* 1698-1702.

Greenspan, S. (1997). *The growth of the mind.* Reading, MA: Addison Wesley Pub.

Greiner, B. M., Czerniecki, J. M., & Deitz, J. C. (1993). Gait parameters of children with spastic diplegia: A comparison of effects of posterior and anterior walkers. *Archives of Physical Medicine and Rehabilitation, 74,* 381-385.

Hadders-Algra, M. (2000). The neuronal group selection theory: Promising principles for understanding and treating developmental motor disorders. *Developmental Medicine and Child Neurology, 24* (10), 707-715.

Hadders-Algra, M., Brogren, E., & Forssberg, H. (1996a). Ontogeny of postural adjustments during sitting in infancy: Variation, selection and modulation. *Journal of Physiology, 493,* 273-288.

Hadders-Algra, M., Brogren, E., & Forssberg, H. (1996b). Training affects the development of postural adjustments in sitting infants. *Journal of Physiology, 493,* 289-298.

Hall, K. G., & Magill, R. A. (1995). Variability of practice and contextual interference in motor skill learning. *Journal of Motor Behavior, 27,* 299-309.

Hartbourne, R. T., Giuliani, C., & MacNeela, J. (1993). A kinematic and electromyographic analysis of the development of sitting posture in infants. *Developmental Psychobiology, 26,* 51-64.

Hayes, M. S., McEwen, I. R., Lovett, D., Sheldon, M. M., & Smith, D. D. W. (1999). Next step: Motor control, motor development and motor learning as they relate to services for children with developmental disabilities. *Pediatric Physical Therapy, 11* (4), 164-182.

Heitman, R., Erdmann, J., Gurchiek, L., Kovaleski, J., & Gilley, W. (1997). From the field. Constant versus variable practice in learning a motor task using individuals with learning disabilities. *Clinical Kinesiology, 51,* 62-65.

Heriza, C. B. (1988). Organization of leg movements in preterm infants. *Physical Therapy, 68,* 1340-1346.

Heriza, C. (1991). Motor development: Traditional and contemporary theories. In M. Lister (Ed.), *Contemporary management of motor control problems. Proceedings from II Step Conference. Foundation for Physical Therapy* (pp. 99-126). Alexandria, VA: American Physical Therapy Association.

Hesse, S., Bertelt, C., Schaffrin, A., Malezic, M., & Mauritz, K. H.(1994). Restoration of gait in nonambulatory hemiparetic patients by treadmill training with partial body-weight support. *Archives of Physical Medicine and Rehabilitation, 75,* 1087-1093.

Higgins, S. (1991). Motor skill acquisition. *Physical Therapy,* 71, 123-139.

Higgins, J. R., & Spaeth, R. K. (1972). Relationship between consistency of movement and environment conditions. *Quest, 17,* 61-69.

Hodges, P. W., Cresswell, A. G., & Thorstensson, A. (2001). Perturbed upper limb movements cause short-latency postural responses in trunk muscles. *Experimental Brain Research, 138,* 234-250.

Hodges, P. W., & Richardson, C. A. (1997). Feedforward contraction of transversus abdominis is not influenced by the direction of arm movement. *Experimental Brain Research, 114,* 362-370.

Hopkins, B., & Westra, T. (1989). Maternal expectations and motor development: Some cultural differences. *Developmental Medicine and Child Neurology, 31,* 384-408.

Hopkins, B., & Westra, T. (1990). Motor development, maternal expectations and the role of handling. *Infant Behavior and Development, 13,* 117-122.

Horak, F. B. (1991). Assumptions underlying motor control for neurologic rehabilitation. In M. Lister (Ed.), *Contemporary management of motor control problems. Proceedings from II Step Conference. Foundation for Physical Therapy* (pp. 11-28). Alexandria, VA: American Physical Therapy Association.

Horn, E. M., Warren, S. F., & Jones, H. A. (1995). An experimental analysis of neurobehavioral motor intervention. *Developmental Medicine and Child Neurology, 37,* 697-714.

Howell, M. L. (1956). Use of force-time graphs for performance analysis in facilitating motor learning. *Research Quarterly, 27,* 12-22.

Howle, J. W. (1999). Cerebral palsy. In S. K. Campbell (Ed.), *Decision making in pediatric neurologic physical therapy* (pp. 23-83). Philadelphia: Churchill Livingstone.

Humphrey, T. (1978). Function of the nervous system during prenatal life. In U. Stave (Ed.), *Perinatal physiology* (pp. 651-683). New York: Plenum.

Jackson, J. H. (1958). *Selected writings.* London: Staples Press. (Reprinted from *Selected writings of John B. Hughlings* [vols. I, II], by J. H. Jackson & J. Taylor, Eds., 1932, London: Hodder, Stoughter).

Jantz, J. W., Blosser, C. D., & Fruechting, L. A. (1997). A motor milestone change noted with a change in sleep position. *Archives of Pediatrics and Adolescent Medicine, 151,* 565-568.

Jenison, R. L. (1997). On acoustic information for motion. *Ecological Psychology, 9,* 131-151.

Jorgensen, H. S., Nakayama, H., Raaschou, H. O., & Olsen, T. S. (1995). Recovery of walking function in stroke patients: The Copenhagen Stroke Study. *Archives of Physical Medicine and Rehabilitation, 76,* 27-32.

Kamm, K., Thelen, E., & Jenson, J. L. (1990). A dynamic system approach to motor development. *Physical Therapy, 70* (12), 763-775, 1990.

Kahn-D'Angelo, L., & Unanue, R. A. (2000). The special care nursery. In S. K. Campbell (Ed.), *Physical therapy for children* (2nd ed., pp. 840-880). Philadelphia: W. B. Saunders.

Kandel, E., Schwartz, J., & Jessell, T. (Eds.). (1991). *Principles of neural science* (3rd ed.) New York: Elsevier Press.

Keele, S. W., Cohen, A., & Ivry, R. (1990). Motor programs: Concepts and issues. In M. Jeannerod (Ed.), *Attention and performance XIII* (pp. 77-110). Hillsdale, NJ. Erlbaum.

Keele, S. W., & Summers, J. J. (1976). The structure of motor programs. In G. E. Stelmach (Ed.), *Motor control: Issues and trends* (pp. 161-186). New York: Academic Press..

Kelso, J. A. S. (1976). Two strategies for investigating action. In G. E. Stelmach (Ed.), *Motor control: Issues and trends* (pp. 283-287). New York: Academic Press.

Kelso, J. A. S. (1984). Phase transitions and critical behavior in human bimanual coordination: Regulatory, integrative and comparative physiology. *American Journal of Physiology, 15,* R1000-R1004.

Kelso, J. A. S. (1992). Theoretical concepts and strategies for understanding perceptual-motor skill: From information capacity in closed systems to self-organization in open, non-equilibrium systems. *Journal of Experimental Psychology, General, 121,* 260-261.

Keshner, E. A. (1991). How theoretical framework biases evaluation and treatment. In M. Lister (Ed.), *Contemporary management of motor control problems. Proceedings from II Step Conference. Foundation for Physical Therapy* (pp. 37-48). Alexandria, VA: American Physical Therapy Association.

Keshner, E. A., Campbell, D., Katz, R., & Peterson, B. W. (1989). Neck muscle activation patterns in humans during isometric head stabilization. *Experimental Brain Research, 75,* 335-364.

Klapp, S. T., Anderson, W. G., & Berrian, R. W. (1973). Implicit speech in reading, reconsidered. *Journal of Experimental Psychology, 100,* 368-374.

Kohl, R. M., Ellis, S. D., & Roenker, D. L. (1992). Alternating actual and imagery practice: Preliminary theoretical considerations. *Research Quarterly for Exercise and Sport, 63,* 162-170.

Kugler, P. N., Kelso, J. A. S., & Turvey, M. T. (1980). On the concept of coordinative structures as dissipative structures: I. Theoretical lines of convergence. In G. E. Stelmach & J. Requin (Eds.), *Tutorial in motor behavior* (pp. 3-47). New York: Elsevier Science Publishing Co., Inc.

Kuypers, H. G. (1981). Anatomy of the descending pathways. In J. M. Brookhart & V. B. Mountcastle (Eds.), *Handbook of Physiology. Volume II: Motor Control.* Bethesda, MD: American Physiological Society.

Kyllo, L. B., & Landers, D. M. (1995). A research synthesis to resolve the controversy. *Journal of Sport and Exercise Psychology, 17,* 117-137.

Larin, H. (2000). Motor learning: Theories and strategies for the practitioner. In S. K. Campbell, D. W. Vander Linden, & R. J. Palisano (Eds.), *Physical therapy for children* (2nd ed., pp. 170-197). Philadelphia: W. B. Saunders.

Latash, M. L. (1998). *Progress in motor control: Bernstein's traditions in movement studies.* Champaign, IL: Human Kinetics.

Lee, D. N., & Lishman, R. (1975). Visual proprioceptive control of stance. *Journal of Human Movement Studies, 1,* 87-95

Lewthwaite, R. (1990). Motivational considerations in physical activity involvement. *Physical Therapy, 70,* 808-819.

Lin, K., Wu, C., & Trombly, C. A. (1998). Effects of task goal on movement kinematics and line bisection performance in adults without disabilities. *American Journal of Occupational Therapy, 53,* 179-187.

Logan, L., Byers-Hinley, K., & Ciccone, C. (1990). Anterior vs. posterior walkers for children with cerebral palsy: A gait analysis study. *Developmental Medicine and Child Neurology, 32,* 1044-1048.

Maruishi, M., Mano, Y., Sasaki, T., Shinmyo, N., Sato, H., & Ogawa, T. (2001). Cerebral palsy in adults: Independent effects of muscle strength and muscle tone. *Archives of Physical Medicine and Rehabilitation, 82,* 637-641.

Massery, M. P. (1996). The patient with neuromuscular or musculoskeletal dysfunctions. In D. L. Frownfleter & E. Dean (Eds.), *Principles and practice of cardiopulmonary physical therapy* (3rd ed., pp. 679-702). St. Louis, MO: Mosby Year Book.

Massery, M., & Moerchen, V. (1996, November/December). Coordinating transitional movements and breathing in patients with neuromotor dysfunction. *NDT Network,* 1-7.

Massion, J. (1992). Movement, posture and equilibrium: Interaction and coordination. *Progress in Neurobiology, 38* (1), 35-36.

Mayston, M. J. (1992). The Bobath concept: Evolution and application. In H. Forssberg & H. Hirschfeld (Eds.), *Movement disorders in children* (vol. 36, pp. 1-6). Basel, Switzerland: Medicine and Sport Science/Karger.

Mayston, M. J.(2001). People with cerebral palsy: effects of and perspectives for therapy. *Neural Plasticity,* 8, 51-69.

McCarty, M. E., Clifton, R. K., Asmead, D. H., Lee, P., & Gojubet, N. (2001). How infants use vision for grasping objects. *Child Development, 72* (4), 973-87.

McGraw, M. (1963). *The neuromuscular maturation of the human infant.* New York: Hafner. (Original work published 1945, Columbia University Press.)

Milani-Comparetti, A. (1967). Pattern analysis of motor development and its disorders. *Developmental Medicine and Child Neurology, 9,* (5), 625-630.

Morris, M. E., Summers, J. J., Matyas, T. A., & Lansek, R. (1994). Current status of the motor program. *Physical Therapy, 74* (8), 738-752.

Muir, R. B., & Lemon, R. H. (1983). Corticospinal neurons with a spinal role in precision grip. *Brain Research, 261,* 312-316.

Newell, K. M., & Carlton, L. G. (1985). On the relationship between peak force variability in isometric tasks. *Journal of Motor Behavior, 17,* 230-241.

Newell, K. M., Carlton, M. J., & Antoniou, A. (1990). The interaction of criterion and feedback information in learning a drawing task. *Journal of Motor Behavior, 22,* 536-552.

Padula, W. V., & Argyris, S. (1996). Post trauma vision syndrome and visual midline shift syndrome. *NeuroRehabilitation 6,* 1665-1671.

Pehoski, C. (1995). Cortical control of skilled movements of the hand. In A. Henderson & C. Pehoski (Eds.), *Hand function in the child: Foundations for remediation* (pp. 3-15). St. Louis, MO: Mosby.

Perry, S. B. (1998). Clinical implications of a dynamical systems theory. *Neurology Report, 22,* 4-10.

Prechtl, H. F. R. (1997). The importance of fetal movements. In K. J. Connoly & H. Forssberg (Eds.), *Neurophysiology and neuropsychology of motor development. Clinics in Developmental Medicine 143/144* (pp. 42-53). London: McKeith Press.

Quinton, M., & Wilson, J. (1981). Competition of movement patterns applied to the development of infants. In D. Slaton & J. Wilson (Eds.), *Caring for special babies.* Chapel Hill: Division of Physical Therapy, University of North Carolina-Chapel Hill.

Quinton, M. (2002). *Making the difference with babies: Concepts and guidelines for baby treatment.* Albuquerque, N.M.: Clinician's View.

Rast, M. (1986). Play and therapy, play or therapy. In *Play: A skill for life* (pp. 29-41). Rockville, MD: American Occupational Therapy Association.

Rast, M. (2000, January/February). NDT in continuum: Micro to macro levels in therapy. *NDT Network,* 1, 4-7.

Reed, D. L. (1996). The effect of the saddle seat on seated postural control and upper extremity movement in children with cerebral palsy. *Developmental Medicine and Child Neurology, 38,* 805-815.

Ronnqvist, L., & Hopkins, B. (2000). Motor asymmetries in the human newborn are state dependent, but independent of position in space. *Experimental Brain Research, 134* (3), 378-84.

Rosenbaum, D. A. (1977). Selective adaptation of "command neurons" in the human motor system. *Neuropsychologia, 15,* 81-91.

Ross, S.A., Engsberg, J. R., Wagner, J. & Park, T. S. (2002). Changes in gait and gross motor function measure at 8 months after selective dorsal rhizotomy. *Developmental Medicine and Child Neurology. Supplement* 91 (44), 23-24.

Ryerson, S., & Levit, K. (1997). *Functional movement reeducation.* Philadelphia: Churchill Livingstone.

Salmoni, A. W., Schmidt, R. A., & Walter, C. B. (1984). Knowledge of results and motor learning: A review and critical reappraisal. *Psychological Bulletin, 95,* 355-386.

Schindl, M. R., Forstner, C., Kern, H., & Hesse, S. (2000). Treadmill training with partial body weight support in nonambulatory patients with cerebral palsy. *Archives of Physical Medicine and Rehabilitation, 81,* 301-306.

Schmidt, R. A. (1976). More on motor programs. In G. E. Stelmach (Ed.), *Motor control: Issues and trends* (pp. 189-217). New York: Academic Press.

Schmidt, R. A. (1991). Motor learning principles for physical therapy. In M. Lister (Ed.), *Contemporary management of motor control problems. Proceedings from II Step Conference. Foundation for Physical Therapy* (pp. 49-64). Alexandria, VA: American Physical Therapy Association.

Schmidt, R. A., & Lee, T. D. (1999). *Motor control and learning. A behavioral emphasis* (3rd ed.). Champaign, IL: Human Kinetics.

Scholz, J. P. (1990). Dynamic pattern theory: Some implications for therapeutics. *Physical Therapy, 70* (12), 827-843.

Schotland, J. (1992). Neural control of innate behavior. In H. Forssberg & H. Hirschfeld (Eds.), *Movement disorders in children* (vol. 36, pp. 159-168). Basel, Switzerland: Medicine and Sport Science/Karger.

Shea, C. H., & Kohl, R. M. (1990). Specificity and variability of practice. *Research Quarterly for Exercise and Sport, 61,* 169-177.

Sherrington, C. S. (1947). *The integrative action of the nervous system* (3rd ed.). New Haven, CT: Yale University Press.

Sherwood, D. E. (1996). The benefits of random variable practice for spatial accuracy and error detection in a rapid aiming task. *Research Quarterly for Exercise and Sport, 67,* 35-43.

Shumway-Cook, A., Baldwin, M., Pollisar, N., & Aruber, W. (1997). Predicting the probabilities of falls in community dwelling older adults. *Physical Therapy, 77,* 812-819.

Shumway-Cook, A., & Woollacott, M. H. (2000). Attentional demands and postural control: The effect of sensory context. *Journal of Gerontology Series A. Biological Sciences and Medical Sciences, 55* (1), M10-16.

Shumway-Cook, A., & Woollacott, M. H. (2001). *Motor control. Theory and practical applications* (2nd ed.). Philadelphia: Lippincott Williams and Wilkins.

Sochaniwskyj, A. E., Koheil, R., Bablich, K., Milner, M., & Lotto, W. (1991). Dynamic monitoring for sitting posture for children with spastic cerebral palsy. *Clinical Biomechanics, 6,* 161.

Sporns, O. (1994). Selectionist and instructionist ideas in neuroscience. *International Review of Neurobiology, 37,* 3-26.

Sporns, O., & Edelman, G. M. (1993). Solving Bernstein's problem: A proposal for the development of coordinated movement by selection. *Child Development, 64,* 960-981.

Sporns, O., Tononi, G., & Edelman, G. M. (2000). Connectivity and complexity: The relationship between neuroanatomy and brain dynamics. *Neural Networks, 13* (8-9), 909-922.

Stack, D. M., & Arnold, S. L. (1998). Changes in mother's touch and hand gestures influence infant behavior in face-to-face interchanges. *Infant Behavior and Development, 21* (3), 451-468.

Stelmach, G. E. (1976). Motor control and motor learning: The closed loop perspective. In G. E. Stelmach (Ed.), *Motor control: Issues and trends* (pp. 93-115). New York: Academic Press.

Sveistrup, H., & Woollacott, M. H. (1997). Practice modifies the developing automatic postural response. *Experimental Brain Research, 114* (1), 33-43.

Sweeney, J. K., Heriza, C. B., & Mrakowitz, R. (1994). The changing role of pediatric PT: A 10-year analysis of clinical practice. *Pediatric Physical Therapy, 6,* 113-118.

Taub, E., & Berman, A. J. Movement and learning in the absence of sensory feedback. In S. J. Freedman (Ed.), *The neuropsychology of spatially oriented behavior* (pp. 173-192). Homewood. IL: Dorsey.

Thelen, E. (1985). Developmental origins of motor coordination. Leg movements in human infants. *Developmental Psychobiology, 18* (1), 1-22.

Thelen, E. (1986). Development of coordinated movement: Implications for early human development. In M. G. Wage & H. T. A. Whiting (Eds.), *Motor development in children: Aspects of coordination and control* (pp. 107-120). Boston: Martinus Nijhoff Publishers.

Thelen, E. (1992). Development of locomotion from a dynamical systems approach. In H. Forssberg & H. Hirschfeld (Eds.), *Movement disorders in children* (vol. 36, pp. 169-173). Basel, Switzerland: Medicine and Sport Science/Karger.

Thelen, E. (1994). *A dynamic systems approach to the development of cognition and action.* Cambridge, MA: Bradford Books/MIT Press.

Thelen, E. (1995). Motor development: A new synthesis. *American Psychologist,* 50, 79-95.

Thelen, E. (1998). Self-organization in developmental processes: Can system approaches work? In M. Gunner & E. Thelen (Eds.), *System and development* (pp. 77-117). Minnesota Symposium on Child Psychology. Hillsdale, NJ: Erlbaum.

Thelen, E., Corbella, D., Kamm, K., Spencer, J. P., Schneider, K., & Zernicke, R. F. (1993). The transition to reaching: Mapping intentional and intrinsic dynamics. *Child Development, 64,* 1058-1098, 1993.

Thelen, E., Kelso, J. A. S., & Fogel, A. (1987). Self-organizing systems and infant motor development. *Developmental Review, 7* (1), 39-65.

Thelen, E., & Ulrich, B. (1991). Hidden Skills. *Monographs of the Society for Research in Child Development, 56* (1, Serial No. 223).

Thorpe, D. E., & Valvano, J. (2002). The effects of knowledge of performance and cognitive strategies on motor skill learning in children with cerebral palsy. *Pediatric Physical Therapy, 14,* 2-15.

Toglia, J. P. (1990). Generalization of treatment: A multicontext approach to cognitive perceptual impairments in adults with brain injury. *American Journal of Occupational Therapy, 45* (6), 505-516.

Toglia, J. P. (1991). Generalization of treatment: A multicontext approach to cognitive perceptual impairment in adults with brain injury. *American Journal of Occupational Therapy, 45,* 505-516.

Treisman, A. (1988). Features and objects: The Bartlett Memorial Lecture. *Journal of Experimental Psychology, 40A,* 201-237.

Tscharnuter, I. (1993). A new therapy approach to movement organization. *Physical and Occupational Therapy in Pediatrics, 13* (2), 19-40.

Tscharnuter, I. (2002). Clinical application of dynamic theory concepts according to Tscharnuter Akademie for Movement Organization (TAMO) Therapy. *Pediatric Physical Therapy, 14,* 29-37.

Tuller, B., Turvey, M. T., & Fitch, H. L. (1976). The Bernstein perspective: II. The concept of muscle linkage or coordinative structure. In G. E. Stelmach (Ed.), *Motor control: Issues and trends* (pp. 253-270). New York: Academic Press.

Ulrich, D. B. (1997). Dynamic systems theory and skill development in infants and children. In K. J. Connolly & H. Forssberg (Eds.), *Neurophysiology and neuropsychology of motor development. Clinics in Developmental Medicine, 143/144* (pp. 319-345). Philadelphia: J. B. Lippincott.

Valvano, J., & T. Long. (1991). Neurodevelopmental Treatment: A review of the writings of the Bobaths. *Pediatric Physical Therapy, 3* (3), 125-129.

van der Weel, F. R., van der Meer, A. L. H., & Lee, D. H. (1991). Effect of task on movement control in cerebral palsy: Implication for assessment and therapy. *Developmental Medicine and Child Neurology, 33,* 419-426.

Van Sant, A. (1991). Neurodevelopmental treatment and pediatric physical therapy: A commentary. *Pediatric Physical Therapy 3* (3), 137-141.

Van Vliet, P., Sheridan, M., Kerwin, D. G., & Fentem, P. (1995). The influence of functional goals on the kinematics of reaching following stroke. *Neurology Report, 19* (1), 11-16.

von Hofsten, C. (1982). Eye-hand coordination in the newborn. *Developmental Psychology, 18* (3), 450-461.

von Hofsten, C. (1991). Structuring of early reaching movements–A longitudinal study. *Journal of Motor Behavior, 23* (4), 280-292.

von Hofsten, C., & Ronnqvist, L. (1993). The structuring of neonatal arm movements. *Child Development, 64* (4), 1046-1057.

von Hofsten, C., Vishton, P., Spelke, E. S., Feng, Q., & Fosander, K. (1998). Predictive action in infancy: Tracking and reaching for moving objects. *Cognition 67,* 255-285.

von Hofsten, C., & Woollacott, M. (1989). Anticipatory postural adjustments during infant reaching. *Neuroscience Abstracts, 15,* 1199.

Wade, M. G., Linquest, R., Taylor, J. R., & Treat-Jacobson, D. (1995). Optical flow, spatial orientation and the control of posture in the elderly. *Journal of Gerontology, 50B,* 51-58.

Walshe, F. M. R. (1961). Contributions of J. Hughlings Jackson to neurology. *Archives of Neurology,* 119-131.

Weiner, A. S., Long, T., DeGangi, G., & Bataile, B. (1996). Sensory processing of infants born prematurely or with regulatory disorders. *Physical and Occupational Therapy in Pediatrics, 16* (4), 1-16.

Whiting, H. T. A. (Ed). (1984). *Human motor actions–Bernstein reassessed.* New York: Elsevier Science Publications.

Wilson, J. (1989). Outpatient-based physical therapy program for children with cerebral palsy undergoing selective dorsal rhizotomy. In T. S. Park, L. H. Phillips, & W. J. Peacock (Eds.), *Management of spasticity in cerebral palsy and spinal cord injury. Neurosurgery: State of the Art Reviews, 4* (2), 417-429.

Wimmers, R. H., Savelsbergh, G. J. P., Beek, P. J., & Hopkins, B. (1998). Evidence for a phase transition in the early development of prehension. *Developmental Psychobiology, 32* (3), 235-248.

Winstein, C. J. (1991). Designing practice for motor learning: Clinical implications. In M. Lister (Ed.), *Contemporary management of motor control problems. Proceedings from II Step Conference. Foundation for Physical Therapy* (pp. 65-76). Alexandria, VA: American Physical Therapy Association.

Woodruff, N. (2000). *Someone Else's Child.* (p. 105). N. Y: Simon & Schuster.

Woollacott, M. H., & Shumway-Cook, A. (1989). *Development of posture and gait across the life span.* Columbia: University of South Carolina Press.

Woollacott, M., & Shumway-Cook, A. (1990). Changes in posture control across the life span: A systems approach. *Physical Therapy, 70,* 799-807.

Woollacott, M., & Sveistrup, H. (1992). Changes in the sequencing and timing of muscle response coordination associated with developmental transitions in balance abilities. *Human Movement Science, 11,* 23-36.

World Health Organization. (1999). *ICIDH-2: International classification of functioning and disability. Beta-2 draft, short version.* Geneva, Switzerland: Author.

Wu, C., Trombly, C. A., Lin, K., & Tickle-Degnen, L. (2000). A kinematic study of contextual effects on reaching performance in persons with and without stroke: Influences of object availability. *Archives of Physical Medicine and Rehabilitation, 81* (1), 95-101.

Zernicke, R. F., & Schneider, K. (1993). Biomechanics and developmental neuromotor control. *Child Development, 64* (4), 982-1004.

Chapter 2

Movement Dysfunction

"The main problem of patients with lesions of the upper motor neurone...is abnormal coordination of movement patterns. Problems of the strength and activity of individual muscles and muscle groups we see as secondary to that of the coordination of their action. The assessment and treatment of the patient's motor patterns is the only way of leading directly to functional use." (B. Bobath, 1990, p. xiii)

Introduction

Like all persons, individuals with central nervous system (CNS) pathology develop movement from the need to solve motor problems in a specific context by using whatever neural and body systems are available to them. The Neuro-Developmental Treatment (NDT) approach recognizes that atypical movements in individuals with CNS pathology result from (a) damage to specific (discrete or diffuse) neural tissue, (b) the attempt of the many remaining subsystems distributed throughout the nervous system to compensate for the initial lesion, (c) the linkage of body systems and environmental factors to a damaged neural system, producing ineffective interactions, and (d) the inability of the CNS to adapt to opportunities afforded by the environment. These factors lead to a decrease in function and disability in daily life. Analysis of these interrelationships in a model of enablement/disablement allows the NDT clinician to classify movement disorders as they affect the individual's life, guide clinical decision making, develop strategies for client examination, implement treatment, and measure outcomes.

This chapter examines the enablement/disablement model that provides an overall framework in NDT for organizing, labeling, and categorizing biological and social perspectives on motor dysfunction. The chapter describes in depth the specific impairments that occur in individuals with CNS neuropathology, relating these impairments to posture, movement, and functional activities in various contexts, demonstrating the problem-solving method and clinical reasoning that constitutes the NDT approach.

NDT Enablement Model of Health and Disability

NDT Focus: NDT has always emphasized the individual as a whole person with competencies and limitations. The NDT modification of the ICF taxonomy adds a fourth dimension focused on motor functions in the attempt to answer the questions, What does the client do? How does the client do it? and, Why does the client do it?

In 1998, the Instructors Group of the NDT Association (NDTA) adapted the International Classification of Impairments, Disabilities, and Handicaps (ICIDH-2) taxonomy developed by the World Health Organization (1999; currently International Classification of Function, ICF; World Health Organization, 2001) by adding a fourth dimension–motor functions–as part of the decision-making process in NDT to help plan interventions directed to specific functional outcomes and ascertain the individual's participation in society. This four-level enablement model (see Table 2.1) classifies function and disability in four dimensions: (a) system integrity/impairments, (b) effective/ineffective posture and movement, (c) individual functional activities/activity limitations, and (d) participation/participation restrictions in clients with cerebral palsy (CP) or stroke. Each dimension addresses the entire continuum from function to disability, consequently each dimension has a positive and a negative domain. This model was selected for very sound reasons. It mirrors the NDT problem-solving process that began with Mrs. Bobath: to observe *what* the client does, record *how* the client does it, and hypothesize *why* the client does it, paying specific attention to posture and movement in all steps of this process (Diamond and Cupps, 2002). The model is compatible with the current NDT assumptions and theoretical foundation, which propose that pathology or dysfunction in the nervous system, or the body systems, affects the individual's ability to solve motor problems in a specific environmental context and therefore affects the overall function of that individual in society, including how he or she is perceived by others in the community (see Table 2.1).

The NDT Enablement Classification of Health and Disability

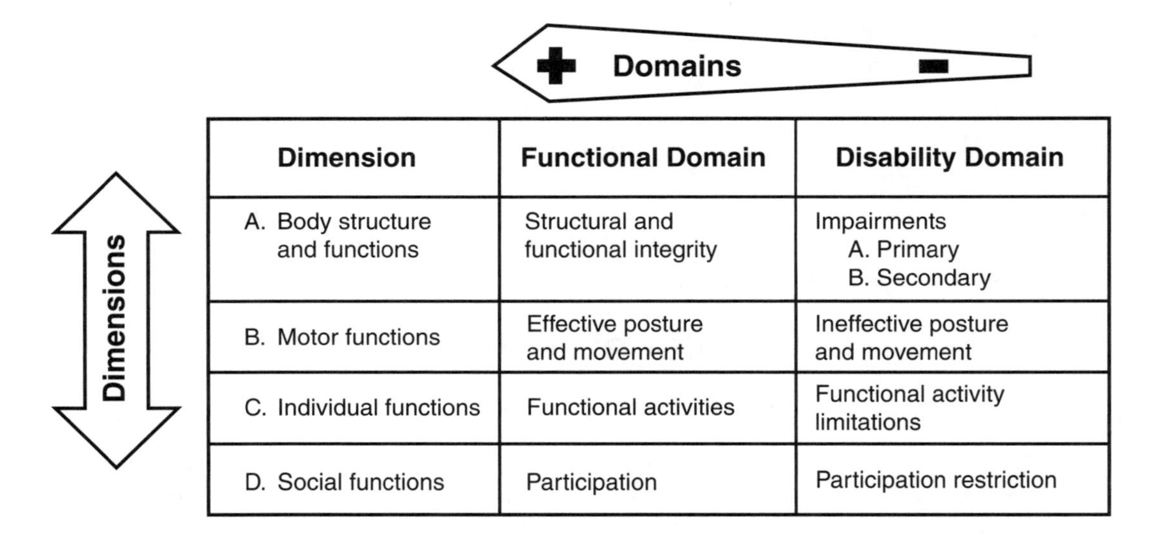

Dimension	Functional Domain	Disability Domain
A. Body structure and functions	Structural and functional integrity	Impairments A. Primary B. Secondary
B. Motor functions	Effective posture and movement	Ineffective posture and movement
C. Individual functions	Functional activities	Functional activity limitations
D. Social functions	Participation	Participation restriction

Table 2.1. The NDT enablement classification of health and disability illustrates relationships among four dimensions to the domains of function and disability (based on the ICF Model, World Health Organization, 2001).

A further advantage of the modified ICF model is the inclusion of environmental context as a factor in disability (see Figure 2.1). This model acknowledges that the extent of physical disability cannot be determined solely by intrinsic neural and body factors, but takes into account the effects of the environmental context on the disabling condition. NDT currently uses this model for classifying and describing the posture and movement problems in individuals with CP, stroke, and traumatic brain injury (TBI)* and also when developing examination and intervention strategies. This chapter examines only those issues related to classifying and describing movement dysfunction. Chapter 3 and 4 applies this taxonomy to the principles of examination, treatment, and outcomes.

* NDT therapists who work with clients with neuropathology often include individuals with traumatic brain injury (TBI) in their practices. For simplicity, the terms stroke and CP will be used throughout this book to refer to clients with neuropathology.

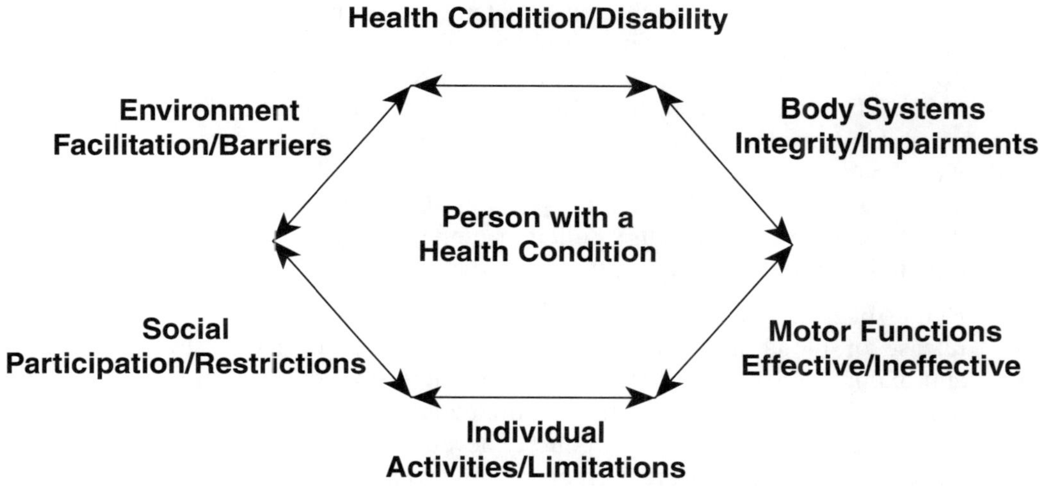

Figure 2.1. The interactions among the all dimensions of the NDT enablement model, depicted as the sides of a hexagon, include the environmental context and the health condition or neuropathology.

Health Condition/Pathophysiology of Disorder or Disease

Pathophysiology is the underlying medical or injury process, at the cellular or tissue level of either neural or body structures, that interrupts or interferes with normal physiological and developmental processes in any dimension of the individual.

Stroke

Stroke or cerebral vascular accident (CVA) is a sudden, focal, neurological deficit resulting from disruption to the blood supply in the brain that persists for at least 24 hours.

Two different neuropathological conditions result in stroke in adults–hemorrhage or ischemia. Although stroke does occur in infancy and childhood (Nicolaides & Appleton, 1996), NDT classifies this condition as hemiplegic CP because impairments, motor functions, and functional limitations are influenced by growth and development, as are all other types of CP.

1. Ischemic strokes account for three-quarters of the total incidence of stroke and are diffuse or localized depending on cerebral blood flow. Ischemic strokes are related to thrombotic, embolic, or hemodynamic factors. Thrombotic infarction in large vessels occurs when a thrombus forms on an atherosclerotic plaque. Embolic infarction results when an embolus occludes an artery or arteriole. Hemodynamic infarction occurs when a severe stenosis or occlusion of a proximal artery to the brain is uncompensated by collateral flow (Flick, 1999; Post-Stroke Rehabilitation Guideline Panel, 1995; Stewart, 1999). An infarction of the ventral posterior and lateral posterior nuclei of the posterolateral thalamus and its cortical projections seems to be responsible for impairments in the control of upright body posture and produces what is called "pusher syndrome" (Karnath, Ferber, & Dichgans, 2000a, 2000b). This specific ischemic syndrome was first described by Davies (1985). The name derives from the most striking system impairment, characterized by the individual pushing strongly toward the hemiplegic side in all positions and resisting any attempt at passive correction of the posture. MRI scan investigations have indicated that these clients have a neural deficit leading to an altered perception of the body's orientation in relationship to gravity (Karnath et al., 2000b).

2. Hemorrhagic strokes result from rupture of the vessels of the brain and subsequent release of blood into the extravascular space. Hemorrhagic strokes constitute approximately 10% of all strokes and are either intracerebral or subarachnoid in location. Hypertension is the most common cause of brain hemorrhage. Signs and symptoms develop acutely with altered levels of consciousness, severe headache, and elevated blood pressure. Cerebellar hemorrhage usually occurs unilaterally and is associated with dysequilibrium, nausea, and vomiting. Persons with brainstem syndrome can exhibit hemiparesis or quadriparesis. Subarachnoid hemorrhage is also characterized by sudden severe headache and stiff neck. The cause of subarachnoid hemorrhage is usually a ruptured sacular aneurysm (Stewart, 1999).

The characteristic functional limitations of individuals with stroke are numerous and vary with the site and extent of the lesion (Flick, 1999; Stewart, 1999):

1. Limitations in walking. This is a more significant problem in the acute stage of stroke than in the later stages. Most studies have reported that approximately 85% of adults with stroke are able to walk independently after 6 months (Wade & Hewer, 1987).

2. Limitations in self-care skills of daily living that require upper-extremity coordination and dexterity, including dressing, bathing, feeding, toileting, grooming, and transfers from one support to another (Nakayama, Jorgensen, Raaschon, & Olsen, 1994).

3. Limitations in communication, including aphasia, dysarthria, and apraxia.
4. Limitations in neuropsychological functions, including reasoning, planning, and problem-solving skills; visual-spatial perception; appropriate levels of alertness and attention; and affective functions (depression, anger, crying).

These activity limitations are caused by impairments in multiple systems, most notably the neuromuscular, musculoskeletal, perceptual/cognitive, sensory, and regulatory systems.

1. Neuromuscular system impairments produce hemiplegia. "Right" or "left" hemiplegia is the standard terminology for describing the major motor impairments of individuals following stroke. Hemiplegia is a presenting symptom in three-quarters of clients with stroke. Hemiplegia describes the distribution of motor problems on the side of the body opposite the brain lesion. NDT recognizes that asymmetric brain lesions can produce generalized motor symptoms, and the terms *more involved* and *less involved* are more appropriate when describing the motor impairments resulting from neuromuscular system impairments (Thillmann, Fellows, & Garms, 1990).
2. Sensory system impairments range from loss of the single sensory modalities of vision or hearing to complex sensory impairments including visual-spatial deficits, homonymous hemianopsia, pain, numbness, and somatosensory deficits.
3. Perceptual/cognitive system impairments and regulatory system impairments initially can produce confusion, emotional volatility, inattention, and decreased arousal levels that can interfere with the ability to benefit from rehabilitation.

Cerebral Palsy

CP is commonly classified by clinical types and topographic distribution of movement impairments. This classification from the American Academy for Cerebral Palsy and Developmental Medicine remains the most widely used descriptive system of classification and provides common terminology among clinicians and parents (Scherzer, 2001). However, adding a standard classification system based on abilities and limitations, such as the Gross Motor Function Classification System (GMFCS; Palisano et al., 1997) can clear up disagreements about the classifying types of CP and provide information for prognosis of gross motor functions and helps establish the value of intervention. The clinical types of CP include:

1. **Spastic or hypertonic CP,** characterized by muscles that are stiff and in which velocity-dependent resistance to passive movement produces increased muscle tone; selective control is limited, producing abnormal and limited movement synergies; excessive co-activation of muscular activity leads to limitation in range of motion (ROM); and the timing of muscle activation and postural responses is abnormal (Campbell, 1991; Feldman, Young, & Koella, 1980). Children who have stiff muscles that are not velocity sensitive, are classified as hypertonic CP.

Spastic CP is the most common type of CP. Diplegic CP is the most common type of spastic CP. Combined with spastic hemiplegia and quadriplegia, this group makes up 75% of all children with CP. In all cases of CP, a correlation between clinical findings and neuroanatomy is possible only to a limited degree. A white matter infarct in the periventricular areas caused by hypoxia can lead to spastic diplegic CP. Hypoxic-ischemic events lead to damage to the corticospinal tracts and other nervous system pathways traveling through the periventricular areas (Scherzer, 2001). Periventricular atrophy is the most common abnormality found in preterm infants who develop hemiplegic cerebral palsy (Wiklund & Uvebrant, 1991). Cioni et al. (1999) identified four main types of lesions related to hemiplegic CP, including periventricular white matter abnormalities, cervical-subcortical lesions, brain malformations, and nonprogressive postnatal injuries.

2. **Dyskinesia,** a group of disorders in which movements appear to be uncontrolled and involuntary even though the client has intent and purpose. Dyskinesia includes athetosis, rigidity, and tremor. *Athetosis* always involves involuntary movement; movements that are abnormal in timing, direction, and spatial characteristics; impairments in postural stability; abnormal coordination in reversal of movement and latency of onset of movement; and oral-motor dysfunction involving feeding and speech production. *Rigidity* is a much less common type of dyskinesia. The primary problem in children who have rigidity is resistance to both active and passive movement. This resistance continues throughout the range of movement in both the agonists and antagonists and is not velocity dependent. *Tremor* rarely occurs as an isolated type in CP, but is seen in combination with athetosis or ataxia. Tremor often occurs in clients with TBI. Dyskinesia results from impairment of the basal ganglia and their connections to the prefrontal and premotor cortices (Cote & Crucher, 1991; Guyton & Hall, 1996).

3. **Ataxia,** primarily a disorder of balance and control in the timing of coordinated movement. Ataxia, representing less than 10% of the cases of CP, results from deficits in the cerebellum. Because of the cerebellum's inputs and outputs connected with the motor cortex and the brainstem, ataxia often occurs in combination with spasticity and athetosis (Esscher, Flodmark, Hagberg, & Hagberg, 1996).The specific symptoms correspond to the area of the cerebellum that is affected. Whereas the neuropathology is extremely heterogeneous, the primary characteristic of ataxic CP is impaired postural control, which can manifest as ineffective postural alignment, anticipatory postural adjustments, and abnormal postural stability. Often there is hypotonia, impaired force during active movement, and tremor (Howle, 1999b; Montgomery, 2000).

4. **Hypotonia,** which can be permanent, but more often is a transient condition in the evolution of athetosis or spasticity and might not represent a specific type of CP. Hypotonia is characterized by diminished resting muscle tension, a decreased ability to generate voluntary muscle force, excessive joint flexibility, and postural instability. Researchers have not been able to correlate hypotonia with a particular neural lesion (Lesny, 1979).

The second component of the descriptive classification of CP describes the topographic distribution of abnormal tone, posture, or movement. There are three primary categories of CP: *diplegia,* involving the lower body and legs to a greater degree than the upper body and arms; *hemiplegia,* involving primarily one side of the body; and *quadriplegia,* involving the entire body, with equal or greater involvement of the arms and upper body. Clinicians sometimes use the term *double hemiplegia* to indicate a type of quadriplegia in which the arm and leg on one side are significantly more impaired than those on the other (Mutch, Alberman, Hagberg, Kodama, & Perat, 1992; Scherzer, 2001).

Classification of severity is useful in providing clues for reliable prognosis. Clinicians are using the Gross Motor Function Classification System (GMFCS) (Palisano et al., 1997) to describe and predict severity of motor impairments in young children with CP (Bower, Mitchell, Burnett, Campbell, & McLellan, 2001; Howle, 1999a, Sterba, Rogers, France, & Vokes, 2002) and correlate this with restrictions in social integration. Beckung and Hagberg (2002) found that functional limitations in mobility, as reported by the GMFCS, were important predictors for participation restrictions in children with CP. This system provides an objective classification of the child's current gross motor function. The focus is on self-initiated movements with particular emphasis on sitting and walking. The authors describe a five-level ordinal grading system with clinically meaningful distinctions in motor function among levels. The distinction between levels is focused on the functional limitations and need for assistive technology, including mobility devices and wheeled mobility, rather than quality of movements (Palisano et al., 1997). Children in level 1, at one end of this continuum, have the most independent motor function. This level includes children with mild neuromotor impairments, whose functional limitations are less than those typically associated with CP. Children in level 5, at the other end of the continuum, lack the most basic antigravity postural and movement control. This classification system, based on abilities and limitations in gross motor functions, assists clinicians in describing the development of children with CP, making management decisions based on level of functional limitations (Campbell, 1999a; Howle, 1999a, 1999b), and determining the efficacy of intervention on motor function.

Beckung and Hagberg (2002) also described a Bimanual Fine Motor Function Classification System (BFMFCS), which is similar to the GMFCS. This five-level scale corresponds to the levels of the GMFCS and includes single-hand and bimanual functions. Distinctions among the different levels focus on bimanual functional limitations. The correlation between the GMFCS and the BFMFCS is very strong, indicating that severity of gross and fine motor function runs in parallel.

The NDT therapist's responsibility is to understand the signs and symptoms that verify a diagnosis and to correlate the recovery process (both natural and interventional) to the basic health condition. The goal of the NDT approach is to target a population that has a CNS neuropathology; however, this does not mean that the client does not have other pathophysiologies contributing directly or indirectly to the impairments and activity limitations. For example, the child with CP shows increasing problems as the developing (albeit abnormal) nervous system interacts with other maturing systems, as the child develops upright against the forces of gravity, and as the body changes and develops with growth and maturation. Beckung & Hagberg (2002) studied additional neuroimpairments that occur in children with CP. They reported that 40% of the children had learning disabilities, 35% had epilepsy, and 20% had visual impairments. Thirteen percent of the children exhibited a combination of two impairments, and 15% had a combination of three. Additional impairments were most commonly seen in children with quadriplegic CP and least often in children with hemiplegic CP. Children with CNS malformations and those with peri/neonatal intraventricular hemorrhage and hypoxic-ischemic encephalopathy frequently had significant additional neuroimpairments compared with those with prenatal CNS lesions or no identifiable antecedents.

In addition to the interactions of primary and secondary system neuroimpairments, growth and development in specific contexts can limit full participation in social contexts. Scherzer (2001) identified six life stages that present specific implications for the individual with CP: birth to 3 years, preschool, school age, adolescence, adult, and senior adult. These various life stages require different focuses for identification, care, and management. The management of the person with stroke changes with (a) the age and activity level at the time of onset (not all clients with stroke are elderly), and (b) stage of recovery, acute or chronic. A therapist must also remember, for example, that complaints of pain along with joint malalignment in a 4-year-old child with CP can be the result of CP but might have another cause as well, such as juvenile rheumatoid arthritis. Fatigue can be related to asthma. Intolerance or refusal of oral feeding can occur with bronchial pulmonary dysplasia (Bergman & Farrell, 1992) or reflux (Heine, Jaquiery, Lubitz, Cameron, & Catto-Smith, 1995).

In the person with stroke, abnormal postural alignment could result from osteoporosis or earlier sports injuries; intermittent confusion could be related to poorly controlled diabetes; poor balance might be due to cataracts, decreased visual acuity, visual field deficits, auditory deficits, or vestibular problems. Weakness might result from post-polio syndrome or a sedentary life style prior to the stroke. Sorting out which symptoms are directly related to the neuropathology and which are not is an ongoing challenge to the clinician.

Dimensions and Domains of the NDT Health and Disability Model

Body Dimension: Domain of Structural and Functional Integrity/Impairments

The NDT enablement model separates the structure and function of the nervous system from those of the other body systems. Because the population of individuals treated in NDT all have neuropathology, the clinician is able to focus on the various neural subsystems and their interactions with other body systems that contribute to posture and movement impairments and activity limitations. Impairments are divided into primary and secondary body system impairments.

Primary impairments are either "positive" signs, behaviors that are *present* because of the brain pathophysiology, or "negative" signs, behaviors that are *absent* because of the pathophysiology. Primary impairments can occur in a single system or in multiple systems. For example, decreased force production, a "negative" sign, could be a neural system impairment, the result of insufficient descending input to bring motor neurons to the high-frequency discharges necessary for titanic contraction, or multisystem neuromuscular and musculoskeletal impairments, which involve additional changes in the motor units themselves with decreases in the number and type of motor units recruited. In stroke or CP, primary impairments include, but are not limited to, problems in detecting, registering, modulating, and organizing sensory information; selecting, activating, sequencing, and executing coordinated movement synergies; regulating anticipatory postural strategies; producing appropriate levels of co-activation; and force production (Campbell, 1992; Davies, 1985; Girolami, Ryan, & Gardner, 2001; Olney & Wright, 2000; Ryerson & Levit, 1997). Although classifications are flexible and vary, depending on the particular view of the person using the model, primary impairments for persons with CNS pathology most often occur in the neuromuscular, musculoskeletal, and sensory systems.

Secondary impairments do not result directly from the original pathophysiology and generally develop over time. The effects of the brain lesion interacting with other body systems and environmental contexts influence the development of secondary impairments. Secondary impairments most frequently occur from atypical interactions between the neuromuscular system and structural or functional changes in the musculoskeletal systems. They can coexist as a result of pathology in body systems quite separate from these systems, such as the cardiopulmonary, cognitive-regulatory, gastrointestinal, or metabolic systems. Secondary impairments have an impact on the client's level of disability by contributing additional physical, cognitive, or emotional problems that affect the person's ability to cope with the primary impairments. Examples of secondary impairments include weakness or muscle atrophy from overuse of orthotics, epilepsy, visual system impairments, decreased endurance due to impairments in the cardiopulmonary system, limited selection of patterns of activation due to limited practice in multiple contexts, inability to allocate attention to multiple motor tasks due to cognitive system impairments, and joint or muscle pain from abnormal mechanics during movement or prolonged abnormal joint alignment (Campbell, 1997).

Primary or secondary impairments can be temporary or permanent and are subject to change over time. For example, positive changes can arise because of recovery from nervous system pathology, such as decreased cerebral swelling occurring after the acute stage of stroke, associated with spontaneous return of function. Negative changes occur because of complicating problems in other body systems, which affect the original impairments. For example, mechanical ventilation that is necessary because of bronchopulmonary dysplasia in a premature infant, necessitates prolonged positioning in supine with extension of the head and neck, producing secondary, atypical somatosensory experience and abnormal body alignment (Kahn-D'Angelo & Unanue, 2000).

The presence of impairment necessarily implies a cause; however, the cause might not be sufficient to explain the resulting impairment. For example, two children born at 28 weeks' gestation with perinatal leukoencephalopathy and periventricular hemorrhage, grade III confirmed with cranial ultrasound, might present with quite different impairments contributing to functional limitations. One child might show low postural tone with trunk instability, combined with excessive co-activation in the extensors and adductor muscles of the lower extremities (LEs) producing abnormal alignment in sitting, yet might be able to selectively control reciprocal movements in the legs for crawling. The second child might show quite normal tone in the trunk muscles with a vertical pelvis and normal spinal alignment for stability in sitting postures, evidence of spasticity with velocity-dependent movement, and the inability to time and activate interlimb coordination, which results in a "bunny-hopping" pattern for locomotion. The multiple systems contributing to or constraining function, along with individual experiences and selection of preferred movement synergies, complicate the cause and consequent relationship of a particular pathology to impairment. On the other hand, a client can have a long list of impairments, yet some of those impairments might not limit how the person functions on a daily basis (Bierman, 1998). For example, Winstein, Merians, and Sullivan (1999) found that individuals with stroke-related damage in the sensorimotor areas were able to accurately and consistently learn rapid actions with the upper limb ipsilateral to the lesion with augmented feedback practice conditions and concluded that damage to the sensorimotor areas affects the processes underlying the control and execution of motor skills, but not the learning of those skills.

Motor Dimension: Domain of Posture and Movement Function/Dysfunction

NDT Focus: The continuum from effective to ineffective posture and movement in a dimension of motor function is unique in the NDT enablement model. The NDT approach identifies and analyzes patterns of posture and movement that link functional abilities with underlying systems.

Effective or ineffective postures and movements are observable conditions of motor functions, but are not, in themselves, either functional limitations or system impairments. The inclusion of the domain of effective/ineffective posture and movement is unique in the NDT model of enablement and illustrates the NDT focus on the importance of posture and movement in the overall performance of persons with stroke or CP. NDT defines effective motor function as actions that are flexible yet reliable, accurate, quick and fluid and that efficiently solve motor problems for the individual at any time across the life span. Effective movement is based on the client's individual neural and body systems, experiences, values, and preferences. Ineffective movement, therefore, is inefficient and energy consuming and limits and constrains movement options. These motor impairments are observable symptoms of posture and movement and are components of functional skills or activity limitations. For example, an adult post stroke might have adequate concentric control in the LEs to climb stairs in a reciprocal manner, but inadequate eccentric control to descend the stairs. A child with CP demonstrates a heel-toe sequence when walking slowly in therapy, but cannot produce this pattern quickly enough to use it at normal walking speeds throughout the day. In both cases, these ineffective movements can be observed and constrain the overall ambulation skills of the client.

This domain is an important link between functional limitations and underlying system impairments and describes symptoms of motor function or dysfunction. This domain includes: effective or ineffective alignment, weight bearing, coordination, balance and postural control; the temporal and spatial components of motor planning; description of tone and movement combinations. Mrs. Bobath taught clinicians to use a problem-solving process that focused specific attention on the problems of posture and movement as a way to answer the question, Why does a client move or stabilize posture in a particular way? Analysis of these movement components leads to a deeper understanding of how functional limitations develop and how multiple system impairments interrelate to produce these limitations.

Individual Functions: Domain of Functional Activity/Functional Activity Limitations

Functional activities and functional activity limitations are observable and reportable performances of the tasks or actions that matter in the life of the individual in the context of his or her culture (Gray & Hendershot, 2000). Functional activities can range from simple tasks, involving one hand (such as holding onto a spoon) to complex bimanual skills (such as manipulating two pieces of silverware for cutting, stabbing, or scooping while eating) (Krageloh-Mann et al., 1993). Functional activity always implies a goal or purpose, and the purpose is included in the statement of the function. For example, an adult with hemiplegia can stabilize a glass with the more involved hand while pouring from a container (activity) but cannot maintain grasping while lifting the glass to drink with the more involved hand (activity limitation). The functional activity limitation, then, is classified by the extent to which the individual has difficulty performing a specific task. Functional activity limitations are usually related to a combination of system impairments; however, the same observed functional limitation might derive from different underlying impairments. For example, several researchers, working with adults with stroke have associated nonuse of the paretic hand with different impairments. Garland, Stevenson, and Ivanova (1997) related poor use of the paretic arm to poor anticipatory control mechanisms. Pai, Rogers, Hedman, and Hanke (1994) associated the nonuse of the arm and hand to fear of falling and inadequate balance. The subjects simply chose to use the unaffected arm as the safest way to reach for items and reduce their fear of falling. Kusoffsky, Apel, and Hirschfeld (2001) found that lack of spontaneous use of the paretic hand results primarily from difficulties in planning the hand trajectory in space as reflected by atypical temporal and spatial parameters during task performance. Trombly and Wu (1999) found that the organization of upper-extremity movements depended on the use of goal-directed, object-present activities. Clients reached for preferred food more easily than when they were reaching with an abstract, object-absent goal (e.g., "reach forward to here.”). These findings imply that observing a functional limitation does not support any one specific system impairment.

> ***NDT Focus: In an NDT approach, it is the specific job of the clinician to identify functional limitations, then to theorize which motor dysfunctions and system impairments are responsible for limitations in the client's behavior.***

Because functional activities are organized around behavioral goals, descriptions of movement patterns, such as poor head control, poor postural control, or asymmetry in posture, are important clinical observations, but do not constitute functional limitations. A functional activity limitation might be the inability to cut up meat, dress independently, sit in a regular classroom chair, or get on and off the toilet unassisted (Stamer, 2000). Functional activities and functional activity limitations are grouped in the following categories:

1. gross motor control of the body posture and movement in and through space (i.e., sitting, standing, movement in and between positions, crawling, walking)
2. communications (i.e., speaking, reading, comprehending, writing, arm and hand gesturing [pointing, signing], facial expressions and body posturing)
3. fine-motor task-directed functions (i.e., reaching, exploration and manipulation of objects for play, self-care, work, school, leisure activities)
4. social, behavioral, and emotional skills (i.e., self-regulation, attentional skills, age-appropriate interpersonal interactions, social appropriateness)

The NDT enablement model uses the ICF description of performance and capacity to further classify functional activities and functional activity limitations. *Performance* describes what an individual does in his or her current environment. *Capacity* describes the individual's ability to execute a task or an action using modifications of the task or environment, physical assistance, or verbal or nonverbal cues. The gap between capacity and performance reflects the effects of various conditions and provides a useful guide to the ability of any given environment to improve the individual's performance. A problem with performance can result directly from the structure of the environment, even when the individual has minimal impairments. For example, Belanger, Boldue, and Noel (1988) showed that when clients returned home following stroke, fewer than 18% used a technical aid to move around the house, but this proportion increased to just over 31% when the individuals left their homes. Rather than suggesting a increase in system impairments or deterioration in function, use of a mobility aid or support outdoors might reflect an individual's greater sense of insecurity in dealing with the varying contact surfaces and unpredictable environmental elements (such as unidentified noise or the appearance of moving people and vehicles), compared to a greater sense of familiarity and safety indoors, with accessible stable supports, such as furniture, walls, door frames, banisters, and railings. In this case, 82% of the clients had the *capacity* to walk without aids, but only 69% *performed* at this level when going out of the home.

> ***NDT Focus: NDT examination focuses on difference in performance and capacity as it relates to function in various settings and uses this information to determine strategies for intervention that might bridge the gap between the two.***

Social Dimension: Domain of Participation/Participation Restrictions

Participation and *participation restrictions* refer to the nature and extent of a person's involvement in life situations and represent the complex interactions of health condition, impairment, functional activity, and context. The functional activity limitations become more specific in this dimension. The social dimension takes into account the *expected* performance, activity, and roles within physical and social contexts. For example, walking independently but slowly allows functional autonomy for an individual following stroke, in that the person can be independent in the home and safe from falling. However, this level of skill becomes a participation restriction if the individual cannot walk quickly enough to cross a street with a traffic light in order to go to the grocery store to maintain independent living. Identification of participation and participation restrictions relies heavily on identifying the environmental context, the functions, and anticipated roles for the individual, given the person's age and cultural and personal expectations.

Examination of participation and participation restrictions takes into account the ability to take part in changing life roles, which vary with the client's age and need for function, as well as underlying motor impairments. For example, using this model to examine the development of a child with CP, the NDT clinician must consider the following. A 9-month-old baby enjoys being held for play, therapy, dressing, and feeding. A natural environment is the mother's lap, which is appropriate for evaluating the child's ability to participate in dressing. Participation includes visually attending to appropriate body parts and items of clothing; offering a leg or arm in anticipation of dressing; processing and following the commands of "push" or "pull," "straighten" or "bend;" reaching for the body part or clothing item; and maintaining a level of interest and motivation to engage in the interaction. On the other hand, dressing for a 10-year-old involves selecting, organizing, and putting on socially appropriate clothes and outer garments depending on the setting (school, sports events, or social gatherings) and climate, with minimal supervision. Dressing also includes accomplishing the task within a given time frame (such as before breakfast on school mornings), in the presence of other visual or auditory distractions. An adult also faces these more demanding circumstances, which require allocating attention to more than the posture and movements needed to accomplish dressing. The definition of "successful participation" takes on an entirely new meaning. Clinicians must be sensitive to what the client needs at the moment, as well as across the life span to maintain effective intervention and prevent secondary impairments or functional limitations due to inattention to the client's changing needs.

In NDT Baby Courses, Mary Quinton taught students to examine and treat the past, present, and future simultaneously, working on a function while keeping in mind past experiences and preparing for complexities of that function in the future. This remains one of the principles of treatment to ensure that the client is prepared for full participation throughout life (Bly, 1999).

Contextual Factors

Facilitators/Barriers or Hindrances

Contextual factors represent the complete background of an individual's life. They include *environmental factors* and *personal factors* that could affect the individual with a health condition. Environmental factors make up the physical, social, and attitudinal environment in which people live and conduct their lives. These factors are external to individuals and can have a positive or negative influence on the individual's performance as a member of society.

Environmental factors include two elements.

1. **Individual factors** are elements in the immediate personal environment of the individual, including but not limited to settings such as home, workplace, community, and school. Individual factors include the physical and material features of the environment with which an individual comes in direct contact, as well as other people in the individual's environment, such as family, acquaintances, peers, and strangers. An *individual contextual facilitator* is a person or structure in the environment that will enhance participation in life, such as a brother who provides transportation to stores and appointments, or a high school that is all on one level with wheelchair access. *An individual contextual barrier or hindrance* might be a wife who does everything for the client, thus limiting practice and autonomy, or the lack of assisted-care restrooms in the airport or shopping mall.
2. **Services and systems** include formal and informal social structures and services in a community that affect the individual, such as organizations and services related to the work environment, community activities, government agencies, communication and transportation services, and informal social networks. This category also includes laws, regulations, attitudes, and ideologies. For example, an *environmental facilitator* might be a community pool that sets aside a particular time each week for swimming for persons with disabilities, a state law that permits persons with disabilities not to stand in the line at the Division of Motor Vehicles or the post office, or a requirement for a specific number of parking places for persons with disabilities outside all businesses. An *environmental barrier* might be locker rooms and showers at the community pool that cannot accommodate a personal assistant or parent of the opposite sex to assist with changing clothes, or a community pool that schedules the "special time" late in the evening when most persons with disabilities are too fatigued to take advantage of this service.

Personal factors are the particular background of an individual's life, the features of the individual that are not part of a health condition (but certainly can be affected by it). These factors include age, race, gender, educational background, culture, aptitudes, fitness, lifestyle, habits, upbringing, coping styles, social background, profession, place in the family and community, and personality and character style. *Personal facilitators* might include strong sense of self worth, determination, and sense of humor. Kirk Douglas's leading role in the movie *Diamonds* following his stroke certainly demonstrates his sense of humor, strong sense of self-esteem, and self-determination. *Personal barriers* can include depression, fearfulness, dependency, and low frustration tolerance. NDT intervention does not directly address these personal factors, but therapists agree that personal factors often determine the successful outcome of intervention. No matter how well a therapist knows what to do and how to do it, success will be severely limited if the client lacks motivation because the goal or strategies selected are not consistent with the expectations of the person's personality, attitude or outlook.

The NDT model of enablement supports the changes in the ICIDH-2 model from the 1980 version to the ICF model of 2001, reinforcing the hypothesis that a person's functioning and disability depend on a dynamic interaction between health conditions and contextual factors. Environmental factors are essential components that interact with all the domains of function and disability and play important roles in dimensions of individual participation, functional activities, and system integrity (see Figure 2.2). The basic construct of environmental factors is the facilitating (or hindering) impact of the physical, social, and attitudinal worlds (World Health Organization, 2001).

NDT Focus: NDT focuses on the impact of the specific environment in shaping the patterns of movement that develop in individuals with neuropathology. This focus provides additional avenues for intervention strategies. This attention to the dynamic interactions between the individual and the environment reflects a change in NDT focus.

The enablement model of NDT systematically classifies the consequences of health conditions in the individual's life and provides a framework for analyzing movement disorders, beginning with functional activity limitations in the social context and working to hypothesize which impairments are linked to the functional limitations. This was an early part of the Bobaths' teaching and continues to be a basic principle of NDT. Mrs. Bobath was never content with describing postures and movements in her clients, but always searched for explanations to understand **why** the client had limitations in function. NDT has modified the ICF classification to show more specific relationships between the neuropathology of CP and stroke and the consequences of these health conditions in functional limitations and disability. This taxonomy provides standard classification and terminology to describe and categorize the dimensions of disability that can then lead directly to developing effective strategies for implementing treatment. Acceptance and use of this enablement framework is a first step allowing the clinician to evaluate the effect their intervention has on the client's outcome (Barry, 2001). The NDTA Theory Committee designed the schematic depicted in Figure 2.2 to demonstrate the importance of these relationships in an NDT approach. This diagram is useful as a therapist examines the issues confronting each client, formulates hypotheses about these interactions, and plans treatment strategies to test the hypotheses.

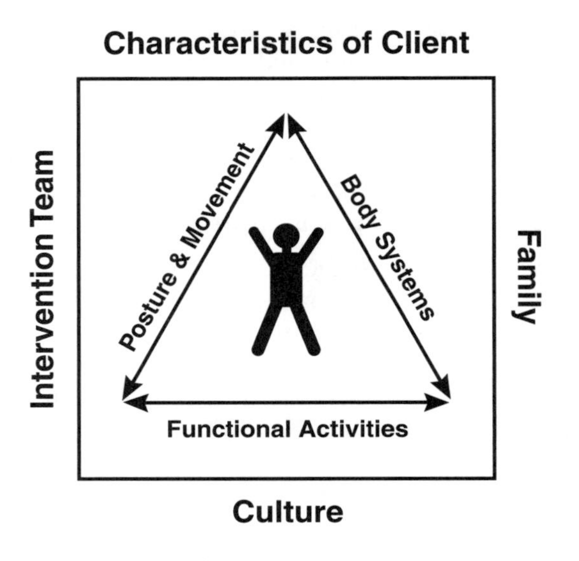

Figure 2.2. The triangle represents the dynamics of posture and movement, individual systems, and the changing relationships to function. The square represents relationships among personal and environmental factors including the characteristics of the client, the family and culture, and the members of the intervention team. (Illustration by Claire Wenstrom.)

The current NDT understanding of motor dysfunction in clients with neuropathology (Figure 2.2) reflects the changes and evolutions that have taken place in the approach as a result of experience and additional knowledge in the neurosciences. In the early days, the Bobaths assumed that the motor problems of CP and stroke arose fundamentally from CNS dysfunction. The lesion in the brain interfered with the development of coordination of movement patterns, led to atypical amounts and distribution of tone, produced abnormal sensory feedback, and impeded typical motor development or recovery of motor function after brain injury. Although theorists and clinicians still accept that the main problem of these clients is abnormal coordination of movement synergies, motor dysfunction is now understood to be produced by impairments in any of the body systems, experience, learning, practice, and the specific cultural and environmental context. For example, dysfunctional movements in children with CP can arise from biomechanical alterations in the musculoskeletal system (such as contracture of the hamstrings) along with hyperextensibility of the quadriceps, which leads to a short stride and knee flexion, excessive lumbar lordosis, and hip flexion during stance phase (Bleck, 1987). In another example, allowing or encouraging individuals with stroke to overcompensate with their sound side produces "learned nonuse" and greater asymmetry, which leads to atrophy in the hemiplegic side (Gardiner, 1996; Woll & Utley, 2001).

NDT Assumptions of Motor Dysfunction

NDT views motor dysfunction within the enablement framework. This perspective has led to the following assumptions:

1. Movement dysfunction emerges from (a) discrete or widespread neuropathology leading to primary impairments, (b) secondary impairments from atypical interactions within and between the neural and body systems, (c) the inability to identify and resolve constraints created by the atypical interactions between the environment and the systems contributing to posture or movement, and (d) the individual's desire to solve motor problems in specific environments.
2. All individuals have competencies and strengths. Identification of posture and movement dysfunction implies identification of posture and movement competencies as well.
3. Motor dysfunction affects the whole individual–the person's functional activities, place and participation in the family and community, independence, and overall quality of life. Primary sensory and motor impairments, along with the secondary biomechanical impairments of the musculoskeletal system, create an abnormal appearance in posture and movement that are expressed in the individual's self-image, adaptation in the environment, and motor behavior.
4. Individuals with CNS dysfunction have limited ability to explore and develop a wide, flexible range of movement strategies, which leads to limited repertoires of movement and an inability to discover efficient motor solutions.
5. Individuals with CNS pathology present with somewhat predictable and identifiable primary sensory and motor impairments in multiple systems that can limit the person's ability to carry out meaningful life functions.
6. Impairments are identified in body structures and functions. Primary impairments include both "positive" and "negative" signs of the underlying neuropathology. Positive signs are those characteristics that are present because of the pathophysiology and include sensory systems and sensory processing impairments, spasticity, abnormal co-activation, abnormal reciprocal relationships, impaired muscle activation, abnormal muscle synergies, abnormal intra- and interlimb dynamics, and impaired motor execution. Negative signs are those characteristics that are absent because of the lesion, such as insufficient force generation, impaired temporal qualities (such as slowness and paucity of movement), impaired anticipatory postural control, and loss of independent joint movements.
7. If unresolved, primary impairments contribute to secondary impairments in various body systems and subsystems. Secondary impairments are not the direct

result of the nervous system pathology but occur as a consequence of the interactions of primary impairments with other body systems or environmental influences. Secondary impairments further complicate the individual's functional ability and lead to disability in life roles.

8. Impairments, primary or secondary, include changes in the neuromuscular, musculoskeletal, sensory, regulatory, perceptual/cognitive, integumentary, respiratory, cardiovascular, and gastrointestinal systems.
9. Clinicians identify limitations to functional activities by observing what a client can and cannot do, integrating this with the knowledge of the consequences of the health condition and using problem-solving analysis to answer the question, What impairs the individual's daily functions? (K. Bobath & B. Bobath, 1984).
10. Identifiable impairments can be permanent or temporary and can change, either improving or deteriorating with such things as CNS recovery, intervention, growth, development, experience, additional impairments, or environmental modifications.
11. Effective and ineffective posture and movement serve as a link between the individual's functions and the system impairments.
12. If atypical patterns of motor dysfunction can be identified and treatment begun before the individual begins to practice compensations, the person has a greater chance to benefit from intervention aimed at reducing the impact of these atypical patterns on functional skills. However, because neural and muscle plasticity continues in response to activity in a functional context across the life spectrum (Sporns & Edelman, 1993), it is possible for a client to benefit from intervention at any time.
13. Knowledge of the process and comparison of atypical movements to more typically organized movement provide the foundation for analysis of the client's performance and contribute to effective treatment planning. For children, clinicians must understand the norms of functioning at different ages and the developmental processes underlying attainment of motor milestones. For adults, the clinician must understand the typical effects of aging in a life-span approach.
14. The facilitating or constraining impact of environmental factors, including the family and the community, influence the domains of function and disability and play important roles in determining the level of participation and independence in functional activities and the consequences of a potentially disabling condition.

How Do Impairments in Body Systems Contribute to Movement Dysfunction?

Classifying Impairments to Function

It is often not clear exactly how specific impairments fit into categories of primary and secondary impairments in the model of enablement that NDT uses. It can be argued that remaining true to a systems perspective, each impairment could be classified as a multisystem impairment, recognizing that the neural and body systems and the environment all affect the final functional activity and provide reasons for dysfunction. However, this is not a useful organizational strategy when formulating hypotheses or determining causal relationships. During an examination, the therapist sees a person–an infant, a child, or an adult with competencies and limitations. The therapist observes the person's functional skills or lack of skill and wonders, What contributes to these limitations? To help answer that question, NDT organizes impairments into categories that seem the most useful in describing constraints on function in persons with CP and stroke. The important issue is to include *all* possible impairments in an analysis of a client's functional problems, to broaden the understanding of the impact of stroke or CP on the individual. In the NDT model of enablement, the dimension of motor functions adds a stronger link between the functional limitation and system impairments.

NDT Focus: NDT classifies impairments by the system we believe offers the best explanation for limitations on function. Therapists can then formulate hypotheses that describe the relationships between neural and body systems and motor impairments and determine intervention that can be directed at reducing these impairments and thereby improve motor function.

Primary Neuromuscular System Impairments—Positive Signs

Primary impairments encompass a diverse group of problems that represent major constraints on movement and postures. Impairments of the neuromuscular and musculoskeletal systems can occur as "positive" or "negative" signs of pathology.

The positive impairments related to neuropathology are well described in both stroke and CP. Primary positive impairments include spasticity; impaired muscle activation; excessive coactivation and ineffective, stereotyped muscle synergies, and impaired motor execution; atypical scaling of muscle forces, excessive overflow of intra-and interlimb contractions, timing and sequencing impairments.

Spasticity

NDT defines spasticity as the component of an upper motor neuron disorder that is characterized by velocity-dependent increases in tonic stretch reflexes with exaggerated tendon jerks and clonus resulting from hyperexcitability of the stretch reflex (Lance, 1980). Clinically, spasticity is confirmed by the increased resistance to rapid passive lengthening of individual muscles at rest. In the past, the term *spasticity* referred to a wide range of abnormal manifestations related to movement dysfunction. Dr. Bobath (1980) used this term to describe the extreme end range of hypertonicity and included both velocity-dependent increases in tonic stretch reflexes, as well as exaggerated postural tone resulting from excessive co-activation expressed in atypical and stereotyped patterns that occurred during active movement (see Chapter 5). Katz and Rymer (1989) provided a critical review of the mechanisms underlying spasticity in individuals with CNS pathology. The current understanding is that, in addition to neural elements producing spasticity, abnormal tone involves changes in the biomechanics of muscle structures and musculoskeletal variables (Campbell, 1991; O'Dwyer, Ada, & Neilson, 1996). Dietz, Quintern, and Berger (1981) and Dietz and Berger (1983) presented evidence that altered mechanical properties of muscle fibers contribute to hypertonia. For this reason, spasticity is considered a primary neuromuscular impairment, while abnormal muscle and postural tone are classified in the dimension of motor function/dysfunction

The anatomical basis of spasticity is still unclear, however, the predominant hypothesis is that the neuropathology underlying spasticity is the net result of superspinal and spinal inputs that produce changes in descending activity, resulting in abnormalities within the segmental stretch reflex (Berger, Quintern, & Dietz, 1987; Katz & Rymer, 1989). The basic neural circuit is the segmental reflex arc consisting of muscle receptors, their central connection with spinal cord neurons, and motorneuronal output to muscle. Within this arc, the alpha motor neuron is the final conduit for motorneuronal outflow. Ia afferent fibers arise from the muscle spindle and carry information about muscle length and speed of stretch to the spinal cord via the posterior spinal nerve roots. The Ia fibers make excitatory synapses with alpha motor neurons in the spinal cord to produce contraction in the stretched muscle. Ia fibers also innervate antagonist muscles and cause reciprocal inhibition in antagonist muscles. Normally, the outflow is the sum of the many different synaptic and modulating influences, each contributing to the final level of excitation. Normal muscle tone is the result of this balanced facilitation and inhibition of alpha motor neurons. Alpha motor neuron hyperexcitability exists if motorneuronal recruitment and/or increased discharge are elicited with smaller-than-normal levels of excitatory input. Clinically, this means that a smaller stretch amplitude or slower-than-usual stretch velocity would excite the motor neurons. A state of increased excitability would arise if motor neurons are continuously depolarized more than normal so that they are very close to their threshold for excitation. In this situation, a very slight increase in synaptic input would achieve activation. These changes could decrease the stretch reflex threshold and/or alter the gain of the stretch reflex in response to stretch in individuals with CP or stroke (Kershner, 1991; Lin, Brown, & Brotherstone, 1994a, 1994b; Ryerson & Levit, 1997; Shumway-Cook & Woollacott, 2001).

Two different mechanisms exist by which the nervous system could produce enhanced reflex response to muscle stretch: enhancement of excitatory synaptic input and reduction of inhibitory input. The conditions that enhance excitatory input include (a) increased depolarization from segmental afferents, (b) enhanced regional excitatory interneurons, and (c) enhanced monosynaptic descending pathways (Katz & Rymer, 1989). The three conditions that produce reduced inhibitory input are (a) reduced reciprocal inhibition of antagonist motor neuron pools by Ia afferents, (b) decreased presynaptic inhibition of Ia afferents, and (c) decreased nonreciprocal inhibition by Ib afferents (Berger et al., 1987; Olney & Wright, 2000).

Both of these mechanisms permit higher-than-normal co-activation rather than the expected reciprocal inhibition. There is considerable evidence indicating that reciprocal inhibition is reduced in CP (Hallett & Alverez, 1983; Leonard, Hirschfeld, Moritani, & Forssberg, 1991; Leonard, Moritani, Hirschfeld, & Forssberg, 1990). In addition, in a study comparing muscle response to passive stretch in individuals following stroke, researchers found a velocity-dependent increase in stretch reflex in all individuals with spastic paresis, indicating that spasticity was related to decrease in stretch reflex threshold and reflex hyperexcitability (Thillmann, Fellows, & Garms, 1991; Levin & Hui-Chan, 1993). Researchers have also proposed that enhanced stretch reflex activity can occur because the alpha motorneuronal pool at the segmental level is hyperexcitable, due to loss of descending inhibitory input or postsynaptic denervation supersensitivity (Mayer, Esquenazi, & Childers, 1997; Noth, 1991). The affected inhibitory pathways are unknown, and it is also not known whether the same mechanism is the basis of spasticity in different clients (von Koch, Park, Steinbok, Smyth, & Peacock, 2001). Brouwer and Ashby (1991) provided evidence of simultaneous activation of the antagonistic muscle groups through abnormal alpha motor neuron innervation using transcranial magnetic cerebral stimulation. The role of decreased presynaptic inhibition of Ia afferents in spasticity has been supported by studies showing that vibration-induced inhibition of the H-reflex is much lower in spastic than in normal muscles (Leonard et al., 1991). Other investigators have studied both passive muscle conditions and active contracting muscles in subjects of typical ability and individuals with stroke and have hypothesized that although neural mechanisms might be responsible for altered tone in response to stretch during passive conditions, changes in muscle properties are more likely responsible for stiffness in actively contracting muscles (Ibrahim, Berger, Trippel, & Dietz, 1993; Sinkjaer & Magnussen, 1994).

Obviously, the mechanism of spasticity is complex. Additionally, there is not a direct relationship between spasticity and constraints on motor impairments or functional performance, as the Bobaths first proposed. For example, Neilson and McCaughey (1982) used a biofeedback system to train young adults with CP to reduce their spasticity. These individuals were able to regulate their spasticity, but only one (an individual with spasticity and athetosis) showed any improvement in functional activities. Children with CP who have undergone selective dorsal rhizotomy show a measurable reduction in spasticity (Cahan, Adams, Beeler, & Perry, 1989; Engberg, Ross, & Park, 1999; Kundi, Cahan, & Starr, 1988). However, functional changes depend more on voluntary strength, selective control of movements (including reduction in co-activation of antagonists), and the ability to learn new movement patterns (Giuliani, 1991; Subramanian, Vaughan, Peter & Arnes, 1998; von Koch et al., 2001).

NDT Focus: NDT views spasticity as one symptom of impairment in the neural system that contributes to increased tone and skeletal muscle stiffness. NDT attributes abnormal muscle tone to a <u>composite</u> of abnormal motor behaviors resulting from impairments in many interacting systems. Abnormal tone, therefore, is classified as an ineffective component of posture and movement rather than a primary impairment.

Impaired Muscle Activation

CNS pathology can produce impairments that affect how posture and movement look during active functional tasks based on musle activation patterns. These impairments have both positive and negative signs. Positive signs of impaired muscle activation include (a) excessive co-activation, (b) atypical synergies, and (c) excessive overflow of intra- and interlimb contractions. NDT views disturbances in muscle activation as arising primarily from neural pathology while recognizing complex contributions of sensory system and body system impairments to the final patterns of activation.

Excessive Co-activation

Inappropriate levels of co-activation (co-contraction) are a positive expression of impaired muscle activation. Muscle co-activation is the simultaneous activation of agonist and antagonist muscle groups crossing the same joint and acting in the same plane (Olney, 1985). Mechanically, co-activation increases joint stiffness and is a normally occurring mechanism in both eccentric and concentric contractions when an individual needs increased joint stability or precise motor accuracy. Although co-activation is a common motor control strategy from a mechanical standpoint, co-activation is an inefficient utilization of muscle forces because it prevents the normal flexible response patterns needed to adapt to changing conditions (Horak, Nutt, & Nashner, 1992). Excessive co-activation does not occur during skilled posture and movement control; rather, the neuromuscular system scales the amount of agonist and antagonist activation, adjusted by sensory information, in order to grade the motor response to the demand of the task (Diener, Horak, & Nashner, 1988; Woollacott et al., 1998).

Excessive use of co-activation, which impairs efficient, adaptive movements, occurs in adults and children with CNS pathology (Berger et al., 1982; Farmer et al., 1998; Knutsson & Richards, 1979; Nashner, Shumway-Cook, & Marin, 1983). Children with CP commonly use co-activation during both over-ground and treadmill walking and during isometric maximal exertions (Damiano, Martellotta, Sullivan, Granata, & Abel, 2000). The negative effects of co-activation included greater total muscle activation during force production and altered movement quality and quantity because of joint stiffness. Because co-activation occurs in the early stages of learning a skilled movement and in children developing posture, Shumway-Cook and Woollacott (2001) suggested that this characteristic is not a neurological impairment, but is an early form of coordination as the body attempts to control the degrees of freedom to produce stable posture. However, if these patterns of co-activation persist and do not give way to flexible coordinative structures (see Chapter 1), co-activation will occur under conditions that are not typically selected by a normal neural system, contributing to overall stiffness, limiting the adaptability of muscles for the variations needed for skill development, and contributing to fatigue and decreased endurance. Overuse of co-activation as a muscle activation strategy has the cost of decreased energy, which could affect the functional potential for a person who is already physically or neurologically compromised (Damiano, 1993).

Impaired Muscle Synergies

Ineffective muscle synergies are stereotyped patterns of movement based on limited movement repertoires that are resistant to change or adaptation to more flexible movement repertoires that the individual needs to meet specific task requirements (B. Bobath, 1990; Hadders-Algra, 2000; Shumway-Cook & Woollacott, 2001). Normally, synergies represent the way muscles are organized for efficient movement and represent functional coupling or linkage of groups of muscles, often spanning several joints, coordinating them to act together as units (Lee, 1983; Sporns & Edelman, 1993; Tuller, Turvey, & Fitch, 1976; Turvey, Fitch, & Tuller, 1976).

Functional synergies simplify the demands on the CNS by linking the timing, order, and force relationships of the neuromuscular and musculoskeletal systems with experience and sensory information to form a secondary repertoire of functional movements. The more frequently the individual selects and uses the synergy, the stronger the interconnections become. This permits linking groups of muscles with sensation and perception to produce adaptive movement that meets specific task requirements efficiently. Bernstein (Tuller et al., 1976) first hypothesized muscle linkage in general body movements, however, more recently, Kelso and Tuller (1984) demonstrated flexible muscle synergies also supporting speech production. Normal muscle synergies represent the best possible solution for functional motor problems. However, as Girolami et al. (2001) and Hadders-Algra (2000) have pointed out, synergies in children with CP can be so strongly linked that they produce movement synergies that are stereotypical, restricted in range, and limited in variety. Children with CP can produce functional movement with inefficient synergies, but they are often unable to adapt to specific conditions that require altering velocity, force, timing, and sequencing of muscle execution demanded by the task (Olney & Wright, 2000).

For example, a 4-year-old child with diplegic CP experiments and gets into a standing position at a table by pulling to stand with a pattern that includes flexion of the arms and upper trunk. The legs follow with a bilateral, symmetrical extension pattern. This is a familiar pattern for any therapist who treats young children with CP. As illustrated in the case study in Chapter 4, a more flexible, effective synergy uses the LEs to push into the support surface so that the child can rise to stand either through a half-kneeling or a squat position, freeing the arms from weight bearing. However, if a child uses the symmetrical extension synergy daily and is encouraged to pull up to standing by family members who have been anxiously waiting for the child to walk, this synergy becomes efficient for the child, is extremely difficult to change, and limits variability in movements that can be selected to gain standing. The goal of getting into standing drives the abnormal synergy. The opposite synergy, extension of the UEs and flexion of the LEs, contributes to "bunny-hopping" and "W-sitting," typical patterns in children with diplegic CP. The formation of effective yet atypical synergies demonstrates the dangers of allowing a child to practice atypical muscle synergies that might effectively meet an immediate goal (of getting into standing or developing sitting) yet interfere with development of flexible movement repertoires that prepare the individual for more complex functional movements. Continued use of strongly linked synergies limits the ability to adapt to various task requirements and interferes with developing broader movement experiences.

A variety of impaired synergies that prevent efficient function occur in adults with hemiplegia (B. Bobath, 1990; Davies, 1985; Ryerson & Levit, 1997). One example is rising to stand by placing all the weight on the sound side. The client pulls the less involved leg back under the chair, the more involved leg remains in front of the less involved one (perhaps because the individual cannot isolate knee flexion on the more involved side), and the less involved leg therefore takes the entire body weight as the person rises to stand. Just as in the case of children with CP, highly motivated adults often acquire these limited, ineffective synergies through independent experimentation (Ryerson & Levit). Movement synergies that do not integrate both sides of the body to meet the posture and movement requirements demand greater energy to perform and interfere with retrieval of the broad repertoire of movements that the individual used before the stroke (Davies; Ryerson & Levit).

The Bobaths described these atypical patterns of coordination of posture and movement (synergies) in CP and adults with hemiplegia (B. Bobath, 1990; B. Bobath & K. Bobath, 1975). Although the Bobaths hypothesized that stereotypic synergies, which they called abnormal patterns of coordination, resulted directly from neural pathology (B. Bobath, 1990; K. Bobath & B. Bobath, 1984), NDT currently classifies atypical synergies as primary or secondary neuromuscular or musculoskeletal impairment based on problems arising in multiple systems. For example, if the damaged neural system contains only limited movement repertoires and these limited synergies occur repeatedly when the individual attempts a task, the options for movement combinations will be limited. In this case, the impaired synergy results directly from the neural pathology and is considered a primary impairment (Campbell, 2000b; Hadders-Algra, 2000). However, changes in alignment and restrictions in joint and soft tissue mobility that occur in older children and adults also produce additional mechanical constraints on movement, forcing movement substitutions and creating ineffective synergies as secondary impairments (Ryerson & Levit, 1997). Ryerson and Levit and Gordon (2000) described abnormal synergies in adults with stroke as inappropriate patterns of muscle activation based on learned substitutions and compensations due to biomechanical changes in alignment and musculoskeletal properties rather than abnormal neural mechanisms.

NDT Focus: NDT recognizes that impaired synergies can be classified as either primary or secondary neuromuscular impairments because they result from problems that are a direct result of the neuropathology or arise secondarily from interactions of the neural and body systems.

Impaired Motor Execution

Impaired Modulation and Scaling of Forces

Adults with stroke and children with CP demonstrate poor modulation and adaptability of the forces needed for specific tasks. Various researchers have described the inability of these persons to execute the appropriate amount of force and tension needed for accurate grasp or control of acceleration or deceleration phases of ambulation (Damiano et al., 2000; Levin, 1996; Valvano & Newell, 1998). Eliasson et al. (1992) found that children with CP coordinated grip and load forces sequentially rather than simultaneously. In addition, these children had excessive and oscillatory grip forces. This impairment leads to over-reaching and inability to decelerate for the target approach phase of reach or to modulate the forces to accommodate the specific characteristics of the target. The inability to modulate forces for execution reduces accuracy and interjoint coordination. A separate study found that children with hemiplegic cerebral palsy had difficulties replacing and releasing an object (Eliasson & Gordon, 2000). These children abruptly replaced an object and showed prolonged and uncoordinated release of their grasp of the object. Individuals with stroke of CP can produce too much or too little muscle activation in anticipation of movement, select too many muscle groups during a movement, or use inappropriate types of muscle contraction, demonstrating excessive co-activation rather than reciprocal patterns for eccentric or concentric muscle execution.

Timing and Sequencing Impairments

Temporal impairments. Latency in initiation, slowness in performance, and problems terminating muscle contractions are common problems resulting in the inability to turn on and off patterns of muscle execution, impairing the adaptation of movement for function. (Farmer, Swash, Ingram, & Stephens, 1993; Howle, 1999a; Stamer, 2000). *Reaction time* is the interval between the individual's decision to move and the actual initiation of the movement itself, resulting in latency in initiation. Shumway-Cook and Woollacott (2001) listed the following factors in the neuromuscular, musculoskeletal, and cognitive systems that affect reaction time: (a) inadequate force generation, including the inability to overcome gravity, inertia, or antagonist muscle restraint, (b) inability to generate adequate force within a specific time period or for a specific action, (c) insufficient ROM to allow movement, (e) reduced motivation to move, and (e) abnormal postural control to stabilize the body in anticipation of destabilizing movements. Several studies of individuals with stroke have reported slower-than-normal performance of actions, such as walking and sit-to-stand (Ada & Westwood, 1992; Giuliani, 1997). Eliasson, Gordon, and Forssberg (1992) reported abnormalities in the temporal parameters with long delays between sensory signals and muscle activation in manipulative grasping in children with spastic diplegic or hemiplegic CP. In a separate study, Eliasson and Gordon (2000) found prolonged and uncoordinated release of the grasp. B. Bobath and K. Bobath (1975) described latency in initiation as part of the movement problems in children with athetoid CP.

Movement time is the time required to execute a task-specific movement once it has been initiated. Slowed movement times during upper-extremity functions and gait occur in adults following stroke (Cirstea & Levin, 2000; Levin, 1996), as well as in children with various types of CP (Bohannan, 1989; Steenbergen, Hulstijn, Lemmens, & Meulenbroek, 1998). Prolonged movement times were associated with disruptions of the spatial and temporal coordination between the elbow and shoulder in persons with hemiparesis following stroke. Levin (1996) used pointing movements to study upper-extremity control and found that movement times were significantly longer in the more affected arm than in the less affected arm. The author concluded that regardless of the location of the lesion, the CNS might not be able to determine the optimal set of relationships between upper-extremity segments to perform timely, coordinated reaching movements.

Steenbergen et al. (1998) studied children with hemiplegic CP and found that total movement time (the sum of the time *to* contact and the time *in* contact with an object) was longer in the involved hand than in the non-involved hand. They concluded that the increased time to contact arose from problems in the transport phase of the movement, and the increased time in contact was the result of impaired sequencing to grip forces. In children with ataxic or athetoid CP, Forsstrom and von Hofsten (1982) found longer transport phases than their peers who were developing typically.

Difficulty in terminating muscle contractions can manifest itself as the inability to stop or change the direction of a movement. Sahrmann and Norton (1977) investigated isotonic, isometric, and passive ROM in the upper extremities (UEs) of adults with hemiplegia. They reported limited and prolonged recruitment of agonist muscles at the beginning of a movement and delayed cessation of agonist contraction at the end of the movement. They proposed that this difficulty results from the inability to dampen the forces of the agonist at the end of a movement. The inability to terminate a movement can also result from inadequate timing and force generation in the antagonist muscles necessary to brake a movement. Most often this problem occurs in children with ataxic or athetoid CP in association with cerebellar disorders. However, many children or adults with spasticity or hypertonia find that the quickness and adaptability of the movements break down with repetition, such as when children with CP try to skip, perform dance steps, play basketball, or roller skate. Active ROM decreases and co-activation increases to compensate for the inability to coordinate the spatial and temporal components of ongoing reciprocal movement (Howle, 1999a; Milner-Brown & Penn, 1979).

Sequencing impairments. In addition to problems in timing, researchers have shown that adults with stroke and children with CP activate muscles in the wrong sequences. Knutsson and Martensson (1980) observed premature or prolonged hamstring hyperactivity in the wrong phase of the gait cycle in clients with hemiplegia. O'Sullivan et al. (1998) found poor timing and sequencing along with overflow of muscle contraction into the antagonist muscles during upper-extremity movements in children with CP. Berger, Quintern, and Dietz (1982) found abnormal reciprocal activity between agonist and antagonist muscles during gait. Children with CP and adults with hemiplegia demonstrate distortions in movement patterns that result from an impaired ability to initiate movement with the appropriate body part for the task (Ryerson & Levit, 1997; Shumway-Cook & Woollacott, 2001; Stamer, 2000). Crenna and Inverno (1994) have suggested both segmental and supraspinal mechanisms as causes of this impairment.

Excessive Overflow of Intra- and Interlimb Contractions

Overflow of contractile activity in multiple muscles produces widespread motor responses in muscles of the same body segment and in muscles far removed from the prime movers. Overflow occurs in normal control systems when movements either are first being learned or are performed with effort, but this contractile overflow can be overridden and dampened as needed to permit just the right amount of movement that serves the goal. These "associated movements," described by the Bobaths (B. Bobath, 1985), frequently occur when a person is learning a new skill. For example, when children are first learning to print or write, they often clench the hand not holding the pencil as though they were holding a pencil in that hand as well. In addition, they may clench their jaw or protrude their tongue and drool with the effort. When they tire, they shake both hands to reduce the tension. In the presence of CNS pathology, overflow contractions can inhibit the normal reciprocal relationships between agonists and antagonists during active movement, preventing intra- or interlimb coordination (Bierman, 1998; Nashner et al., 1983; Knutsson & Martensson, 1980; Leonard et al., 1991). Fowler, Ho, Nwigwe, and Dorsey (2001) described this characteristic in children with spastic CP during strength training. When asked to extend one knee forcefully against resistance, children with CP were apt to extend the other knee as well. The inability to produce isolated muscle control when exerting effort can make it impossible for the individual to move the muscles around one joint without moving the muscles of the entire extremity. The inability to override the tendency to use many more muscles than needed for the task contributes to the abnormal quality of self-initiated movements and muscle tone, particularly when the client uses excessive effort to reach a goal.

The "confusion response" is another clinical sign of overflow. When the individual attempts to flex the hip against maximal resistance, ankle dorsiflexion occurs in the ipsilateral leg (Bleck, 1987). The Bobaths recognized this feature in their clients with stroke or CP. They observed that clients were not able to produce selective action of muscle groups, but that movement at one joint produced an increase in muscle tone, or even movement in neighboring muscle groups (B. Bobath, 1948). They called this abnormal increase in tone "associated reactions," following the description of Walshe (B. Bobath, 1985). They believed that associated reactions were responsible for many of the deformities that occurred in children and adults with hemiplegia as the effort of walking or using the less involved UE increased the flexor tone of the more involved UE, which remained in flexion due to the increase in flexor tone. Early in the development of treatment methods, the Bobaths developed and used "reflex-inhibiting postures" to inhibit the overflow of activity from one muscle group to another. They later abandoned this treatment strategy because it did not prepare the client for active movement, and there was no carryover into self-initiated, spontaneous movement, as the Bobaths had hypothesized there would be. It did, however, control abnormal overflow (K. Bobath & B. Bobath, 1984).

Primary Neuromuscular System Impairments—Negative Signs

Increasing evidence provides further confirmation that the "negative" signs of neuropathology are major constraints to functional movements (Burke, 1988; O'Dwyer, et al., 1996). These impairments include (a) insufficient force generation; (b) impaired anticipatory postural control; (c) hypokinesia; and (d) loss of fractionated movements.

NDT Focus: NDT now focuses equally on the positive and negative signs of nervous system pathology when hypothesizing causes of motor dysfunction. The Bobaths originally focused strongly on the "positive" signs as major impairments to function.

Insufficient Force Generation–Weakness

In the last 10 years, there has been increasing emphasis on the examination of strength in individuals with CNS lesions. New treatments, including selective dorsal rhizotomy and continuous intrathecal baclofen infusion, have made it possible to better evaluate problems in strength without the interference of spasticity. (Giuliani, 1991; Milla & Jackson, 1977; von Koch et al., 2001). New findings reflect the awareness that weakness, a negative sign of CNS dysfunction, can be a more important factor in impaired functional performance than spasticity or other positive signs (Campbell, 2000b; Carr & Shepherd, 2000; Sahrmann & Norton, 1977). Research appears to demonstrate a relationship among muscle strength, recovery of function in selected muscle groups, and functional outcomes in individuals with CP and stroke (Andrews & Bohannon, 2000; Berman, Vaughn, & Peacock, 1989; Bourbonnais & Vanden Noven, 1989; von Koch et al., 2001).

Weakness is the inability to generate sufficient levels of force in a muscle for the purposes of posture and movement. It is a major primary neuromuscular impairment in persons with upper motor neuron lesions. Weakness in these individuals can result from insufficient input from descending motor pathways that converge on the final motor neuron pool, either to shape complex movements by recruiting graded activation of coordinating muscles, or to bring motor neurons to the high-frequency discharges necessary for titanic contraction strength (Ghez, 1991). This insufficiency results in loss of strength of voluntary muscle action. Muscle force is dependent on the number and type of motor units recruited and the characteristics of motor unit discharge and of the muscle itself. Increasing the number of active motor units and the firing rates of those units increases muscle force. Many studies have documented alterations in the physiology of motor units (notably reduced number of motor units, impaired motor unit activation and recruitment, and decreased firing rates of available motor units) in individuals with cerebral cortex lesions and resultant hemiparesis (Bourbonnais & Vanden Noven, 1989; Frascarelli, Mastrogregori, & Conforti, 1998; Yan, Fang, & Shahani, 1998a, 1998b). Frascarelli et al. found significant differences in the patterns of recruitment between the paretic side and the nonparetic side. They maintained that this was consistent with the observation that, following a cerebral cortex lesion, the CNS loses its ability to modulate firing frequency during voluntary movements, a finding that is more often true in distal than in proximal muscles. This characteristic has been investigated in both upper- and lower-extremity muscles and in the ipsilateral and contralateral sides (Dietz, Ketelson, Berger, & Quintern, 1986; McComas, Sica, Upton, & Aguilera, 1973; Rosenflack & Andreasson, 1980; Tang & Rymer, 1981; Andrews & Bohannon, 2000).

Insufficient force generation is generally considered a primary impairment, but it can also result from secondary changes in the musculoskeletal system. Prolonged primary or upper motor neuron weakness produces changes in the morphological and mechanical properties of the muscles, which show atrophy of fast (type II) and slow (type I) muscle fibers (Castle, Reyman, & Schneider, 1979; Ito et al., 1996; McComas et al., 1973). Children with CP exhibit varying degrees of atrophy and hypertrophy of type I and type II fibers that appear to be dependent on muscle group, severity of CP, and age of the child. Ito and colleagues reported type I fiber predominance in the gastrocnemius muscle of children with diplegic or hemiplegic CP. They also noted a greater variation in fiber size in older children and in the more severely involved limb. Rose et al. (1994) found that children with spastic diplegic CP who had a predominance of type I fibers expended more energy and had more prolonged EMG activity during walking than children with CP who had a predominance of type II fibers. Both Rose et al. and Ito et al. speculated that spasticity might produce structural changes in the developing muscle. Gajdosik and Gajdosik (2000) suggested that if this is so, controlling the spasticity in the very young child might be a way of promoting more typical muscle development, which might in turn allow for more efficient expenditure of energy and better function and prevent secondary impairment complications. This is consistent with treatment methods used in an NDT approach.

Changes in muscle and tissue length can also contribute to weakness. Muscles that are maintained in a constant lengthened position can be more difficult to contract than they would in a midrange or shortened position (Ryerson & Levit, 1997). The contraction of muscles also becomes more difficult when soft tissue shortening or inappropriate muscle activity (hypertonicity) is present in the antagonist muscles. In these situations, addressing the biomechanical constraints to muscle contractions can resolve the apparent weakness of voluntary muscle contraction. For example, positioning premature infants in sidelying, or prone with flexion of the trunk and limbs, promotes active hand-to-mouth movements and shoulder protraction with a decrease in the general hypotonia associated with constant supine posture (Sweeney & Chandler, 1990).

Impairments and imbalances in muscle strength are important to NDT therapists because of their effects on function. Muscle weakness and imbalance between agonists and antagonists leads to an inability to perform movement sequences and encourages reliance on compensatory movement patterns, which in turn leads to disuse, more weakness, joint deformities, and soft-tissue contractures that produce disability (Damiano, Vaughan, & Abel, 1995). Various investigators have shown that it is possible to increase strength in specific muscle groups without additional detrimental effects overall (Damiano, MacPhail, & Kramer, 1995; Fowler et al., 2001). These same studies showed only a low correlation between strengthening and improved movement skills.

Impaired Anticipatory Postural Control

Anticipatory control is the production of the forces *prior* to the intended movement that are crucial to setting the posture to maintain the body upright against the force of gravity while allowing tasks to be accomplished in an efficient, coordinated manner within an environmental context (Eliasson et al., 1992). Campbell (1999b) hypothesized that postural responses are a necessary part of the formation of Edelman's secondary repertoire, adding the postural component to the movement synergy needed to anticipate the particular force, velocity, and direction-specific adjustments for adaptive movement against gravity. Thus posture becomes inextricably linked with movement and sensations to create efficient and effective actions. Researchers have demonstrated that the ability to anticipate and prepare for movement is necessary for transitions, balance, and skilled UE movement. Nashner & Woollacott (1979) and more recently Hadders-Algra, Brogren, Katz-Salamon, and Forssberg (1999) have shown that children with CP have serious postural dysfunction, lacking direction-specific postural adjustments. Both clinical and pathophysiological data suggest that these children lack functionally relevant activity in the primary cortical and subcortical neuronal networks, resulting in problems with initiating and timing anticipatory postural muscle activity for balance (Hirschfeld, 1992). These children demonstrated difficulty in sequencing appropriate strategies for muscle activation during sitting and standing balance activities. The strategies they selected were limited, inefficient, and very different from those used by children without disabilities. Their efficiency was also compromised by co-activation of antagonists, which limit movement strategies necessary to produce adequate balance reactions (Nashner et al., 1983). Individuals with hemiplegia due to CP or stroke are also unable to activate postural muscles in anticipation of voluntary arm movements. In a number of studies, muscle activity in the arm on the hemiplegic side preceded that of the postural muscles or required greater contralateral forces to gain postural stability (Bertrand & Bourbonnais, 2001; Horak, Esselman, Anderson, & Lynch, 1984; Nashner et al., 1983). Levin, Michaelsen, Cirstea, and Roby-Brami (2002) found that, during reach in persons following stroke, there was a stereotyped recruitment of the arm and trunk, in that the trunk began moving simultaneously with or before the hand and stopped moving after the end of the hand movement, suggesting that there were abnormal temporal aspects of trunk recruitment for anticipatory control. In a separate study, abnormal trunk recruitment for postural stability limited the elbow and shoulder movements during reaching. Providing trunk restraint allowed clients with hemiparetic stroke to use the arm joint ranges that were present, but not normally recruited, when anticipatory proximal control was limited (Michaelsen, Luta, Roby-Brami, & Levin, 2001).

Hypokinesia: Poverty of Movement

Poverty of movement was described by Prechtl et al. (1997) and Prechtl (2001) in premature and term infants who later were diagnosed with CNS pathology. This characteristic has also been observed and reported by Campbell (1999b) in this same population. In older infants and children with brain dysfunction, spontaneous movements have a monotonous quality, lacking fluidity, adaptability, variety, and complexity. The child is unable to adapt movements to natural situations and instead activates movement synergies with the same body segment in a variety of settings. The ranges of movement are small and often are limited to flexion or extension without rotation. Prechtl et al. found that a specific quality of movement, which they named *cramped synchrony,* is most predictive of spastic CP when it appears in the early weeks of life and persists on repeated examinations.

Hypokinesia also produces stereotypic movements in children with CP (B. Bobath & K. Bobath, 1975; Howle, 1999a; Stamer, 2000). These children are unable to initiate movement with the body part that adapts the posture and the movements for a specific task. Repetition of these limited synergies limits exploration and elaboration of secondary repertoires. For example, the child with diplegic CP uses the head and upper trunk to move from supine to sitting while the legs simply follow without making appropriate postural adjustment, or using the support surface to most effectively adapt the movements during this transition. There is often long latency at the onset of movement that others can perceive as a lack of understanding or motivation. In addition, children with CP exhibit poor anticipatory control and do not change their posture to accommodate to different task requirements. Hypertonus or hypotonus can contribute to paucity of movement when the effort to move against the force of gravity or overcome inertia takes too much effort. Children with hypotonia usually have limited synergies with which to produce movement, and the movement lacks variety. It is unclear whether the limited synergies are due to the neural lesions that limit the selection and activation of muscles, or whether certain movement patterns are used and strengthened in response to hypotonia.

This poverty of movement also occurs in adults with hemiplegia following stroke. For example, seated in a wheelchair, they do not attempt to scoot their hips back, equalize weight distribution across the hips, or orient to the midline (Davies, 1985). An individual might ride all the way from the hospital room to the therapy department without making any adjustment whatsoever. This lack of movement can involve primary or secondary impairments in postural control, sensory processing difficulties in the vestibular and visual systems, hypotonia or insufficient force generation, depression, and cognitive impairments.

Loss of Fractionated or Dissociated Movements

Loss of fractionated movement manifests as difficulty making precise, independent joint movements, particularly of the fingers, thumb, and hand, resulting in poor dexterity for fine manipulation tasks. Theorists have long considered hand function as one of the major responsibilities of the motor cortex. Lesions in the sensorimotor cortex and corticospinal tracts produce impairments in dexterity because of the control that these structures exert on precise and accurate grip and independent finger movements (Muir & Lemon, 1983). Dexterity depends on the sustained and rapid transfer of sensorimotor information between the cerebral cortex and spinal cord and exteroceptive and somatosensory feedback (Darien-Smith, Galea, & Darien-Smith, 1996). Jeannerod (1990) found very different reach and grasp abnormalities, depending on the location of the lesion. Lesions at the brainstem level affected the hand ipsilateral to the lesion. Without vision, finger grip was either absent or incomplete; but with vision, grasp was normal. Parietal lobe lesions produced impairment in grip formation, even with visual feedback. Jeannerod concluded that loss of sensory information results in abnormal grip forces and problems in the control of fine movements of the hand.

Because the intricate control of manipulatory forces relies heavily on sensory input, abnormalities in the sensory mechanisms (such as sensory awareness and processing and interpreting of sensory information) also contribute to loss of dexterity (Ryerson & Levit, 1997).

The primary function of visual feedback in reaching appears to be related to timely deceleration and sensing the position of the hand simultaneously with the position of the target to attain final accuracy (Lee, Georgopoulos, Clark, Craig, & Port, 2001; van der Meer, van der Weel, & Lee, 1996). Wing and Frazer (1983) hypothesized that constancy of thumb position relative to the wrist is necessary as part of a strategy providing visual feedback regarding the end point of the limb. Eliasson et al. (1992) concluded that sensory deficits are a major factor in impaired precision grip in children with CP. These researchers found impaired tactile regulation of isometric fingertip forces during grasping and concluded that children with CP can form internal representations of the object's properties only after considerable practice because they are not able to extract adequate information during manipulatory experiences.

Abnormal coordination of isometric force generation and abnormal temporal patterns have been associated with loss of dexterity in children with hemiplegic and diplegic CP, as described above. Jeannerod (1990) found very different hand grasp patterns when comparing the less affected and more affected hands in children with hemiplegic CP. These children exhibited exaggerated opening of the hand during the entire movement, no anticipatory grasp formation, abnormal finger shaping, and hand closing that was dependent on contact with the object. Erhardt (1994) confirmed these patterns in the development of hand grasp patterns in children with different types of CP. Van Heest, House, and Putnam (1993) reported that 58% of children with CP have abnormal grasp and 60% have abnormal release.

Sensory Systems and Sensory Processing Impairments

Specific sensory impairments and difficulties in processing sensory information occur frequently in individuals with CNS pathology (Carey, Matyas, & Oke, 1993; Carr & Shepherd, 2000; Cioni et al., 2000; Guzzetta, Cioni, Cowan, & Mercuri, 2001; Guzzetta, Mercuri, & Cioni, 2001; Stamer, 2000). All the sensory systems contribute to motor control. Successful treatment of motor impairments depends on knowledge and understanding of the impairments in individual sensory systems (Erhardt, 1998; Nelson, 2001; Shumway-Cook & Woollacott, 2001). For example, vision is critical in regulating gait. Loss of vision affects stability and adaptation aspects of gait, as well as route finding and obstacle avoidance (Shumway-Cook & Woollacott, 2001). Infants rely heavily on visual information and processing for orientation, posture, reaching, and forming attachment to caregivers (Bradley, 2000; DeGangi, DiPietro, Greenspan, & Porges, 1991). A central lesion affecting vision will impair the ability to locate objects or persons in space, affect parental recognition, and limit the child's interaction with and appreciation of the surroundings (Erhardt, 1998; Lee, 1978). Specific impairments in the visual and auditory systems are frequently associated with both CP and stroke. Numbers vary tremendously, but approximately 30-35% of children with CP have various degrees of visual impairments. Guzzetta, Frazzi, et. al. (2001) reported 80% of children with hemiplegic CP had at least one abnormal visual test. Primary impairments include cortical visual impairments, strabismus, nystagmus, binocular fixation, visual tracking, retinopathopy of prematurity, and refractory errors (Hagberg, Hagberg, Olow, & Wendt, 1996). Visual impairments are frequently cited as associated impairments in stroke (Post-Stroke Rehabilitation Guideline Panel, 1995; Powell, 2001; Ryerson & Levit, 1997) and include both visual acuity and visual field defects (hemianopsia) as well as diplopia and impairments in ocular motility.

Hearing impairments are less frequent and vary with prematurity and birth weight (Borg, 1997; Sutton & Rowe, 1997). Auditory impairments related to aging are common in individuals with stroke. Reduction of information from these senses is part of the typical aging process, but complicates the options available when motor deficits from stroke further decrease means of gaining information from the environment (Shumway-Cook & Woollacott, 2001). Hearing impairments tend to isolate the individual from people, while visual deficits isolate the individual from objects and the environment. Both deficits affect overall motor control, producing a sense of insecurity and fear of falling (Woollacott, 1989). A great deal of information exists on the various sensory systems and a thorough description is beyond the scope of this publication. The reader is encouraged to investigate the sensory systems from the many sources available relating sensory systems to gross motor and fine motor skills (Corso, 1981; Fisher, Murray, & Bundy, 1991; Van Deusen & Brunt, 1997).

Sensory processing is the ability of the nervous system to perceive, interpret, modulate, and organize sensory input for use in generating or adapting motor responses to interactions with other persons, task parameters, or the environmental context (Miller & Lane, 2000). Tscharnuter (2002) points out that the link between perception and action dictates that posture and movement cannot be separated from the sensoriperception that contributes to their formation. Sensory processing contributes to planning and executing appropriate postural adjustments and purposeful goal-directed actions, contributing feedback to the neural and motor systems about movement correctness and self-regulation. The visual, auditory, vestibular, and somatosensory (tactile and proprioceptive) systems are the primary systems through which individuals perceive and channel specific sensory contributions linking action to sensation (Bly, 1999). (See Chapter 1 for the use of sensory information via feedforward and feedback.)

Sensory processing problems can affect motor control in four ways. First is the *inability to detect and identify incoming sensory information* that influences the general level of CNS activity. Poor sensory detection results in deficits in awareness of incoming sensations from the body or environment and affects the client's ability to plan and execute movements automatically. The classic example is the adult with right-hemisphere, parietal-lobe damage who shows a lack of awareness of the contralateral side (including personal and external space) and neglects to use the left side of the body, even when movement is preserved (Jeannerod, 1990; Montgomery, 1991; Ryerson & Levit, 1997). A second example is deficits in the visual field that contribute to neglect of part of the environment when scanning to detect cues necessary for overall safety as the person moves through space.

The second effect of sensory processing problems on motor control is the *inability to interpret single-sensory or multisensory input,* either in anticipation of movement or during movement resulting in incorrect postural orientation or movements (Lee, 1988; Lee &

Aronson, 1974). Visual and proprioceptive deficits contribute to movement disorders in children. Children depend primarily on vision as a frame of reference when planning and guiding movement, perhaps because their body mass is changing so rapidly during growth years that they do not establish stable or reliable interactions between somatosensory information and gravitational forces to guide movement (Butterworth & Hicks, 1977; Jouen, 1990). The frequency of visual deficits in children with CP and their inability to establish spatial and gravitational orientation from somatosensory information results in their inability to select, attend to, and place value on sensory input produced by their actions. This will limit these children's ability to selectively and actively gather information that can be used as a meaningful guide to posture or movement.

In most instances, adults with CNS pathology are able to adapt to loss of somatosensory information as long as information is available from visual and vestibular senses (Carey, 1995; Horak, Nashner, & Diener, 1990). Changing the visual cues significantly affects stability when somatosensory inputs decrease (DiFabio & Badke, 1991). Individuals who depend on one particular sense for stability become unstable when conditions reduce input from that source (Horak & Diener, 1994; Nasher, Black, & Wall, 1982). Not only do vision and proprioception have to function in an optimal way by themselves in making well-coordinated movements, but the two systems also have to be coordinated and calibrated to each other (Black & Nashner, 1985). Individuals with stroke and children with CP demonstrate sensory selection problems (Shumway-Cook & Woollacott, 2001). In these studies, individuals were unable to select an appropriate sense for postural control in environments where one or more orientation cues inaccurately reported the body's position in space (Shumway-Cook & Woollacott, 2001). These individuals became unstable when there was a discrepancy among the senses, and they were unable to select an orientation reference.

Montgomery (1991) suggested that individuals use specific motor strategies to compensate for sensory deficits. She cited the pattern of asymmetrical weight bearing in individuals with hemiplegia as a possible strategy for the inability to perceive or interpret proprioception. Chaudhuri and Aruin (2000) found that changing somatosensory input by placing a lift on the shoe of the unaffected limb in adults with hemiplegia shifted the weight toward the hemiplegic side, improved symmetry, and provided increased stimuli for muscle activity on this side. Powell (2001) described a client, post-stroke, who used a persistent lateral head tilt to compensate for an unrecognized diplopia. Once the individual began wearing prism lenses, the head tilt resolved.

Third, the *inability to modulate sensory inputs to match changes in task and environmental demands* results in atypical posture and movement. When the threshold for sensory information is abnormally high or low, the client can become confused by sensory input, particularly from somatosensory input (Reeves, 1998; Wilbarger, 1998). If the threshold is too low, the client requires little sensory input, is easily overwhelmed, and can interpret sensory input as uncomfortable, even painful, which causes the person to become fearful of therapy and movement. Clients who do not regain the ability to modulate sensory input correctly avoid movement and protect their involved side, which can result in chronic pain secondary to disuse (Ryerson & Levit, 1997). Boehme (1998) described children who have a low threshold for sensory input: they are easily over-aroused and do not feel in control of themselves or their environment. These children often are hyper-responsive or defensive to touch. They respond with excessive emotional reactions, an increased activity level, distractibility, or behavioral problems such as aggression or crying (Blanche, Botticelli, & Hallway, 1995). Clients who have a low threshold for tactile input do not modulate their posture relative to the support surface because they perceive that the surface might be uncomfortable. (Tscharnuter, 1993). For example, such a client would sit down and contact the back of the chair with minimal body surface rather than relaxing into the support, reducing his or her postural support tone and taking advantage of the external support that the chair provides.

Moore (1984) described three sites of CNS damage that produce sensory-processing dysfunction: the cerebellum, the basal-ganglia-thalamus-cortex loop, and the pyramidal tract. As an example, damage to the cerebellum results in ataxia. Children with ataxic CP often are unable to filter and modulate sensory inputs. They will avoid touch and overreact even to minor displacements in space. Treatment must progress by carefully modulating the sensory input matched to motor functions (Howle, 1999b).

On the other hand, clients who have a high threshold to sensory stimulation are hyporesponsive, exhibit paucity of movement and decreased awareness, and appear unmotivated. Clients who are under-responsive fail to register touch when it is applied, particularly outside the visual range, and "forget" to use the hand for manipulation even when motor functions are intact (Blanche et al., 1995). This occurs in children and adults with hemiplegia. These clients are at risk for injury to the more involved side. Children who are hyporesponsive to sensation can respond with unusual or extreme behaviors, including self-mutilation and dare-devil stunts. Knickerbocker (1980) introduced the term *sensory dormancy* to describe sensory inhibition or the lack of adequate arousal to sensory input, which could produce immature and disorganized behavior.

Fourth, *the inability to relate sensory information to experience, memory, and specific tasks* results in misperceptions of the significance of a particular stimulus in the value it has on the intended action (Bernstein, 1996; Montgomery, 1991). The ability to remember and relate task-specific sensory information to movement is essential for executing purposeful actions (Gibson, 1966). Clients who cannot relate to the sensation of "how it felt" will be unable to remember what they planned and how they achieved their goal. Ryerson and Levit (1997) referred to this as *kinesthetic memory,* which they defined as the body's sensory knowledge of typical movement–what the movement should feel like and how to execute it correctly. Kinesthetic memories allow an individual to replay movements with mental imagery (a motor learning strategy) and to recognize when the body moves in this same way again. Clients with deficits in kinesthetic memory lose the knowledge of the way they moved prior to the onset of their disability, as well as the muscle memory for the patterns and timing of muscle activation. Ryerson and Levit contended that this contributes significantly to the abnormal quality of movements these clients develop.

Secondary Impairments in the Neuromuscular and Musculoskeletal Systems

Secondary impairments do not result directly from CNS pathology but develop as a consequence of primary impairments and environmental influences (World Health Organization, 1999). Secondary impairments contribute to the client's functional limitation and disability just as strongly as primary impairments by contributing additional physical constraints that affect the ability to generate typical movements and functional activities. In growing children with CP, secondary impairments that progressively influence movement account for much of the deterioration in function (Stamer, 2000) and possibly contribute to the low physical and social self-esteem that occurs especially in adolescent girls (Magill-Evans & Restall, 1991).

Problems in Joint and Soft Tissue Flexibility

Problems in flexibility occur in joints, soft tissues, ligaments, tendons, and muscles. Impairments in joint mobility and muscle extensibility are common in children with CP and adults with hemiplegia. Joint mobility problems include *hypermobile* and *hypomobile* joints. *Hypermobility* describes joints that have excessive laxity and greater ROM than normal. Hypermobility often correlates to hypotonia and muscle weakness, soft-tissue wear and tear, and overuse syndromes (Cusick, 1990; Davies, 1985; Ryerson & Levit, 1997). Hypermobility of the midfoot is common in older children with CP and adults with hemiplegia. Chronic stretch occurs in the midfoot as a result of laxity in the longitudinal ligaments of the arch, combined with tendo-achilles hypertonus or contracture along with continued ambulation and weight bearing over a malaligned foot (Cusick). *Hypomobility* is present in joints that have less-than-normal joint mobility for active motion through the full range of the joint. Hypomobility of the joints refers to excessive joint stiffness and decreased ROM. It often occurs in combination with hypoextensibility of the muscle and is a contributing factor to changes in alignment, deformities, and pain.

Flexibility problems occur in soft tissues and muscles as well as joints. Soft tissues lose length and flexibility as a secondary complication of changes in muscle tone and muscle strength and ongoing malalignment, particularly in weight-bearing joints. These changes affect muscles, tendons, skin, fascia, and connective tissue. Various authors have described flexibility problems related to individuals with CNS pathology and techniques for elongating these structures (Manheim, 1994). Tendons can become short and resist lengthening. Often hypomobility in one area will result in a compensatory hypermobility in a connected segment. For example, following hamstring lengthenings in adolescents with CP, there is often hyperextension of the knee associated with secondary shortening of the quadriceps muscles and hypomobility of the patellar tendon (Bleck, 1987). In another example, the lack of quadriceps length, combined with patellar tendon shortening, often produces pain in the knee joint as the client descends stairs. The fear of pain produces a hesitancy to flex the knee while taking full weight on descent, and the client may produce excessive hip flexion to compensate for painful knee flexion or, if secondary weakness has developed, be unable to grade the eccentric contraction to control elongation of the quadriceps.

Flexibility in soft tissue length and muscle length is important in the prevention of orthopedic impairments later in life. Maintaining flexibility in the lower back, legs, and shoulders contributes to reduction of injury, while restrictions in back mobility can contribute to gait abnormalities and limitations in activities of daily living that require trunk rotation (e.g., dressing, turning over, and rising from the bed). Shortening of the muscles and tendons often accompanies similar changes in surrounding skin and fascia, which become tight and adhere to muscles, tendons, and bones. Mobility of the skin is lost in some or all directions (Manheim, 1994). Individuals with low tone and severe weakness can develop length restrictions in the trunk and antagonistic muscles and tissues of the extremity from lack of active movement. Flexibility restrictions also occur following prolonged use of orthotics. Shortening and loss of flexibility in joints and muscles can result from limited movement and joint stiffness if the limb remains in the splinted position for long periods of time (Cusick, 1990). Children with CP who have heel-cord lengthenings and then are splinted to hold this position, lose flexibility in the muscles of the anterior compartment and exhibit decreased plantar flexion ROM. This type of loss can occur when a child crawls with solid ankle-foot orthotics (SAFOs) and is unable to contact the dorsum of the feet against the floor (Figure 2.3).

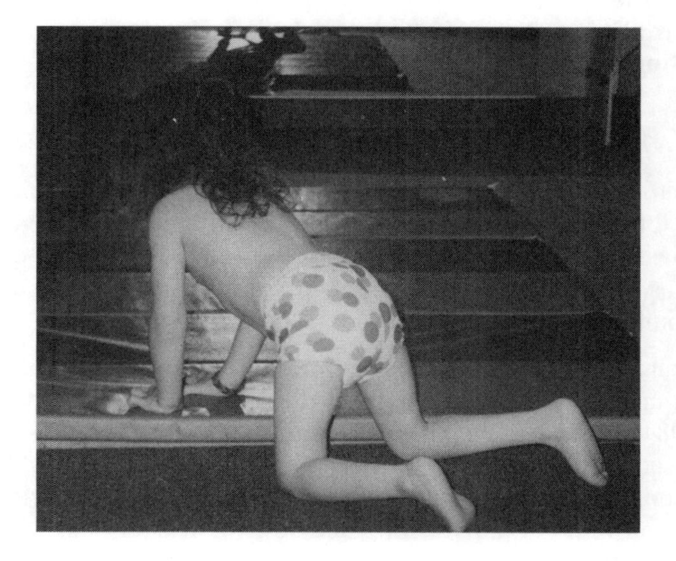

Figure 2.3. The interaction of secondary impairments leading to further decrease in function is shown in this child's inability to contact the dorsum of her feet against the floor when crawling. This is due to loss of range of motion in the muscles of the anterior compartment secondary to weakness of the plantar flexors produced by overuse of positioning with orthotics. The resulting malalignment and loss of flexibility at the ankle shifts the body weight forward onto her knees and hands further limiting functional crawling.

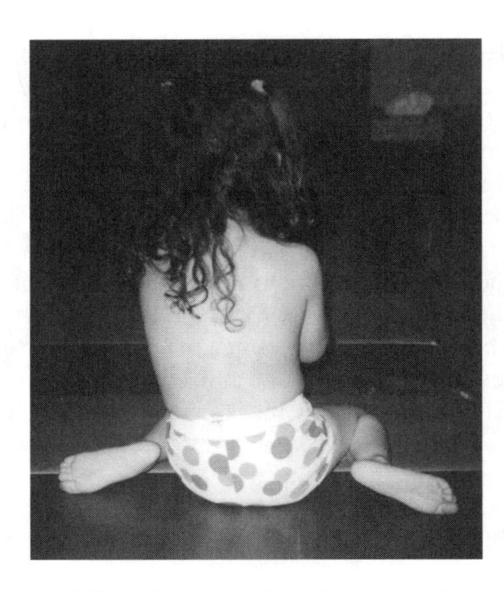

Figure 2.4. This same child who has developed external tibial torsion from W-sitting when wearing AFOs now persists in this pattern due to lack of range of motion and pain when she tries to heel-sit even when she is not wearing her AFOs.

Skeletal Impairments

Campbell, Gardner, and Ramakrishnan (1995) reported that physicians' patterns of referral for physical therapy strongly correlated with their belief that prevention of contractures and deformities was an important benefit for the child. The benefit of contracture prevention (70%) was second only to the benefit of increasing independence through the use of assistive technology (86%).

Various mechanical and neuromuscular forces, including muscle imbalance and spasticity, affect growth and change in the skeletal system (Gajdosik & Gajdosik, 2000; Leveau & Bernhardt, 1984). Skeletal changes in the spine and LEs and their relationship to functional limitations are well-documented in CP (Cusick, 1990; Gage, 1992; Perry & Newsam, 1992). Two common skeletal impairments that occur in children with CP include acetabular changes and femoral antiversion. Buckley, Sponseller, and Maged (1991) reported atypic changes in the shape of the acetabulum and femoral head in children with CP. Beals (1969) found that the acetabula of children with CP are normal at birth, but do not increase in depth as expected by age 2, suggesting that the various impairments in the neuromuscular system might have a negative impact on acetabular development. Once the children are walking, the acetabular depth is comparable to that in the general population of the same age. Scrutton, Baird, and Smeeton (2001) also found that walking by 30 months correlates to hip stability. Beals concluded that the dynamic compressive forces of walking contribute to the increased depth of the acetabulum. Conversely, children who do not walk, or walk late, persist with shallow acetabula and are at greater risk for subluxation or dislocation (Bleck, 1987). Scrutton et al. found that as early as 18 months, hip migration was significantly greater in children with bilateral CP than in the population without CP. The researchers were unable to identify any "CP factor," including type or severity of CP, birth weight, or gestational maturity, as the cause of this early change, suggesting that skeletal changes are secondary to the diagnosis of CP. Torsional changes of the bone also occur in children with CP. Femoral anteversion is present when the proximal femur is rotated anteriorly relative to the transcondylar axis of the femur. In children with CP, the normal decrease in femoral anteversion does not occur, due in part to a lack of the movements of lateral hip rotation and extension (Bleck, 1987). In addition, persistent anteversion supports W-sitting (a functional, albeit atypical pattern that provides a wide, stable base in sitting), which alters the gluteus medius muscle function, placing additional muscle forces on the rotation of the femurs and promoting this malalignment. Skeletal impairments occur in adults with hemiplegia as well, generally as a result of incomplete recovery, persistent weakness, disuse, or habitual compensatory patterns. Depending on age, these individuals are subject to additional complications of osteoporosis and degenerative changes (Williams, Higgins, & Lewek, 2002).

Other Systems Affecting Motor Function

Impairments in the neuromuscular and musculoskeletal systems contribute most directly to movement dysfunction, however, changes in the perceptual/cognitive, regulatory, respiratory, cardiopulmonary, and gastrointestinal systems can affect movement in indirect but significant ways.

Respiratory System Impairments

Smooth coordination of the respiratory system requires intact neuromuscular, musculoskeletal, and cardiopulmonary systems. Impairments in any of these systems affect the development and function of respiratory coordination, which in turn is vital to the smooth execution of sustained posture and transitional movements, including chewing, swallowing, speech, and gait. Respiratory coordination depends on multiple body systems as well as environmental forces. During typical development, respiratory functions, as well as the shape and structure of the rib cage are affected by the recruitment of muscle activity, postures the infant assumes, and the effects of gravity and other outside forces (Alexander, Cupps, & Boehme, 1993). For example, primary impairments of muscle tone, combined with prolonged use of endotracheal tubes, affect the oral-motor coordination in premature infants (Sweeney & Swanson, 1995). Some children with CP do sustain primary damage to the lungs, which interferes with air exchange and produces inefficient respiration. For example, infants with bronchopulmonary dysplasia (BPD) have difficulty maintaining adequate levels of oxygenation during rest. Additional respiratory demands associated with nutritive sucking further disrupt the duration and regularity of their breathing rates (Craig, Lee, Freer & Laing, 1999). These children are at risk for additional impairments in general mobility due to poor cardiorespiratory endurance and failure of the musculoskeletal system to develop (Kelly, 2000; O'Shea et al., 1996).

Primary impairments of the neuromuscular system (involving posture and movement of the head, neck, shoulder girdle, and extrinsic facial and intrinsic tongue musculature) directly affect respiratory coordination. Secondary impairments of the musculoskeletal system prevent or restrict active stability and mobility of the upper rib cage, active use of the abdominals in expiration, and active thoracic expansion for inhalation (Massery & Moerchen, 1996). The pattern of shoulder elevation and the use of a shortened rectus abdominus for stability can result in severe asynchronous breathing with excessive lateral flaring of the lower ribs. This affects the quality, duration, pitch, rhythm, loudness, and rate of phonation.

In children with CP, the ribcage often remains elevated and the spine flexed, leading to immobility or deformities of the rib cage. The ribcage remains immobile and cannot expand with control to increase the volume of air exchange or produce the graded exhalation needed during movement or to support speech. Immobility of the laryngeal areas develops secondary to impairments in muscle tone (either hypotonia or hypertonia) and failure to develop upright posture against the force of gravity. The combination of these primary and secondary respiratory impairments restricts adequate breath support for sound production and adequate coordination among respiration, laryngeal functioning, and oral-motor activity (Alexander et al., 1993).

Perceptual/Cognitive System Impairments

Impairments in interpretation of environmental affordances, problem solving, decision making, and understanding the consequences of actions are examples of perceptual/cognitive influences on the control of posture and movement. In a systems perspective of client-environment interaction, pathology within any body system has a global effect, producing atypical relationships within the various systems and between the body systems and the environmental context. For example, as infants explore their world, they discover how they can act on the world and the consequences of those actions. This is true of infants with CNS pathology, but these infants will develop atypical relationships with the environment as they explore and solve problems with the limited postures and movements available to them (Fetters, 1991). Quintana (1995) identified problems in attention and orientation, inability to focus, inability to perceive and interpret specific stimulus without being distracted, and inaccurate knowledge related to time and place as issues in adults with hemiplegia. Shumway-Cook & Woollacott (2000) found that the inability to allocate sufficient attention under multitask conditions contributed to balance impairments in older adults and suggested that the cognitive disorders might influence posture and balance in significant ways in clients with CNS pathology. These issues are major factors in the lack of progress for many individuals who have CNS pathology (Quintana; Warburg, 1994). In numerous publications, the Bobaths (B. Bobath, 1971, 1977; K. Bobath, 1963; K. Bobath & B. Bobath, 1953, 1984) described the relationships between cognition and motor function in adults with stroke and children with cerebral palsy. They recounted the difficulty each examiner has in determining whether a child had primary mental retardation or secondary retardation due to the inability to move and understand his or her environment. Moving allows children to solve problems that would inevitability arise by moving in and through space, manipulating objects, and communicating with others.

Regulatory System Impairments

The regulatory system is a subsystem of the cognitive-adaptive system and provides the internal capacity to optimize arousal and attention in order to interpret sensory stimulation from individuals and the environment, modulate the intensity of the experience, and remain engaged for purposeful interaction and activity. Als et al. (1994), describing regulatory dysfunction in premature infants, hypothesized that regulatory dysfunction interferes with the infant's ability to make changes in alertness and attention, calm and organize him- or herself, and engage in adaptive functions such as sleep, feeding, mood, and transitions between states. If the infant's energy is consumed with regulatory issues, control of movement will be delayed. Bradley (2000) proposed that infants learn attention as part of the development of typical movement, relating value of experience to repeated activity. This is consistent with development and selection of neural maps linking posture and movement with the appropriate level of attention and arousal (Edelman, 1987).

Greenspan (1997) and DeGangi et al. (1991) described problems of self-regulation in children with various disorders, including CP. Variations in arousal, attention, and motivation can make multiple contributions to the control of movement (Bradley, 2000). For example, Beauregard, Thomas, and Nelson (1988) demonstrated qualitatively better reach in children with CP when reach was part of a game rather than a rote movement condition. During the game, reach was smoother and shorter in duration, and children performed with greater velocity. The researchers concluded that selecting activities in which the child could find meaning and purpose had a significant impact on kinematic characteristics in reach. Van Vliet, Sheridan, Kerwin, and Fentem (1995) found that subjects studied in the early months following stroke were able to improve their reaching kinematics in a reach-to-grasp movement when given the motivating task of picking up and drinking from a glass.

Cardiopulmonary System Impairments

Compared to their peers, who are developing typically, children with CP often exhibit decreased vigor and endurance for daily activities and a general lack of physical fitness. This directly affects the quality of their movements and their ability to maintain well-aligned posture. Physical fitness is multidimensional and involves cardiorespiratory endurance, muscle strength and endurance, flexibility, and conditioning (Stout, 2000b).

Cardiorespiratory endurance is measured in terms of maximal aerobic power. The capabilities of the cardiovascular and pulmonary systems are significant because oxygen supply to the tissues depends on the efficiency and capacity of these systems. Lundberg, Ovenfors, and Saltin (1967) found that the maximal aerobic capacity of children and adolescents with CP is as much as 30% lower than the maximal aerobic capacity of control subjects. In addition, blood flow to exercising muscle after conditioning increases in children with CP, but not in children who are developing typically (Stout, 2000b). The author proposed that the increase in blood flow might result from a decrease in spasticity.

A second component of physical fitness is *muscular strength and endurance.* Strength is necessary for movement and has a direct impact on effective performance. Muscular strength refers to maximal contractile force. Muscular endurance is the ability of muscles to perform work, and muscular power is the ability to release maximal force within a specified time. Strength deficits in children with CP are common (see the earlier discussion on Insufficient Force Generation–Weakness). Wiley and Damiano (1998) compared strength profiles in children with CP with same-age peers who were developing typically and found that children with CP were weaker in all muscles tested. Children with spastic diplegia had strength values from 16% to 71% of same-age peers, depending on the muscle tested. The gluteus maximus and soleus muscles showed the greatest strength deficits. Children with hemiplegic CP showed significant weakness in both LEs. Generally, weakness was greater in distal muscle actions than in the proximal muscle actions, and the hip flexors and ankle plantar flexors were stronger than their antagonist muscles. Andrews and Bohannon (2000) also reported on the distribution of muscle strength impairments in adults with hemiplegia and found bilateral strength impairments but more weakness on the side contralateral to the lesion. However, they found greater impairments in proximal muscle actions than distal muscle actions and greater impairment in flexor actions than extensors, particularly in the UEs. These findings contradict the common clinical assumptions regarding the distribution of strength impairments following stroke. Muscle power is also lower in children with CP. Power production in the plantar flexor muscles in terminal-stance phase provides a key source of power for forward motion during walking. Gage (1991) demonstrated decreased power production in terminal-stance phase in children with CP. Muscular endurance as measured by anaerobic tests in children with CP is also lower (Bar-Or, 1986).

Many studies have reported changes in strength with age (Frontera et al., 2000; Kent-Braun, Ng, & Young, 2000). Lower-extremity muscle strength can decrease as much as 40% between the ages of 30 and 80 years (Aniansson, Hedberg, Henning, & Grumby, 1986), and muscles of older people contain less contractile tissue and more noncontractile tissue than the skeletal muscle of younger individuals (Kent-Braun et al.). Muscle endurance also decreases with age. However, endurance is better preserved with age than strength (Shumway-Cook & Woollacott, 2001). Research has shown that there is a relationship between strength and physical function (Williams et al., 2002). Studies with individuals with stroke have considered muscle strength a reliable predictor of motor recovery, and increases in muscle strength relate to improvements in performance of daily activities (Bohannon, 1989; Bourbonnais & Vanden Noven, 1989).

Physical conditioning is the process by which exercise, repeated over a specified duration, induces morphologic and functional changes in body systems and tissue. These alterations occur in skeletal muscles, the myocardium, adipose tissue, bones, tendons, ligaments, and the CNS (Stout, 2000b). However, adolescents with disabilities can experience a drop in their level of conditioning. The typical increase in body weight and decrease in regular exercise (due to the demands of school and greater use of wheelchairs for quick mobility) result in a decrease in maximal aerobic capacity. Consequently, tasks such as walking become even more difficult (Koop, Stout, Drinken, & Starr, 1989). In addition, during the adolescent growth spurt, muscle mass increases at a faster rate than does muscle strength.

For children with CP, loss of function occurs because the rate of increase in strength is inadequate to support the rate of increase in muscle mass. The goal of physical conditioning for children with CP is to retard or reverse the deterioration of aeroebic capacity that occurs during adolescence. Strength training programs for specific muscle actions in children and adolescents with CP and in adults with hemiplegia produced increased ROM and strength, and improved functional abilities (Damiano & Abel, 1998; Horvat, 1987; Engardt, Knutsson, Jonsson, & Sternhag, 1995).

Gastrointestinal Impairments

The gastrointestinal (GI) system directly and indirectly affects motor function. All body functions, including control of the body in space, require the expenditure of energy, which the body obtains from food sources that the GI system takes in and breaks down into absorbable nutrients. The GI system is also responsible for the absorption of water. Insufficient amounts of water can reduce the body's ability to transport nutrients and metabolic wastes. Inability to take in adequate nutrients will affect the energy available for posture and movement. Poor oral-motor skills and digestive tract dysfunction can influence nutrition. Feeding and swallowing disorders, which interfere with the intake of both foods and liquids, can occur in children with CP and adults with stroke (Davies, 1985; Girolami et al., 2001; Morris & Dunn, 2000; Wolf & Glass, 1992). Stallings, Charney, Davies, and Cronk (1993) related chronic undernourishment to growth failure of children with CP. Improvement in nutrient intake results in weight gain and decreased irritability and spasticity in children with CP (Rempel, Colwell, & Nelson, 1988; Sanders et al., 1990). Even without oral-motor dysfunction, elderly adults often have poor nutrition and reduced caloric and liquid intake, which contribute to reduced energy and overall endurance available for motor functions (Sanders, 1990). Poor nutrition can result from fewer social mealtime opportunities and a decrease in the senses of taste and smell.

The indirect effects of GI impairments arise from the motor responses to pain associated with gastrointestinal reflux, motility disorders, and constipation (Agnarsson, Warde, McCarthy, Clayden, & Evans, 1993; Heine, Reddihough, & Catto-Smith, 1995). These problems can appear as disorders of posture and movement, such as increased extensor arching and high levels of muscle stiffness, as a result of abdominal pain or reflux following feeding (Girolami et al., 2001). Elderly adults with stroke can experience motility disorders and constipation as a consequence of inactivity and change from their typical diet while in the hospital or rehab setting. Often the client considers these problems too personal to discuss and simply refuses to participate in therapy without identifying the source of the problem. Therapists can influence the function of the digestive system with movement and activity and must be alert to the problems that GI impairments contribute to posture and movement.

Multisystem Impairments and Effects on Motor Function

Pain

Pain is a common problem in adults with CP or stroke (Bohannon & Andrews, 1990; Campbell, 1997; Hodgkinson et al., 2001; Murphy, Molnar, & Lankasky, 1995; Ryerson &

Levit, 1997). Pain cannot be classified as an impairment resulting from any one system, but develops from a multifaceted relationship among multiple neural and body systems and external factors. Campbell (1997) listed pain as one of six secondary conditions affecting the quality of life in adults with CP and myelodysplasia. Minor injuries often have a cascading effect, resulting in long periods of increased disability from what would, in persons without disabilities, be a short-term and easily manageable problem (Campbell, 1997). Murphy et al. surveyed adults with CP and reported that nearly 50% reported cervical pain, and 43% of the nonambulatory adults reported back pain. Pain in the weight-bearing joints occurred in 23% of the total population. Joint laxity in the shoulders and wrists also contributed to pain. Overuse syndrome, defined as chronic, repetitive, and atypical use of joints or muscles, resulted in pain.

Pain can arise from primary impairments in the neuromuscular system. Rose and Rothstein (1982) speculated that the loss of fast-twitch fibers (type II) could affect the muscle's ability to protect the joints during sudden loading, and a smaller-than-usual number of slow-twitch (type I) fibers might not be able to preserve the joint integrity when endurance is required. Over time, this could lead to degenerative joint changes and pain (Bohannon & Andrews, 1990; Gajdosik & Gajdosik, 2000). Pain can also arise from pathology unrelated to CNS neuropathology, which then complicates the impairments related to CP or stroke. For example, pain of disease or trauma, such as arthritis or hip fracture can accompany stroke and complicate the neuromuscular impairments of the primary neuropathology. Bohannon and Andrews reported that 70% of individuals with stroke reported shoulder pain in their study. Ryerson and Levit (1997) identified the causes of joint and muscle pain in adults with stroke as complex interactions of abnormal joint alignment, muscle mechanics, trauma, immobility, weakness, and altered sensitivity. They described chronic pain syndromes, including shoulder-hand syndrome, as associated with specific risk factors, including treatment. Pain in very young children or in severely disabled children or adults can be particularly difficult if they do not have a means to communicate this problem (Boehme, 1998).

Edema

Edema is a common problem in adults with hemiplegia. It appears to develop as a consequence of the impairments in (1) neuromuscular and musculoskeletal systems related to loss of movement, decrease in muscle tone, and the loss of the normal physiology of the muscle, (2) the cardiovascular system, including decreased venous return caused by paralysis and decreased activity of the vascular muscle pump (which is normally active during movement and functional use), and (3) environmental factors such as poor posture or positioning of the limbs in dependent positions during acute hospitalization (Burkhardt, 1998). Although edema is most common in the acute stage of recovery from stroke, depending on its cause, it can develop at any time and persist for long periods. Edema in a single limb can result from impingement on the vascular structures from poor positioning. Edema in both LEs can be associated with organ failure. Persistent edema is a significant problem because of its effect on ROM and joint and tissue mobility and its association with pain (Shumway-Cook & Woollacott, 2001). Pain may initially develop in the edematous limb from the pressure that swelling places on the tissues and blood vessels or from trauma to the tissues caused by forced passive-motion exercises. If the client expects a painful response to active or passive movement, he or she will avoid movement, which in turn can delay the resolution of the edema and result in disuse of the limb. Edema, with or without associated pain, will interfere with movement and functional use of the extremity. Ryerson & Levit (1997) recommend manual treatment of pitting edema by massage before it becomes resistant to manual expression.

Motor Planning

Motor planning problems involve multiple body systems and are evident in individuals with CP and stroke as they attempt complex movements requiring a sense of their own position in space, the spatial and temporal characteristics of the task, motor memory, and the gestalt of the completed task. Individuals with motor planning problems often do not develop a sense of "backward space," as shown by the inability to step backward or perform tasks behind their back such as buttoning, hair grooming, putting a belt through belt loops, or fastening a bra. Motor planning deficits are particularly problematic when the individual must plan and perform sequences of skills that depend on memory and learning (e.g., movement toward a goal that is not visible from the start, such as walking to the dining room from the rehabilitation unit). These movements require navigation strategies that depend on memory of spatial knowledge (Palta & Shumway-Cook, 1999).

For the individual to plan a coordinated, sequential motor task correctly, the sensory systems must select and attend to appropriate sensory cues. Sensory input helps to organize position in space relative to objects and persons and provides a reference of correctness as the movement proceeds, such as moving through a group of students in a busy hallway without bumping into them in order to open a school locker (or bumping into them, making corrections, and still getting to the locker). Much of the research on motor planning and coordination has focused on children with developmental coordination disabilities (DCD). These children, who have slow and laborious movements, rely on sensory feedback rather than sensory feedforward (Rosblad & von Hofsten, 1994). Silver (1988) described the motor incoordination resulting from impairments in children's visual perception and cited inefficient use of visual feedback as a possible cause for poor performance. Neural systems must organize appropriate synergies and time the various movement components with musculoskeletal elements of flexibility and stability. For example, retrieval of correct responses with reliable timing is a major impairment in children with DCD (Henderson, Rose, & Henderson, 1992). The neuromuscular system must generate appropriate force, velocity, and acceleration, then coordinate these elements with the kinematic and kinetic forces of the musculoskeletal system for accuracy of the trajectory and end point of the movement. The cognitive system must understand the task requirements and coordinate arousal, attention, memory, intention, and goals. Deficits affecting memory and attention affect motor planning. Motor planning is a complex problem that can result from impairments in multiple systems, environmental factors, and characteristics of the task. Sequential movement deficits result from the faulty interactions among these systems.

Motor Function/Dysfunction

NDT Focus: One of the unique contributions of the NDT approach is the depth of the analysis of postures and movements that link limitations in functional activities with system impairments.

The components of posture and movement that comprise the dimension of motor function include: alignment, weight bearing, balance and postural control, coordination, muscle and postural tone, biomechanical and kinesiological components of movement. These various motor components arise from multiple systems and directly affect the observable actions that a person executes for a specific task.

Atypical Alignment and Abnormal Patterns of Weight Bearing

Alignment of the body refers to the arrangement of body segments relative to each another with reference to the force of gravity, the base of support, and the nature of the task (Howle, 1999a). In NDT, *normal alignment* is the alignment of the body segments as needed to anticipate and organize the movements for a task. Normal alignment is so fundamental to human behavior that deviations from it are generally easily recognized. However, recognizing and hypothesizing the relationship between subtle malalignments and possible causes require analytical observation and problem-solving skills. In the adult with CNS pathology, asymmetric alignment can be a direct result of the neuropathology, as in pusher syndrome or in unilateral neural lesions produced by a CVA (Duncan & Badke, 1987), or can result from musculoskeletal impairments or compensation for weakness (Shumway-Cook & Woollacott, 2001). Following a stroke, abnormal alignment can develop rapidly (as in shoulder subluxation that responds to the pull of gravity and traction of a paretic limb) or slowly (as in hindfoot pronation as a result of increasing ambulation and incomplete motor recovery).

In children with CP, except for the most severe cases, alignment problems develop over time, in response to growth and changes in body mass, as well as to asymmetric neural lesions. Alignment of the body segments over the base of support determines to a great extent the effort required to support the body against gravity. Burtner, Woollacott, and Qualls (1999) found that children with spastic diplegic CP who habitually stood in a crouched posture showed a marked increase in the co-activation of muscles responding to loss of balance. Children developing typically who stood in the same posture also used antagonistic muscles more often in response to platform perturbations, suggesting that the musculoskeletal constraints (such as hip or knee flexion stiffness or contracture, and excessive plantar flexor muscle weakness) associated with standing in a crouched posture play a significant role in the atypical muscle response patterns in children with diplegic CP, rather than imbalance of muscle strength constraining alignment (Burtner et al., 1999; Woollacott et al., 1998). Abnormal alignment can result from muscle tone changes, strength imbalances, or skeletal problems related to growth. Asymmetric forces affect the shape of the bone by stimulating growth in noncompressed areas, while inhibiting bone development in areas of compression (Gajdosik & Gajdosik, 2000). Skeletal deformities, most often in the spine (scoliosis or kypholordosis) and LEs, are common in adults with CP. Strength imbalances, often caused secondarily by surgery or overuse of orthotics, contribute to problems in alignment. For example, the crouched gait often results from overlengthening of the gastroc-soleus group in the presence of static or dynamic contractures of either the hip flexors or hamstrings, or an attempt to correct an earlier alignment problem due to imbalance of agonists and antagonists at the hip or knee (Gage, 1992).

Atypical patterns of weight bearing are a particular alignment problem arising from the distribution of the body weight at rest in relation to the support surface and in anticipation of movement. For example, in adults with hemiplegia, asymmetric stance, with the majority of weight bearing on the stronger side, minimizes the need to unload the paretic limb before swing phase and contributes to gait abnormalities (Wall & Turnbull, 1986). Persistent asymmetrical weight bearing limits the movement on that side and can contribute to the development of additional structural asymmetries (Howle, 1999a). Efficient contact with the support surface is a necessary foundation for movement from that surface. Children with CP often are not able to conform to the support surface. Consequently, only a very small proportion of the body that is in contact with the surface actually bears weight. This limitation in the pressure distribution between the body part and the surface hinders the child's ability to generate the force necessary to push against the support surface in rising to stand, or in the push-off phase of gait (Stamer, 2000; Tscharnuter, 1993, 2002). Adults with hemiplegia often need to relearn effective utilization of the support surface to regain use of the involved extremities during transitions of turning over or rising to sitting from the bed that require efficient use of the support (B. Bobath, 1990).

NDT Focus: Careful attention to alignment as a critical component of anticipatory postural control has always been a significant part of the NDT treatment approach. Handling of key points on the client's body aligns the trunk and the limbs, giving a mechanical advantage to contracting muscles during active movement and increasing sensoriperception of typical alignment in a specific movement context.

Abnormal Muscle Tone: Hypertonia and Hypotonia

Abnormalities in tone, including both hypertonia and hypotonia, are consistent and predictive findings in young children who have CP (Bartlett & Piper, 1993; Van den Berg-Emons, van Baak, de Barbanson, Speth, & Saris, 1996). Hypertonia is also a major impairment for individuals following stroke (Craik, 1991a; Gardiner, 1996). In premature infants, muscle tone normally changes drastically as development progresses through the first year of life (Amiel-Tison, 1968; Saint-Anne Dargassies, 1977).

Muscle tone is the "stiffness" or tension with which a muscle resists being lengthened. Both neural and nonneural mechanisms contribute to muscle tone (Lin, Brown, & Brotherstone, 1994a, 1994b). Clinically, *hypotonia* is a decrease in the sensation of a muscle's resistance to stretch as the joint is moved through the ROM, and the muscle's inability to recruit adequate force to move against the force of gravity. Hypotonia is associated with lesions involving the cerebellar pathways and often occurs as a transient stage in infants who develop CP and adults with acute stroke (Olney & Wright, 2000; Stamer, 2000). *Hypertonia,* on the other end of the spectrum, is characterized by a sensation of increased resistance to stretch, a feeling of stiffness, and limitation in the range and variety of active movements (Katz & Rymer, 1989). Hypertonia can be either a positive primary impairment associated with neuropathology or a secondary impairment (Lin et al., 1994a, 1994b; Olney & Wright, 2000). For example, a child with ataxia bends over to reach objects on the floor by flexing at the hips and trunk while increasing stiffness in the muscles around the knees in order to decrease the degrees of freedom and increase stability (Montgomery, 2000).

Factors contributing to the impairment of muscle tone include the following, from Lin et al. (1994a, 1994b):

1. *Spasticity* produces velocity-dependent resistance to passive stretch and abnormal muscle tone. Researchers currently view spasticity as only one contribution to hypertonia in individuals with CNS pathology. (See the section in this chapter entitled Neuromuscular Impairments-Positive Signs.)
2. *Changes in muscle properties (hypoextensibility, contracture, and muscle atrophy)* are secondary changes in the musculoskeletal system and are described here because they contribute significantly to changes in muscle tone (Dietz et al., 1986). Tardieu, de al Tour, Bret, and Tardieu (1982) coined the term *hypoextensibililty* to describe muscles that produce more force for a given change in length and therefore feel stiff and resist passive lengthening due to changes in the muscle properties. The muscles of children with CP and individuals with stroke offer resistance to passive stretching at a shorter length than normal muscle. Hypoextensibility is a consequence of abnormal muscle shortness caused by structural shortening of the muscle fibers and a reduction in the number of sarcomeres, changes that result in increased tone in the muscle (Dietz et al., 1981). Hypoextensibility makes it difficult for the individual to move actively through complete ranges of motion and to resist passive lengthening at shorter ranges than those of persons without disabilities. *Contracture* of muscle, in which it is no longer possible to move the joint and muscle through the ROM, is the end result of hypoextensibility. *Atrophy* refers to a decrease in the size of the muscle mass and occurs in chronic disuse syndromes related to CNS pathology and weakness.
3. *Changes in adaptability* of muscles can result in excessive co-activation (co-contraction) or loss of movement flexibility during active movement (Crenna & Inverno, 1994). Co-activation increases the apparent mechanical stiffness or impedance of the controlled joint, thus fixing its posture or stabilizing its course of movement in the presence of external force perturbations (Humphrey & Reed, 1983). Excessive co-activation then contributes to stiffness during active movement

4. *Stiffness* describes the characteristics of elastic materials. Like spasticity, stiffness is a measure of the resistance to motion. Stiffness is defined as the amount of force a muscle must produce to cause a change in length. If a great amount of force is required to produce a change in length, then the muscle is said to have increased stiffness (Herbert, 1988; Holt, Butcher, & Fonseca, 2000). Normally, muscles exhibit spring-like characteristics. The physical property of muscle is compliant or "springy," and tension results by purely mechanical means as the muscle's length increases. This change in tension is instantaneous with any stretch. The increase in tension has the effect of opposing the perturbation, bringing the system back to the original position. This kind of adjustment is necessary when the body or limbs are maintaining a relatively static position for posture and also to keep an ongoing movement on course (Nashner & Woollacott, 1979; Sears & Newsom-Davis, 1968). Dr. Bobath (1980) frequently used the example of palpating the muscles of the thigh as an individual prepared to shift from two-foot stance to one-foot stance to illustrate the normal changes in muscle stiffness adapted to postural requirements. If the muscles are less compliant (stiff), they will respond more quickly to passive stretch and feel stiffer to the examiner. Excessive stiffness interferes with the adaptability of muscle to prepare for active movements.

5. *Abnormal force production* that occurs in active movement also contributes to both hypo- and hypertonia. The neural aspects of force production reflect the number and type of motor units recruited and the discharge frequency. Hypotonia is evident when a disruption of the recruitment patterns causes inefficient muscle activation or abnormal timing in recruitment of agonists and antagonists, producing ineffective muscle contractions (Carr & Shepherd, 2000). (This chapter's section on Insufficient Force Generation–Weakness describes these influences in greater detail.) Muscles that are hypotonic create a problem in effective motor execution because they are unable to reach threshold for muscle fiber firing or are unable to recruit enough motor units to initiate movement.

Ryerson and Levitt (1997) described increased muscle stiffness during volitional movement with abnormal patterns of muscle activation. They proposed that the increase in muscle tension results when the patient activates the wrong muscles for the attempted task or activates these muscles with excessive force. Kershner (1991) proposed that increased tone resulted from depolarized motor neuron pools due to a net increase in tonic excitatory synaptic inputs from descending pathways and local interneuron signals. If the threshold is lowered, a smaller or slower motion than usual will result in resistance to manual stretch and an increased muscle force with an increased joint angle. Force production also responds to changes in musculoskeletal properties, such as abnormal joint alignment, changes in muscle elasticity, and tissue length (hypo- or hypermobility or muscle atrophy) (Dietz et al., 1981, 1986).

Abnormal Postural Tone

Postural tone is the distribution of muscle tone among specific muscle groups that must be constrained to act together to maintain posture against the force of gravity and simultaneously adapt stiffness to allow the flexibility necessary for movement (K. Bobath & B. Bobath, 1952; Shumway-Cook & Woollacott, 2001). Postural tone is recognized in the muscles of the trunk and supporting extremities. The amount of tone and the muscle groups constrained at any one time change with the individual's position, counteracting the force of gravity for orientation and stability. For example, a catcher on a baseball team requires a specific distribution of postural tone (and alignment) to be stable in a squat position. The guard on a basketball team requires quite a different distribution, with the trunk fully extended and arms up. A sprinter's postural tone includes both the upper and lower extremities, as well as the muscles of the trunk. Yet all individuals require a high state of readiness to change quickly from static posture to flexible, rapid movement once play is in motion. Muscles throughout the trunk and extremities generate the forces to support body weight against gravity and maintain the body in a vertical position (Basmajian & deLuca, 1985; Schenkman & Butler, 1992).

In individuals with CNS pathology, alterations in postural tone can result from abnormalities in a variety of underlying systems, such as (a) abnormal mechanical properties of muscles (Stockmeyer, 2000), (b) inability to organize and integrate somatosensory input from muscles of the neck (referred to as tonic neck reflexes) so that moving the head changes the pattern of tone (Shea, Guadagnoli, & Dean, 1995), (c) inability to utilize visual and vestibular inputs, including labyrinthine and visual righting reflexes or orientation in space, and (d) excessive use of muscles in patterns of co-activation as a postural strategy to maintain stability (Campbell, 1991; Ryerson & Levit, 1997). Children with CP often show increased postural tone at the expense of movement against gravity.

> ***NDT Focus: Currently, NDT recognizes that multiple systems contribute to the amount and the distribution of postural tone in a task-specific context. Clinicians recognize appropriate postural tone through observation of alignment and by feeling the readiness of muscles to change from static posture to flexible movement.***

Balance and Postural Control Problems

The complexity of balance and postural control problems is evidenced by the fact that various investigators have classified balance and postural control as primary, secondary, or composite impairments or patterns of compensation (Ryerson & Levit, 1997; Shumway-Cook & Woollacott, 2001). The Bobaths initially viewed balance difficulties as a secondary problem resulting from impairments in muscle and postural tone and selective motor control. NDT currently classifies these problems as a component of posture and movement.

Postural control consists of (a) proactive or postural orientation, which anticipates the appropriate relationship between body segments in a task specific context, (b) postural stability or steady-state balance, which is the ability to maintain the center of mass within the limits of the BOS and (c) reactive postural adjustments or equilibrium reactions, which are flexible and varied responses to perturbations from the environment, self-initiated movements, or a moving support surface (Shumway-Cook & Woollacott, 2001). Appropriate postural control depends on inputs from visual and somatosensory receptors (tactile and proprioceptive) and the vestibular system, and on the ability of the CNS to interpret the relative importance of each input. The relative roles of the different sensory inputs remain controversial. The neural mechanisms must activate, time, and execute synergistic muscles at mechanically related joints to ensure stability while permitting mobility at other joints to allow movement, all while comparing the executed movement with the intended action. For these reasons, problems in balance are viewed as components of posture and movement with the goal to support standing, walking, reaching, or other functional tasks. It is not surprising that individuals with stroke or CP have difficulties with balance.

There is a vast amount of evidence describing problems in the various components of postural control and balance (Hirschfeld, 1992). (The development of postural control and balance is described in Chapter 1.) Nashner et al. (1983) first examined issues of postural control in children with CP when the children experienced a change in the BOS. The researchers found differences in the timing and sequences of activation patterns in response to platform sway. These children were unable to recruit and regulate the firing frequency of motor neurons and did not exhibit the normal ascending pattern, from ankles to hips, in response to perturbations to stance balance. Other investigators have confirmed this finding (Badke & DiFabio, 1990; Burtner et al., 1999). A disruption in the recruitment order also occurs in muscles responding to the loss of balance in the seated position (Brogen, Hadders-Algra, & Forssberg, 1998). Nashner et al. (1983) and, in a separate study, Horak et al. (1984) described the inability to activate postural muscles in anticipation of self-initiated perturbation in children with CP and adults with stroke. Individuals with cerebellar lesions are unable to scale the muscle forces needed to respond appropriately to the degree of instability. *Scaling* refers to appropriately matching the size of the muscle response to the size of the perturbation. Postural responses are often too large for the displacement, creating still another balance problem (Horak & Diener, 1994). Abnormal delays in the onset of postural responses, which contribute to instability, have been reported in adults with hemiplegia (Diener, Dichgans, Guschlbauer, & Mau, 1984) and in children with CP (Holt et al., 2000). Problems in alignment, which affect balance, also occur, but this will be discussed as a secondary impairment of the musculoskeletal system.

Kinesiological and Biomechanical Components of Movement

NDT Focus: NDT recognizes that the kinesiological and biomechanical components of the musculoskeletal system, anthropometric changes, and movement experiences in various gravitational contexts account for many of the differences in postures and movements that occur between infancy and adulthood.

The infant's musculoskeletal system is incomplete, and organization of the system is driven by spontaneous movement exploration–and the sensory feedback from those actions–within the physical laws of the environment (Bly, 1999; Jensen, Schneider, Ulrich, Zernicke, & Thelen, 1994). Very young babies do not have full ROM at all of their joints. Under 4 months of age, limitations in spinal extension, hip extension, hip internal rotation, and shoulder flexion constrain the coordination of movement patterns of reciprocal kicking, stepping, and reaching (Heriza, 1991a, 1991b; von Hofsten & Ronnqvist, 1993). Infants gradually increase the ROM at each of their joints by practicing a variety of movements in all three planes of movement–sagittal, frontal, and transverse. Bly (1999) wrote that infants experiment with flexion and extension in supine; extension and flexion in prone; lateral weight shifts to each side in supine, prone, sitting, and standing; and rotation around the body axis in all positions. Flexion and extension occur on the sagittal plane; lateral movements, abduction, and adduction occur on the frontal plane; and rotation occurs on the transverse plane. As the constraints on joint range and muscle strength become more flexible, so do the movements and muscle activity involved in motor control (Stout, 2000b).

Infants with CNS pathology do not practice movements on all three planes. They maintain a few positions and rarely alternate between positions (described earlier as cramped synchrony). Movement within a position is limited in variety. This poor variation manifests as a limited repertoire of general movements (Hadders-Algra, 2000; Prechtl, 1990). These infants move primarily on the sagittal plane and subsequently develop stereotyped, limited secondary repertoires because of limited experience and limited sensory feedback. Because they do not expand their movement repertoires, they have difficulty activating and elongating all of their muscles; consequently, they might never experience full ROM of their joints. If they do not develop full ROM and do not elongate their muscles fully, they are vulnerable to muscular contractures and skeletal deformities (Bly, 1999).

In the acute phase of stroke (flaccid stage), the adult can have a similar experience. The first movements the client makes are from the supine position in bed. Trunk and extremity movements to change position or find a comfortable position occur only as excursions in the sagittal plane using lateral weight shift and pushing with extension (usually with the uninvolved side), with limited excursions of trunk rotation and flexion. Movement is particularly difficult because the entire body is the BOS and the extremities are long and heavy; consequently any activity other than shifting in bed must resist both friction and gravity (B. Bobath, 1990; Ryerson & Levit, 1997).

In addition to the constraints of muscle strength and joint extensibility, body composition also constrains the movements of infants and young children. The body grows during the first 18 years of life, particularly during the first 3 years; but as Shumway-Cook and Woollacott (2001) pointed out, changes in body configuration continue with the aging process. Changes in the anthropometric relationships of the body parts influence the development of upright posture. Campbell (2000a) described the influence of the size of the head, relative to the overall body size, on head lifting. She contended that each child produces a unique and specific pattern of head lifting in prone, based on individual anthropometic characteristics, muscle strength, and limb compliance, as well as previous experience and interest. Thelen and Fisher

(1982) hypothesized that the disappearance of early stepping in infants relates to the increased size of the infant without a concomitant increase in muscle strength.

Changes in spinal flexibility can lead to a stooped or flexed posture in elderly people, which in turn leads to reduced stability in standing and changes in motor strategies for ambulation (Lewis & Bottomley, 1990). Loss of musculoskeletal flexibility (particularly thoracolumbar and cervical-thoracic) and ankle mobility necessarily put mechanical constraints on an individual's capability for the appropriate postural responses used in balance control (Schenkman, 1989). Declining postural and balance abilities (along with reduced proximal muscle strength) are factors in the rate of falling in elderly adults (Lipsitz, Jonsson, Kelley, & Koestner, 1991).

NDT therapists select techniques to use in treatment and to teach the family that encourage the client to alternate actively between positions and move on all three planes, combining flexion, extension, and rotation through a wide variety of positions to discover unique and preferred ways to accomplish self-initiated movement goals.

Coordination Problems

Coordination is the quality of the temporal-spatial execution of a task. Quality includes accuracy, reliability, efficiency, quickness, and adaptability. Impaired coordination refers to movements that appear awkward, uneven, clumsy, or inaccurate and can result from pathology in a wide variety of neural structures. Impaired coordination commonly results from lesions in the motor cortex, basal ganglia, and cerebellum (Shumway-Cook & Woollacott, 2001). In addition, coordination requires an efficient musculoskeletal system, including the properties of the muscles and tendons. Impaired coordination results from the disruption of the activation, sequencing, timing, and scaling of muscle activity, all of which have been discussed as primary impairments in CNS pathology.

Normally, in performing daily activities, an individual produces coordinated actions easily, generating different actions at the same time (e.g., using a knife and fork, climbing stairs while carrying a child, opening a door while holding bags of groceries, breathing while eating and drinking). Coordinated movement involves multiple joints and muscles that activate at the appropriate time, in the right sequence, and with the correct amount of force so that smooth, efficient, and accurate movement results. In addition to multisegment movements, coordination needs to occur in a single body segment among the agonists, antagonists, and synergists, grading the outcome to match the task.

One of the major sources of interference in interlimb coordination involves the temporal structures of the actions that the individual is attempting to coordinate. Actions with the same temporal organization are easy to coordinate (e.g., tapping the same rhythm with both hands), whereas activities with different temporal organization are more difficult to produce (e.g., playing the piano) (Heuer, 1974). In addition, the type of task (discrete or continuous) is an important factor in coordination. Discrete tasks have definite start and end points, and considerable planning goes into preparing the body to move. Even quite simple movements require the organization of various independently moving parts of the motor system. Aiming movements involve the coordination of the eyes and head, arm and hand when perception and action are visually guided. Reach-grasp actions represent discrete movements in which the limb-transport component of the movement is distinct from the object-manipulation component. Evidence suggests that although these components seem to be separable, their actions are highly interdependent (Biguer, Jeannerod, & Prablanc, 1982). The temporal coordination among the eye, head, and limb movements represents a flexible coupling, adapting to the nature of the task.

During reach in adults with hemiplegia and children with CP (Levin, 1996; Levin et al., 2002; Steenbergen et al., 1998), the movement trajectory often displays a loss of coordinated coupling between synergistic muscles and joints, which affects the timing and trajectory of movements (Shumway-Cook & Woollacott, 2001). There is also a spatially impaired coordination during reaching in individuals with CNS pathology that manifests as interjoint incoordination and abnormal movement trajectories (Bastian, Martin, Keating, & Thach, 1996). Manual aiming is more accurate when the head is free to move than when head position is fixed. Individuals who do not develop flexible synergies involving the head, eyes, and limbs will show impaired coordination in discrete movement tasks.

Coordination of gait is an example of a continuous task that requires a high degree of selectivity of muscle activity and interlimb coordination. The basic neural organization and function that underlie locomotion receive both descending and peripheral input to select and organize the activation and firing sequence of intra- and interlimb coordination. In addition to the neural elements, adequate ROM, strength, configuration of skeletal structures, and the specific context affect the coordination of gait (Stout, 2000a). Constraints on any of the musculoskeletal components can change the pattern of muscle activity. While the interlimb timing during gait is easily coordinated for preferred walking speed for each individual, coordination of gait is context-dependent in real-life situations. Feedback, error detection, and error correction play a dominant role in adapting locomotion in functional contexts (Holt, Obusek, & Fonseca, 1996).

A wide variety of neuromuscular and musculoskeletal impairments contributes to coordination disorder in gait. These include abnormal muscle synergies, disordered patterns of activation, ineffective reciprocal activation of agonist and antagonist muscles for eccentric and concentric actions, ineffective muscle execution, loss of ROM, changes in alignment, BOS, muscle hypoextensibility, and joint contracture. Each of these difficulties can occur alone or in combination, which makes gait disorders a particularly complex problem. Ineffective synergies occur in individuals with hemiplegia following stroke, resulting in stereotyped and relatively fixed patterns of movement. The presence of these tightly constrained synergies prevents isolated movements, such as extension of the knee while flexing the hip (see Gage, 1992; Perry, 1992 for further discussion). Lesions in the CNS result in limited selection of muscle activation. The loss of the ability to selectively recruit the anterior tibialis during gait in individuals with hemiplegia is a common problem (Perry, 1992). Premature or prolonged activation of the hamstrings can also occur in children with CP and adults with stroke (Knutsson, 1994; Knutsson & Richards, 1979). Excessive co-activation of the lower-extremity muscles is a common finding among children with CP. Various researchers have found increased co-activation beginning at the end of swing phase and continuing throughout the stance phase of gait (Crenna & Iverno, 1994; Knutsson, 1994; Perry, 1992).

Musculoskeletal problems (e.g., weakness, loss of ROM, and joint contracture and change in the BOS) contribute to problems in coordination of gait. Children with CP and adults with hemiplegia can develop ankle dorsiflexion or plantar flexion contractures, knee and hip flexion contractures, and reduced pelvic and spinal mobility that contribute to disordered gait. Soft-tissue contractures and bony constrictions limit ROM and constrain movement. For example, ROM limitations at the ankle decrease joint mobility during stance, which restricts the smooth progression of the body over the support foot. In swing, decreased joint mobility reduces foot clearance, affecting progression and foot placement for stability. Limited ROM also affects the individual's ability to modify movement strategies to address changing environmental conditions, such as stepping over or around obstacles. Hip flexion contractures, usually combined with knee flexion contractures, result in inadequate extension during midstance that affect alignment and stability in stance and reduce the effect of extension power for forward progression. This produces a gait pattern that is disordered, arrythmical, energy consuming, and inefficient, all characteristics of poor coordination.

The Problem-Solving Process Applied to a Clinical Example

It should be obvious to the reader from the extent of the discussion in this chapter that systems impairments and their relationships to motor functions are complex and multifaceted. Sorting out which impairments might be responsible for functional limitations requires both knowledge and experience. Since NDT assumes that dysfunction in the neural and body systems affects the individual's ability to solve motor problems which, in turn, affects specific functions of that individual, it is important to thoroughly understand this thought process. NDT uses a problem-solving process based on the enablement model to first, examine functional limitations, and second, propose causation in order to systematically apply intervention methods to change function. The following brief example illustrates how this thought process is applied to a very specific functional problem. Chapters 3 and 4 apply this problem-solving process in examination and treatment decision-making.

Pathophysiology:

Mr. Dunlap had a left cerebral artery infarction 4 months ago with resulting right hemiplegia.

A. Participation Restriction

Mr. Dunlap would like to be independent in all areas of self-care, in order to feel better about himself and reduce the daily burden on his wife.

B. Functional Limitation

Mr. Dunlap is unable to lift and cross his right leg over his left to put on his shoes while seated without taking excessive time and exerting a great deal of effort.

C. Posture and Movement Limitations

1. He cannot adjust his posture to anticipate the change in his COM to his BOS needed for this activity.
2. He cannot effectively shift his weight to his left side and balance in this posture sufficiently to raise his right leg and cross it over his left leg.
3. He cannot rotate and flex his trunk to the left and maintain this posture for the length of time needed to get his shoe on.
4. He cannot fully straighten his right elbow, which makes it difficult to reach for his right foot.
5. He cannot coordinate his hands to simultaneously stabilize his shoe and maneuver it onto his foot.

D. System Impairments

The therapist hypothesizes that Mr. Dunlap has the following system impairments:

Neuromuscular System

1. Loss of anticipatory postural control underlies his inability to initiate lateral weight shift prior to crossing his leg.
2. Both hypotonia and inactivation of postural muscles of the trunk interfere with trunk rotation and produce lateral trunk flexion.
3. Loss of fractionated movements limit two-handed dexterity and manipulation of his shoe and limits his ability to wiggle his forefoot and toes into the shoe.
4. Abnormal timing and impaired muscle synergies prevent accuracy in the precise degrees of flexion and abduction of the right hip combined with flexion of the right knee to cross his leg, as well as timing the coordinated action between the hands for stabilizing and manipulating.
5. Weakness in the right LE makes lifting this leg to cross it over his left difficult.

Musculoskeletal System

1. Stiffness, around the right ankle due to muscle hypoextensibility and limitation in joint ROM, prevents movement of the ankle and requires him to manipulate the shoe around his foot rather than adapting the foot to the placement of the shoe.
2. Limited elbow extension of the right arm due to old radial head fracture.

Sensory Systems

1. Decreased tactile discrimination in the fingers of the left hand, contributing to problems in manipulation.

Respiratory System

1. Chronic emphysema with rib cage hypomobility and respiratory compromise limit his ability to breathe easily while flexing and rotating his trunk for the duration of the task.

This is just one example that demonstrates the problem-solving process linking the function of putting on shoes with posture and movement dysfunction and system impairments.

The Process of Recovery and Compensation

The distributed neural model provides a flexible framework within which to explore mechanisms that could account for recovery of function. Chapter 1 discusses the concept of distributed neural control in more detail, but the main ideas are also noted here to relate them to recovery.

In a distributed model, numerous connections exist between and within levels of the nervous system. Information and motor commands flow in ascending, descending, and lateral directions. Function does not reside with a single area, but is a cooperative effort among many regions of the nervous system. The site of control depends on the nature of the task, prior experience, and the need of the moment. A distributive neural model provides a more reasonable framework within which to understand the nervous system's capacity to reorganize following injury, than does the hierarchical model, which included the concepts of localization of function, "top-down" control, and fixed neural pathways dependent on maturation. NDT has adopted a distributed model of the CNS that changes the conceptual framework. Rather than assigning function to the lesioned part and describing impairments produced by the lesion, NDT looks at what the entire nervous system does following injury and how it interacts with other body systems. This approach to recovery helps to explain, first, the variability in functional limitations among individuals despite similar factors (e.g., site and extent of a lesion) and second, the concept that neural damage and recovery can lead to both adaptive and maladaptive behavior (Craik, 1991b).

Recovery and compensation relate to changes in motor function following injury to the CNS. *Recovery* is the reorganization and plasticity changes in the CNS, as well as gradual return of muscle strength and movement control after a deficit occurs following CNS damage. Recovery implies that the individual can perform the function in the same manner and with the same efficiency and effectiveness as before the damage (Held, 2000). *Compensations,* on the other hand, are new strategies of movement that replace normal movements to accomplish a functional goal or task. They are movements the individual adopts to solve movement problems, albeit less efficiently and effectively, and to reduce disability (Stein, 1998).

Research in recovery has shown that the brain has great capacity to change, exhibiting growth and reorganization in the neurons of the adult CNS after injury (Nudo, 1998). No single mechanism accounts for the return of function following injury, but there are a variety of events occurring collectively that could account for recovery. To date, research has not been able to relate a change in a specific neural mechanism to a change in behavior, but has demonstrated that the CNS can and does regenerate, restore, and reorganize and that this is strongly related to the experiences provided (Held, 2000; Craik, 1991b; Vicari et al., 2000).

Cellular Responses to Injury

Focal brain lesions produce two types of functional disturbances: those resulting from actual death of neurons and those resulting from inhibition of intact neurons. *Diaschisis* is the temporary disruption of function produced by the shock of injury to the brain tissue affecting neuronal processes far from the site of the lesion (Craik, 1991b; Luria, Naydin, Tsvetkova, & Vinarskaya, 1969; Stein, Brailowsky, & Will, 1995). Damage to one part of the nervous system deprives other intact regions of normal afferent flow that had previously come from the injured areas, with the result that symptoms arise from the intact distant sites, as well as the injured areas. Because of the interconnections, inhibition of brain regions distant from the primary site of injury can also result from a reduction in blood flow and/or metabolism at the injured site itself. The resolution of diaschisis might therefore account for some of the return of function following injury. If the intact areas recover from loss of some afferent input, symptoms that occurred because of disruption in the distant intact areas will dissipate.

Disruption of neural function can occur as the result of indirect effects of injuries that impair cerebral blood flow, control of the cerebrospinal fluid, or cerebral metabolism. For example, stroke frequently is the result of ischemia (80% of cases). The damage to the CNS depends upon a number of factors, including the extent of collateral circulation, duration and severity of the ischemic event, and relative vulnerability of the specific brain region (Nudo, 1998). Neurons experiencing complete absence of blood flow die within 5 minutes. Surrounding neurons can die from a series of biochemical reactions set off by the initial ischemia, including lack of oxygen and nutrients and build-up of metabolites. For example, glutamate, an excitatory neurotransmitter, accumulates during ischemia. Excessive amounts of glutamate can overstimulate neurons and cause cell death (Nudo).

Many injuries involve interruption of axonal projections from the affected areas. In the zone of injury, there is rapid degeneration of the axon and myelin sheath. The ends of the axons retract and swell. Edema at the injury site can compress axons and produce a physiological block in conduction. The temporary disruption in blood supply can result in loss of function. The term *neural shock* describes the temporary injury to intact areas in the CNS. Resolution of neural shock permits the return of muscle tone following flaccid paralysis in the initial stage of recovery in individuals with stroke.

In addition, there is denervation of the population of neurons innervated by the injured neurons, either orthograde or retrograde (see Figure 2.5). This secondary neuronal death occurs within 2-7 days of the injury and can account for more damage than primary cell death. The degree of atrophy in the pathway during orthograde degeneration correlates to the percent of total input removed from the population of neurons by the lesion. It is possible that the other sources of input can reduce the severity of transneuronal degeneration. Some researchers have proposed that neurons require a certain amount of stimulation to survive. If this critical level of stimulation does not occur, the synaptic terminal releases its trophic substances and dies (Stein, 1998). Aside from the loss of neurons damaged at the site of injury, the synaptic loss from these neurons produces a degeneration along neuronal pathways, including pathways that affect the "other" hemisphere, increasing the extent of neural disruption with time (Steward, 1989; Cioni, Montanaro, Tosetti, Canapicchi, & Ghelarducci, 2001). For this reason, professionals no longer make reference to a nonaffected side and an affected side, but to the more-affected and less-affected sides.

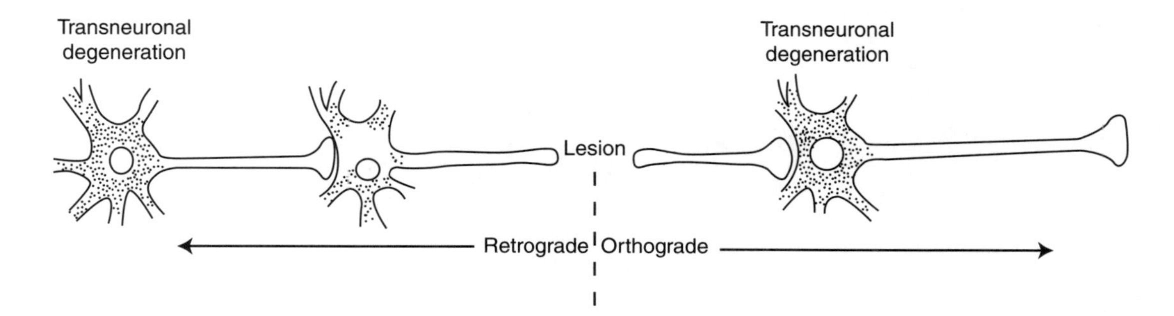

Figure 2.5. Orthograde and retrograde denervation following injury offers an explanation of indirect and direct damage to proximal and distal neurons. (Illustration by Claire Wenstrom.)

Evidence of Neural Reorganization

Two types of sprouting or synaptogenesis occur following damage in the adult CNS. Neural regeneration or regenerative synaptogenesis occurs when injured axons begin sprouting. Although it is now well-established that this does occur in humans, these sprouts must travel over long distances and often do not succeed in reconnecting to their original targets (Aguayo, Clarke, Jelsma, & Wiley, 1996; Bjorklund, 1994; see Figure 2.6). Currently, researchers are trying to find ways of increasing the probability that the regenerative sprouts will reinnervate their usual targets.

Reactive synaptogenesis, a second type of neuronal sprouting, occurs within 4-5 days of injury. Sprouts from nearby undamaged axons innervate synaptic sites that were previously activated by the injured axons. These undamaged axons belong to the same neural system that originally innervated the synaptic sites. Held (2000) suggested that reactive synaptogenesis could be beneficial in two ways: (a) it could prevent dendritic atrophy resulting from denervation, and (b) it could maintain a functional level of excitability so that other inputs would be effective in activating the pathway. Although the exact function of reactive synaptogenesis is still unknown, new synapses can form in the mature CNS, replacing those lost by injury (Held, 2000).

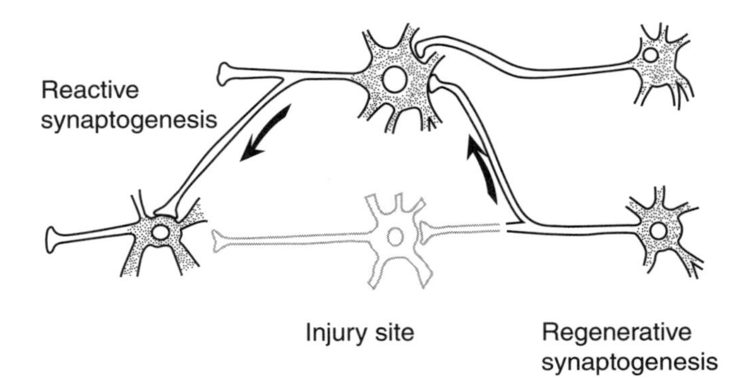

Figure 2.6. Regenerative and reactive synaptogenesis compensates for neuronal injury. Reactive sprouting is depicted here by the extension of the axon on the right to connect to its original target via collaterals and an alternate route. (Illustration by Claire Wenstrom.)

Non-Neural Factors Contributing to Recovery of Function

Age

Many factors affect the results of damage to the CNS, as well as the recovery that occurs afterwards. Age is one of those factors. Until recently, the assumption that brain damage in infancy caused fewer deficits than damage to the adult brain was a guiding principle, based primarily on work with monkeys (Kennard, 1940, 1942). Glassman and Smith (1988) noted this effect in language function in humans. Damage to the dominant hemisphere shows little or no effect on speech in children younger than 2 years, but causes varying degrees of aphasia in persons older than 12 years of age. However, more recent research has revealed a more complex relationship; not all areas show the same capacity for regeneration. Injury to some areas of the brain produces similar deficits whether damage occurs in infancy or adulthood, while damage to other areas shows little effect in infancy, but problems develop later in life (Held, 2000; Shumway-Cook & Woollacott 2001; Stein et al., 1995).

The hypothesis is that the factors determining the effect of the lesion are the maturational status of the damaged area (not the age of the person), the functional status of the remaining systems, the size of the lesion, and the experience of the organism before damage. If an area is mature, the damage will result in comparable deficits, whether in infants or adults. A functionally related area not committed to its own function might take over the function of the damaged tissue during development. If the damaged area had not reached functional maturity at the time of injury, no deficit would be apparent, at first, but would develop at the time when the area would normally assume its own function during maturation (Craik, 1991b; Goldman, 1974; Held, 2000).

Another hypothesis proposes that developmental plasticity might account for changes in functional deficits. Many studies have linked the degree of expressive language deficit with the side of the brain lesion. Children with left-hemisphere damage show greater language deficits. However, Vicari et al. (2000) found that the degree of language deficits following early focal brain lesions depended on the stage of expressive skills rather than the hemispheric damage. Children with left-hemisphere injury had significant delays in expression of single words when compared to children with right-hemispheric lesions, but once they moved to the state of producing at least some sentences, the hemispheric differences were no longer evident. The researchers attributed this to developmental plasticity, suggesting that recovery from initial delays might take place in the early stages of language development.

In addition, the recovery of function brought about by other areas taking over might occur at some cost as the result of a crowding effect of the remaining intact structures as they attempt to subserve more functions than normally required. For example, language functions can be spared in young children with left-hemisphere damage, but this sparing often accompanies a diminished capacity for spatial perception, which is thought to be a function of the right hemisphere (Milner, 1974). In another example, Woods (1980) found that the IQs of children with spared speech following brain damage in the first year of life were well below average and below those of children who sustained brain damage later in life.

Nature of the Lesion

The characteristics of the lesion affect the extent of recovery. A small lesion has a greater chance of recovery, as long as no functional areas have been entirely removed. Slowly developing lesions, such as tumors, appear to cause less functional loss than a sudden insult, such as stroke (Finger & Stein, 1982). However, slow-growing lesions produce more permanent changes than those following a sudden insult.

Environment/Training

Environmental conditions, before and after brain lesions, affect the recovery process. This information comes primarily from animal studies. Rats with lesions, raised in enriched environments, showed changes in brain morphology that included increased brain weight and dendritic branching (Held, 1998; Held, Gordon, & Gentile, 1985). Preoperative environmental enrichment protected animals against certain deficits after brain lesions. Rats that were exposed to enrichment before surgery made fewer errors on maze learning problems. In another experiment with pre- and post-lesion enrichment, the group with preoperative enrichment showed greater recovery after surgery than the group with postoperative enrichment (Held, 1998). An enriched environment might promote development of neural circuitry that is more varied than that of restricted subjects and provide them with a greater ability to reorganize the nervous system after a lesion, or simply to use alternative pathways to perform a task.

Finger and Stein (1982) suggested that nonspecific environmental enrichment could affect the ability to cope with a variety of situations and problems of a general nature. Rats allowed to move freely in the environment and interact with visual cues, showed good recovery of visual function after lesions in the visual cortex, while rats exposed to the same visual cues, but that could not move in the environment, did not show the same degree of recovery (Stein et al., 1995). It appears that environmental stimulation must incorporate active participation of the individual for full recovery of function to occur.

Kalar (1994) looked at the recovery of stroke patients treated in general wards versus those treated in stroke rehabilitation units and found that even though there was less physical and occupational therapy on the stroke units, these individuals recovered sooner and gained greater function than did those treated on the ward. Indredavik, Bakke, Slordahl, Rokseth, and Haheim (1999) found that stroke care units improved survival and functional state and increased the proportion of patients able to live at home 10 years after their stroke.

Training is a distinct form of enriched environment, in that activities are specific. Black, Markowitz, and Cianci (1975) examined the effects of specific motor training in monkeys after removal of the cortical precentral forelimb area. They found that training of the involved hand alone, or training of the involved and normal hands together, was more effective than training of the normal hand alone. Training that started immediately following occurrence of the lesion produced better results than delayed training. In a study designed to evaluate the effect of movement strategies on neural organization using primates, Byl et al. (1997) found that training that utilized variable proximal arm strategies minimized the sensory degradation and preserved motor control, compared to repetitive hand-squeezing strategies, suggesting that changing movement strategies could have an effect on the magnitude of the motor dysfunction. Held (2000) suggested that training after CNS injury leads to improvement, as long as the training is not introduced too early, which ensures a functional level of excitability within the system and perhaps prevents transneuronal degeneration. Specific training might prevent the use of compensation, thus stimulating the remaining intact part of the system to recover. The current thinking is that recovery of function can best be promoted by training or therapy that begins early after injury, is sufficiently intense, is task-specific, provides an enriched environment, is motivational, and takes place when the client is actively participating (Gardiner, 1996; Liepert et al., 2000).

Compensatory Movement Strategies

> ***NDT Focus: NDT treatment strategies emphasize an appropriate balance between promoting and supporting recovery and allowing functional compensations as the client seeks independence in functional activities.***

Individuals can accomplish functional tasks with a variety of movement patterns, but people tend to use the pattern that requires the least amount of energy and is the most efficient for the task goal. Compensations are alternative strategies or movement substitutions that an individual adopts to accomplish a task. Individuals develop compensatory strategies when they cannot produce normal movements because of existing impairments and incomplete recovery from CNS dysfunction. Compensations can occur because the damaged system adopts different receptors, new muscles and new strategies to perform a task (Held, 2000). For example, individuals with stroke involve the muscles of trunk to complete target pointing tasks, recruiting abnormal degrees of freedom not used by healthy subjects, and are unable to recruit the normal arm strategies (Cirstea & Levin, 2000).

Professionals generally consider compensatory strategies to be detrimental to recovery because the CNS has the capacity for recovery and reorganization (Fisher & Woll, 1995; Taub, 1980). However, compensatory strategies can serve to reduce disability and in reality occur in spite of, or during recovery, eliminating the need to recover use of the affected body segments. The question is, when should individuals with CNS dysfunction be allowed or encouraged to use compensatory strategies, and when should therapists encourage individuals to make the effort to modify them?

During recovery, periods of observable change and recovery often alternate with periods of little change and no observable recovery. During the periods of no observable recovery, the client or clinician can often become frustrated with the rate of recovery. Motor learning research has shown that alternating periods of rapid and slow change constitute a normal progression and that, through extensive training and practice, the individual can make substantial gains over the lifetime (Bach-y-Rita, 1980; Fisher & Woll, 1995). Periods of no observable change, as motor learning theory demonstrates, are not permanent but can be followed by a period in which the individual again makes progress. For example, in children with CP who have undergone selective dorsal rhizotomy, quiet periods can precede periods in which gains again occur. Rapid changes usually take place in the first 6 weeks. This is often followed by a 2-4 week period during which the children appear to practice these new movements and do not seem to make additional recovery (Wilson, 1989). However, changes in motor functions, strength, and gait can occur for several years after this procedure (Thomas, Aiona, Buckon, & Piatt, 1997). Wannstedt and Herman (1978) found that 2 1/2 years post stroke, adults with hemiplegia were able to learn to stand with symmetrical weight bearing on their LEs and to shift weight.

There are several other parameters that are relevant in determining whether to encourage compensatory strategies. One important variable is time. For example, during the acute phase of recovery from stroke, the emphasis is on recovery of normal function, while in the chronic phase, the emphasis might need to shift to maximizing function through compensatory strategies. Time is often the factor in the management of children with CP. By the time a child is school-aged, inclusion in a classroom setting with normally developing peers might depend on the child's independence in mobility and self-care as much as intellect, attention, and learning style. Therapists find themselves developing ways for the child to manage independent mobility through mobility aids and wheelchairs, or providing modifications in the bathroom with bars and toilet aids to permit the child to toilet quickly, regardless of the movement pattern. Early on, the Bobaths were quite clear that, if full recovery (or development) were the goal, compensations could not be allowed. However, Mrs. Bobath recognized the impracticality of this approach and acknowledged that there was a difference in movement during treatment and during daily functions. Treatment focused on the capacity of the client to make changes in his or her movements while recognizing that in day-to-day situations, the client performs life functions in ways that allow independence, compensating when necessary to efficiently solve problems (B. Bobath & K. Bobath, 1960; B. Bobath & Finnie, 1958).

A second determinant is the nature of the impairments themselves. If there are permanent, unchanging impairments, regardless of whether the patient is acute or chronic, compensatory strategies are important in decreasing the extent of the disability and preventing the development of additional secondary impairments (Shumway-Cook & Woollacott, 2001). If, for example, there is permanent muscle weakness of the gastroc-soleus group due, perhaps, to lengthening procedures and lack of follow-up after surgery, the child with CP will need to compensate for the loss of strength by wearing solid ankle AFOs to align the tibia over the ankle joint and prevent the development of a secondary impairment of knee flexion that accompanies excessive ankle dorsiflexion during weight bearing. In another example, an individual with permanent loss of vestibular function needs to learn to rely on vision and somatosensory cues for balance.

A third determinant is the characteristics of the compensation pattern. Some compensation patterns closely approximate the normal pattern of movement and can actually preserve function while motor recovery occurs. Clinicians can help to set up functional tasks that the client can practice in ways that promote independence and encourage use of the affected segments (e.g., encouraging the individual to use both arms in a bilateral symmetrical fashion to push up from a chair to gain standing when weakness, poor balance, or insecurity interfere with rising to stand). Teaching an individual to first put the involved arm through a sleeve, even if this was not the side the client dressed first prior to CNS insult, preserves dressing skills and utilizes sequences of posture and movement necessary for many upper-extremity functions. Ryerson and Levit (1997) suggested that using the involved side, even in limited ways, during functional performance helps the individual psychologically to believe he or she is getting better and perceptually to integrate this side into the body scheme. The use of "functional compensations" sends the message that the client can expect recovery. The therapist can develop intervention strategies to retrain movements through functional movement sequences that the individual can remember from before the stroke.

Some compensation patterns do not resemble efficient normal movement patterns. These undesirable compensatory strategies interfere with the recovery of normal muscle function that could allow use of more normal and efficient pattern. For example, many adults with hemiplegia stand and walk with asymmetry. This pattern is made worse by the use of a quad cane, which further displaces the weight outside the base of support. Unfortunately, undesirable compensation patterns develop quickly when the individual is motivated to move.

An individual will sometimes use compensatory strategies even when possessing sufficient motor control to perform the movements in a normal pattern because the person perceives such strategies to be the most efficient and least energy-consuming; the best solution for the moment. Michaelsen et al. (2001) found that clients with hemiplegia extended their reaching movements with compensatory trunk and shoulder girdle movements even when shoulder movements and elbow extension was possible. Adding trunk restraints allowed the client to make use of arm joint ranges that were present but not recruited during unrestrained arm-reaching tasks. This suggests that trunk restraint might be an effective strategy to maximize arm recovery until trunk stability strategies can be recruited separately from upper-extremity movements. The difficulty for the therapist is to determine whether allowing compensatory movements to occur will prevent true recovery and actually increase the level of care the individual will need in the long run.

Implications for Intervention

New scientific information on the nature of motor dysfunction and recovery means that NDT therapists should expect recovery and functional improvements over the life-span and work to prevent transneuronal degeneration and stimulate regeneration. We need to carefully analyze impairments caused both by the CNS pathology and the interaction of the body systems with an impaired CNS. We need to understand the relationships among system impairments, ineffective components of posture and movement, and activity limitations, in order to plan specific intervention strategies that evolve with recovery. We need to offer active, repeated experiences to provide clients with easy access to the appropriate patterns of posture and movement they require to accomplish daily functional tasks in increasingly complex contexts. We must make certain that the environment is both interesting and involving for the client and responsive to the individual needs of the client as a person.

Research in NDT and Evidence-Based Practice

The greatest challenge facing clinicians who believe that NDT improves the lives of their clients is to document outcomes in ways that will demonstrate the efficacy of our interventions. From the beginning, the Bobaths were interested in effective intervention, but their criterion for "effective treatment" was the immediate response of each client to the therapeutic intervention.(K. Bobath & B. Bobath, 1984) However, in today's climate of accountability to clients, their families, and third-party payers, managed care mandates that we justify what we do, beginning with objective observations and then submitting what we believe about our observations to the rigors of experimental research in order to know which interventions work, for whom, and under what conditions (Brown & Burns, 2001; Butler, 2001a). The continuing widespread influence and practice of NDT, as well as the criticism from the professional community, make this a particularly timely issue.

Evaluating outcomes presents a dilemma to therapists involved in treating clients with neuropathology. The dilemma exists because, on the one hand, therapists hold a strong belief that intervention is essential and effective. On the other hand, documenting effectiveness is difficult because of the complex problems characterizing this population and the professions involved in their care. Populations of individuals with neuropathology include infants, children, adolescents, and adults in various stages of development and aging. Various degrees of severity and types of health conditions, from ischemic stroke to cerebellar hypoplasia, are included in the general health conditions related to neuropathology. Even within one specific health condition, such as ataxic cerebral palsy, investigators describe a heterogeneous variety of conditions with either demonstrable brain pathology or undefined micropathology underlying the clinical symptoms (Esscher et al., 1996; Steinlin, Zangger, & Boltshauser, 1998).

Investigators have attempted to control for heterogeneous populations. Gebler, Josefczk, Herman, Good, and Verhulst (1995) compared the response to traditional functional rehabilitation to the response to an NDT approach in clients with specific types of strokes.

Clients with pure motor strokes served as the participants in this study. Josefczyk and Gebler (1995) compared traditional functional rehabilitation to NDT techniques in a group of clients with stroke who had moderate hemiparesis and sensory deficits.

State-of-the-art health care varies throughout the world, and although practice guidelines can exist, individual programs are subject to fiscal and economic pressures to provide the "best" care for the least amount of money. Although randomized clinical trials are powerful techniques for determining the efficacy of rehabilitation interventions, randomized clinical trials have some practical and ethical limitations when applied to many research questions (Ottenbacher & Hinderer, 2001). Withholding treatment is not an option, and comparing treatment in a population in North America with a population in a country that does not have the resources to provide intervention as a standard of care introduces many additional confounding variables, including general level of quality of health care and cultural expectations for recovery or improvement in quality of life.

The multidisciplinary model, which in North America is the standard of care for individuals with CNS pathology, poses additional challenges. The advantage of this care model is its own worst enemy. There is a wide variety of information from different points of view published in a variety of specialty journals, yet, understandably, each discipline tends to read and publish in those journals that support their own profession. Professional journals evaluate and publish research and clinical articles based on what are considered important outcomes by the standard of a specific profession, and there is little consistency among professions in what is measured and how it is measured. This makes it difficult to assess the efficacy of individual interventions and compare the outcomes of one intervention to others (Butler, 2001b).

In the past, studies have been limited by the outcome measures available to examine change. Recent studies have demonstrated that tools such as the Gross Motor Function Measure (GMFM) (Trahan & Malouin, 1999; Knox, & Evans, 2002), the Functional Independence Measure (FIM) (Stinemann, Jette, Fiedler, & Granger, 1997) and the WeeFIM (McAuliffe, Wenger, Schneider, & Gaebler-Spira, 1998) and the Pediatric Evaluation of Disability Inventory (PEDI) (Ketelaar, & Vermeer 1998) are sensitive to changes produced by treatment. New diagnostic tools such as the General Movement Assessment (GMA) (Prechtl et al., 1997) and the Test of Infant Motor Performance (TIMP) (Campbell, Kolobe, Wright & Linacre, 2002) can identify children at risk for CP much earlier and more reliably than has previously been possible. These measures will allow us to measure changes in functional activities; however, additional outcome measures are needed to address movement issues (such as alignment, weight-bearing patterns, and variability of movement synergies) and the client-specific goals and objectives (Mullens, 2001).

Finally, the evolving nature of NDT brings its own set of problems to this general dilemma. The changing nature of NDT principles, the lack of operational definitions in NDT, and the flexible variation in how NDT principles are integrated and practiced in the various specialty fields in different countries, add to the difficulty when evaluating outcomes. Butler and Darrah (2001) compared 10 studies published before 1990 with 11 studies published between 1990 and 2000 and found that the later studies (presumably using contemporary

NDT) had a greater percentage of results that favored NDT than did the earlier studies. When only motor impairment or motor activity measures were considered, NDT showed still more positive results in the later studies. NDT is a problem-solving approach in which intervention addresses the system impairments hypothesized to cause the client's limitations in function. The general aim of NDT intervention is, "leading (clients) to the greatest degree of independence possible and preparing them for as normal an adult life as can be achieved." (K. Bobath & B. Bobath, 1984, p. 6). NDT is not a specific treatment delivered in a standardized manner and, as such, using randomized controlled trial methods to determine if NDT is an effective "treatment" is not appropriate because the question, as posed, is unanswerable (Sharkey, Banaitis, Giuffrida, Mullens, & Rast, 2002). Although it might be possible to set standard treatment settings, such as in a stroke rehabilitation unit or a school setting, other factors (such as the client's family and culture) cannot be standardized. Bower and McLellan (1994) and Zhan and Ottenbacher (2001) suggested that representative series of single-subject research designs with individual goal setting and validated outcome measurement using randomized treatment, would overcome many of the disadvantages of previously published studies and enable more effective group trials to be undertaken to evaluate the impact of providing treatment to a defined population of subjects. Single-subject designs are ideally suited for research in the rehabilitation practice environment and, when properly applied, these designs can help establish the efficacy of practice.

Evaluating the Evidence

Various methods (such as meta-analysis, decision analysis, cost-effectiveness analysis, and systematic review of published research literature) are useful in measuring the effectiveness of evidence-based practice (Scalzitti, 2001). For example, a meta-analysis of the results of nine research studies on NDT found small positive intervention effects (Ottenbacher et al., 1986). A systematic search and review of the relevant published literature by Brown and Burns (2001) produced inconclusive results regarding the evidence of NDT intervention. Currently, studies are more commonly being reviewed by classifying levels of evidence.

Sackett's Levels of Evidence

In order to review the studies that have been done, the American Academy for Cerebral Palsy and Developmental Medicine (AACPDM) has modified the levels of evidence classifications developed by Sackett (Sackett, Rosenberg, & Gray, 1996; Sackett, Straus, Richardson, Rosenberg, & Haynes, 2000) as a framework to categorize various studies in application of NDT to pediatric populations (Butler & Darrah, 2001). Butler (2001a) reviewed 21 studies in which the intervention was stated to be exclusively NDT or NDT combined with other sensorimoter techniques, or could be identified from the description of procedures. The articles by Butler (2001a, 2001b), Butler and Darrah (2001), and Brown and Burns (2001) offer a complete review of the pediatric research literature. The review in this text is not inclusive, but includes examples of research describing the effects of NDT intervention on both the adult and pediatric clients to demonstrate Sackett's level of evidence classification. Focusing only on the levels of evidence does consolidate studies by type and design, but has its own problems of reviewer bias when deciding at which level to place a study with complex, multifaceted treatment outcomes (Butler, 2001a). According to Sackett, (2000), studies are classified in one of five levels.

Level 1 studies have large numbers of subjects randomly assigned to either an intervention group or a control group. The results of these studies can be generalized to clients similar to those studied. For example, Butler (2001a) classified the study completed by Palmer et al. (1988) as a design that meets level 1 criteria. The Palmer et al. study examined the effects of physical therapy on 48 infants with spastic cerebral palsy, randomly assigned to 12 months of physical therapy using an NDT approach or 6 months of physical therapy preceded by 6 months of infant stimulation. The blinded assessment performed at 6 and 12 months showed no motor advantage for the infants in the NDT intervention. Law et al. (1997) used a randomized crossover design to evaluate the difference between intensive NDT plus casting to a less intensive regular OT program for children with CP between 18 months and 4 years of age. Blinded assessments at baseline, 4 months, 6 months and 10 months of intervention, did not demonstrate a beneficial effect of an increased amount of therapy.

Level 2 studies do not involve random group assignment although they are otherwise well-controlled experiments or comparison studies. Both level 1 and level 2 studies include some control group or manipulation of some condition, such as the length or intensity of intervention. Dickstein, Hocherman, Pillar, and Shaham (1986) studied 131 adults following stroke, assigning them to one of three treatment groups comparing therapeutic exercise, Bobath, and Rood neurofacilitation approaches. These persons were not randomly assigned, so this study represents level 2 evidence. Outcome was measured using the Barthel Index, measures of muscle tone, active ROM, and ambulatory status. None of the approaches showed an advantage on any of these measures. In another example of a study classified as level 2, Wright and Nicholson studied 47 children with spasticity under 6 years of age assigned to immediate-treatment, delayed-treatment, or no treatment groups. This study showed no evidence after 1 year that physical therapy affected the range of dorsiflexion of the ankle or abduction of the hip or that PT had any effect on the retention or loss of primitive reflexes. Embry, Yates, and Mott (1990) used a single-subject research design to evaluate the effects of NDT on excessive knee flexion during walking in children with cerebral palsy. There was a no-treatment phase and two treatment phases that evaluated NDT intervention and NDT intervention combined with the use of orthotics. Both treatment phases demonstrated improvements, with greater improvements in the NDT-only phase. Girolami and Campbell (1994) demonstrated that an NDT program for prematurely born high-risk infants could help to attain postural control similar to that of full-term healthy newborns at an equivalent age This study did include a control group, but subjects were not randomized, classifying it in level 2.

Level 3 studies include case-controlled studies, the purpose of which is to establish an expectancy about the outcome in the absence of intervention. Level 3 designs are comparison studies, but one or both of the comparisons is retrospective. Wagenaar et. al. (1990) studied the relative efficacy of NDT versus the Brunstrom method in seven clients with stroke, using a B-C-B-C single-case study design in which the two approaches were alternated. No differences were noted between treatment methods in this level 3 study. Sharkey (1996) compared the effect of early NDT-based intervention in 63 children grouped as early-referred (before 9 months of age) to another group of 63 children late-referred (between 12-15 months of age). She found that the rate of development in the areas of perceptual-fine motor skills, cognition, language, social/emotional and self-care favored the early group, but not at a level that was statistically significant. The early group did have a rate of gross motor development significantly higher (35%) than the late group. Most recently, Knox and Evans (2002) studied the effects of an NDT physical therapy program with 15 children with CP between the ages of 2 and 12 years. The children served as their own control in a repeated measure design. Participants showed significant improvements on the outcome measures (GMFM and PEDI) following NDT therapy for 12 weeks when compared to equal periods before or after NDT intervention

Level 4 designs have no comparison group or condition and are often single-subject or case-series-without-a-control-group designs. Although these studies are based on less convincing evidence because they have no comparison group, they are helpful as a first step in collecting objective evidence so that clinical decisions do not rest solely on beliefs or observations. Zhan and Ottenbacher (2001) proposed that single-subject designs are ideally suited for research in rehabilitation intervention when it is difficult to access a large numbers of clients in a reasonable time. Single-subject designs involve a single subject or a small number of subjects to be observed over time, during which the treatment and outcomes variables are controlled. For example, Adams, Chandler, and Schuhmann (2000) reported on changes in gait characteristics of 40 children with cerebral palsy who participated in an 8-week NDT course. Significant improvements were found in the whole group for stride and step length, foot angle, and velocity. However, because there was no control group or group exposed to different treatment conditions, this design is classified as level 4. Trahan and Malouin (1999) examined changes in gross motor performance in 50 children with various types of CP, who were undergoing NDT-based PT twice a week and demonstrated changes in gross motor skills as measured by the GMFM.

Level 5 designs merely suggest causation; consequently, no conclusions regarding treatment efficacy can be drawn from level 5 evidence. Case reports are examples of level 5 designs. A case report is a documentation of clinical practice for a client and, unlike single-subject designs, they do not provide comparisons across different conditions or phases and the intervention is not systematically controlled (Zhan & Ottenbacher, 2001). Montgomery's (2000) reporting on the achievement of gross motor skills in two children with cerebellar hypoplasia is an example of longitudinal case reports at evidence level 5. Howle's (1999b) description of the effectiveness of an NDT-based physical therapy program for a child with ataxic cerebral palsy is another case study that evaluated changes in functions, as measured with the GMFM and the PEDI. Zacharewicz (2002) reported on the functional changes in a 70-year-old woman 6.5 years post-stroke using an NDT-based occupational therapy program. The NDT intervention addressed the secondary musculoskeletal impairments that interfered with function. All of these reports include objective outcome measures.

The Enablement Model and the Evidence of Outcomes

Despite all the problems of conducting clinical research with this client population and classifying evidence for intervention, clinicians interested in moving their professions forward, and at the same time providing the scientific evidence to support intervention, can now propose hypotheses about the impact of NDT on the different dimensions of disability as defined by the NDT enablement model. The acceptance of this model as part of the NDT framework allows us to provide objective information on the effect that our intervention has on the various dimensions in a person's life.

Using an enablement framework allows the clinician to analyze outcomes based on the dimension of disability that are important to the person. Butler (2001a) summarized outcomes based on the dimension of disability from impairment to societal limitations and compared this to the level of evidence. For example, Palmer et al.'s (1988) level 1 evidence study examined outcomes in 9 areas of impairment and 10 measures of social and contextual dimensions (Butler, 2001a). The level 4 study by Adams et al. (2000) measured six parameters of motor functions related to gait. Trahan and Malouin's level 4 study (1999), evaluated changes in gross motor functional activities. Dickstein et al. (1986) evaluated outcomes in impairments in clients with stroke, including isolated control of the ankle, muscle strength, ROM, ambulation, muscle tone, and activities of daily living, as measured by the Barthel index. This information is important when targeting outcomes in the various dimensions of disablement that are meaningful and make a difference to the clients and their families.

Evidence-Based Practice

The current state of evidence is too inconsistent to support statements that intervention based on NDT concepts and principles has any advantage over other approaches in improving functional outcomes. Brown and Burns (2001) systematically reviewed 17 published research studies that used a randomized research design specific to pediatric clients diagnosed with a neurological impairment in which NDT was used as a treatment approach. They concluded that the current research literature does not clearly demonstrate the efficacy or inefficacy of NDT as a treatment approach. Absence of effectiveness in evidence reports should not be construed as proof that a treatment is not effective, but rather reflects areas in which more meaningful research is needed (Sharkey et al., 2002). To provide clear evidence regarding the efficacy of NDT, Brown and Burns (2001) strongly recommended a multicenter clinical trial of NDT, using a randomized clinical trial protocol with double-blinding. They listed five criteria for such a study:

1. Using consistent NDT techniques with subjects
2. Employing consistent diagnostic groups
3. Including a comparison control group with no neurological dysfunction
4. Using assessment tools with sound measurement properties that are sensitive to change in clinical status

5. Having a large enough sample size for adequate statistical power and meaningful data analysis

This type of study represents a massive undertaking and commitment of time and money. Because clinicians usually do not have the freedom to apply a standard treatment in a predefined way to assign large groups of subjects to treatment and nontreatment groups, Zhan and Ottenbacher (2001) proposed single-subject designs as a method to examine clinical accountability. These designs can provide a systematic approach to documenting clinical change and furnish objective evidence regarding the effect of treatment (Gonella, 1989). While not solving all the problems of randomized clinical trials, single-subject designs provide a method for clinical research and documentation that is practice-based and clinician-oriented.

We cannot answer big questions, such as, "Is NDT the most effective approach for managing individuals with stroke or cerebral palsy?" However, there is evidence for therapists to use when answering smaller yet significant questions that can support their own clinical opinions and expertise and assist families as they make informed decisions about the optimal care they seek. For example, a child with spastic diplegic CP has been asked to participate in an NDT pediatric training course. The parent asks, "Would my child's participation in this course jeopardize the progress she is making toward independent ambulation?" Based on the evidence in the study by Adams et al. (2000) demonstrating changes in gait characteristics, the therapist can say that children in this course showed improvement in gait characteristics. This information can assist the family in making a decision to include their child in this experience. In another example, a physical therapist is trying to make a decision regarding the type of walker to use with a child with spastic CP. Studies by Greiner, Czerniecki, and Deitz (1993), Levangie, Guihan, Meyer, & Stuhr (1989), and Logan, Byers-Hinley, and Ciccone (1990) all demonstrate that children with CP have better alignment and more normal gait characteristics when using posterior walkers than when using forward-support rolling-type walkers. On the other hand, when deciding whether to use horizontal versus vertical hand grips on a walker, one study by Levangie et al. showed no advantage with vertical hand grips over horizontal grips in relationship to posture or gait. If a physician asks, "Does the age of referral for NDT intervention make a difference in developing motor skills for infants with CP?" the therapist can refer to Sharkey's (1996) study, which demonstrated that infants referred before age 9 months achieved the greatest benefit in the area of gross motor skills. If a family explains that academic tutoring is interfering with the therapy schedule and asks, "How many times a week should we have therapy?" the clinician might explain that there is conflicting evidence regarding the intensity of intervention and changes in outcomes. Bower and McLellan (1992) and Bower, McLellan, Arney, and Campbell (1996) demonstrated that increasing the frequency of intervention did have an effect on motor skills, provided they were associated with functional activities understood by the child. However, Law et al. (1997) did not show that increasing the intensity affected UE skills. In addition, Trahan and Malouin (2002) showed that for children with CP (levels IV and V on the GMFM), combining intensive therapy periods (4 times a week for 4 weeks) with periods without therapy (8 weeks) led to functional improvements as measured on the

GMFM. These improvements were maintained during the non-treatment period. The therapist might suggest that the family consider what time commitment will work for their life style and set a definitive trial period to see if the rate of improvement is acceptable.

If a client with stroke asks, "Will additional rehabilitation help, now that I am more than 1 year post-stroke?" the therapist can refer to the study by Tangeman, Banaitis, and Williams (1990), in which clients demonstrated significant improvement in outcome measures of weight shift, balance, and improved ADL scores one year after stroke. Barry (2001) provided additional examples of the application of evidence in practice in pediatric physical therapy. The levels of evidence available do not provide conclusive evidence in the intervention for either stroke or CP, but such information can assist the family so that they can make decisions based on what treatment offers (or doesn't) and how it relates to their own values. It is permissible to explain that we do not have evidence about the ways in which NDT intervention benefits a client with a particular health condition, but only after the evidence has been examined and objectively reported. There is an undeniable art in NDT intervention, but the basis of our practice should be to integrate art and science, making decisions that allow us to provide our clients and their families with the information regarding optimal care.

What is NDT Doing to Achieve Evidence-Based Practice?

Currently, there is no body of evidence that is sufficiently comprehensive or rigorous enough to allow generalization about the effectiveness of NDT. However, therapists can use the evidence available that approximates the client characteristics, apply a therapeutic intervention most like the one the NDT clinician currently provides, and use the most valid results in outcome dimensions that are meaningful to the client. NDTA has taken several steps in working toward evidence-based practice.

1. NDTA established a research committee in 1990 that regularly reviews the pertinent scientific literature, examines the benefits and limitations of the evidence, publishes these findings in the *NDT Network,* and provides guidance to and answers question from the membership.
2. NDTA provides financial support for clinically relevant research studies at all levels of evidence by its members and encourages publication of these results in the professional literature. The research committee reviews the research proposals and supports studies that examine the effects of specific NDT techniques, comparison of NDT to other approaches, pilot studies, and multiple-site studies.
3. NDTA supports advanced clinical training courses for PTs, OTs, and SLPs related to stroke and CP to develop a consistent knowledge base among therapists to ensure that the most current theories and intervention methods are used in clinical practice and research applications. These courses also include information on data collection methods that allow comparison of results.

4. NDTA and the theory committee supported the publication of this book, which defines our philosophy, theoretical basis, and examination and intervention strategies so that the scientific community can answer the question when examining the evidence, "Does this study include current concepts and application of the principles of NDT?"
5. Since 1998, NDTA has accepted an enablement framework for classifying and defining pathology, impairments, ineffective motor functions, functional limitations, and social restrictions in order to analyze the effect this approach has on various dimensions of disability in meaningful contexts.
6. NDTA has developed a web site, www.ndta.org, which regularly includes case studies and relevant articles that combine evidence with clinical expertise.
7. The *NDT Network,* the quarterly publication of the NDTA provides an venue for new writers to publish case studies, single-subject designs, and other clinical research strategies; provides regular columns describing changes in NDT theory and practice; and reviews articles from other professional publications to ensure that the membership receives up-to-date information.

Chapter Summary

1. Like all persons, individuals with CNS dysfunction develop movement in response to the need to solve motor problems within specific contexts, using the best available strategies.
2. NDT has developed an enablement framework based on the ICF model to provide structure for the problem-solving approach used in NDT, to describe and classify functional integrity and impairments, and to identify their relationships to posture and movement and to functional activities and limitations and participation in society.
3. The NDT enablement model includes personal and environmental facilitators and barriers as important contextual factors in evaluating disability.
4. Not all impairments interfere with function. The clinician's task is to cluster impairments that contribute to the same functional limitation, prioritize and sequence the importance of these impairments, and determine which impairments can be addressed in treatment that will relate to the functional limitations of the client.
5. Impairments to function are classified as (a) primary; positive, or negative impairments, those that result directly from the neuropathology, and (b) secondary impairments, those that occur as a consequence of the primary impairments and other environmental influences. Secondary impairments further complicate the individual's functional ability and lead to disability in life roles.
6. In this NDT enablement model, the components of effective or ineffective posture and movement function and dysfunction constitute the link between functional activity and system integrity. Multiple systems contribute to functional limitations,

and a careful analysis of posture and movement can help to identify which system or systems are the most influential in facilitating or impairing movement. It is the therapist's responsibility to observe, evaluate, and analyze the kinesiological, biomechanical, and anthropometric changes in the musculoskeletal system and integrate these findings with missing or atypical functions.

7. One of the unique contributions of the NDT approach is the depth and extent of the analysis of effective and ineffective postures and movements in individuals with CNS pathology. This analysis gauges alignment and patterns of weight bearing, muscle tone, postural control, kinesiological and biomechanical components of posture and movement, motor planning, and coordination.
8. Although NDT recognizes that the motor and sensory systems might be the most important systems contributing to the overall disability of clients with CNS pathology, the perceptual/cognitive, regulatory, cardiopulmonary, respiratory, and gastrointestinal systems also contribute to life functions.
9. The potential for the individual to function successfully in life requires a meaningful examination of the personal, cultural, and life environments.
10. New scientific information on the nature of dysfunction and recovery challenges the clinician to recognize that recovery is an ongoing process, and intervention must seek an appropriate balance between promoting and supporting recovery, and allowing compensation as the client seeks independence in function.
11. Currently there is little evidence in published research studies that demonstrates efficacy or inefficacy of NDT as a treatment approach for children or adults with CNS dysfunction. Although "big questions" cannot be answered at this time, clinicians must accept the responsibility to generate robust studies that systematically evaluate current NDT principles and intervention methods to determine what works for specific types and ages of persons with sensorimotor disabilities. This information will empower clients, their families, and third-party payers with the best information that is available, even if imperfect, as they make informed decisions for optimal care.

References

Ada, L., & Westwood, P. (1992). A kinematic analysis of recovery of the ability to stand up following stroke. *Australian Journal of Physiotherapy, 38,* 135-142.

Adams, M. A., Chandler, L. S., & Schuhmann, K. (2000). Gait changes in children with cerebral palsy following a neurodevelopmental treatment course. *Pediatric Physical Therapy, 12,* 114-120.

Agnarsson, U., Warde, C., McCarthy, G., Clayden, G. S., & Evans, N. (1993). Anorectal function of children with neurological problems: II. Cerebral Palsy. *Developmental Medicine and Child Neurology, 35,* 903-908.

Aguayo, A. D., Clarke, D. B., Jelsma, T. N., & Wiley, M. (1996). Effects of neurotrophins on the survival and regrowth of injured retinal neurons. In *Growth factors as drugs for neurological and sensory disorders* (pp. 135-148). New York: Ciba Foundation Symposium.

Alexander, R., Cupps, B., & Boehme, R. (1993). *Normal development of functional skills.* Tucson, AZ: Therapy Skill Builders.

Als, H., Lawhon, G., Duffy, H., McAnulty, G., Gibes-Grossman, R., & Bleckman, G. (1994). Individualized developmental care for the very low-birth-weight preterm infant. *Journal of the American Medical Association, 272,* 853-858.

Amiel-Tison, C. (1968). Neurological evaluation of the maturity of newborn infants. *Archives of Disease in Childhood, 43,* 89-93.

Andrews, A. W., & Bohannon, R. W. (2000). Distribution of muscle strength impairments following stroke. *Clinical Rehabilitation, 14,* 79-87.

Aniansson, A., Hedberg, M., Henning, G., & Grumby, G. (1986). Muscle morphology, enzymatic activity and muscle strength in elderly men: A follow-up study. *Muscle and Nerve, 9,* 585-591.

Bach-y-Rita, P. (1980). Brain plasticity as a basis for therapeutic procedures. In P. Bach-y-Rita (Ed.), *Recovery of function: Theoretical considerations for brain injury rehabilitation* (pp. 225-263). Baltimore: University Park Press.

Badke, M. B., & DiFabio, R. P. (1990). Balance deficits in patients with hemiplegia: Considerations for assessment and treatment. In P. Duncan (Ed.), *Balance: Proceedings of the APTA Forum* (pp. 73-78). Alexandria, VA: American Physical Therapy Association.

Bar-Or, O. (1986). Pathophysiological factors which limit the exercise capacity of the sick child. *Medicine and Science in Sports and Exercise, 18,* 276-282.

Bartlett, D., & Piper, M. C. (1993). Neuromotor development of preterm infants through the first year of life: Implications for physical and occupational therapists. *Physical and Occupational Therapy in Pediatrics, 12* (4), 37-55.

Basmajian, J. V., & deLuca, C. J. (1985). *Muscles alive: Their functions revealed by electromyography* (5th ed.). Baltimore: Williams and Wilkins.

Bastian, A. J., Martin, T. A., Keating, J. G., & Thach, W. T. (1996). Cerebellar ataxia: Abnormal control of interaction torques across multiple joints. *Journal of Neurophysiology, 76,* 492-509.

Beals, R. K. (1969). Developmental changes in the femur and acetabulum in spastic paraplegia and diplegia. *Developmental Medicine and Child Neurology, 11,* 303-313.

Beauregard, R., Thomas, J. J., & Nelson, D. L. (1988). Quality of reach during a game and during a rote movement in children with cerebral palsy. *Physical and Occupational Therapy in Pediatrics, 18* (3/4), 67-84.

Beckung, E., & Hagberg, G. (2002). Neuroimpairments, activity limitations and participation restrictions in children with cerebral palsy. *Developmental Medicine and Child Neurology, 44* (5), 309-316.

Belanger, L., Boldue, M., & Noel, M. (1988). Relative importance of after-effects, environment and socio-economic factors on the social integration of stroke victims. *International Journal of Rehabilitation Research, 11* (3), 251-260.

Berger, W., Quintern, J., & Dietz, V. (1982). Pathophysiology of gait in children with cerebral palsy. *Electroencephalography and Clinical Neurophysiology, 53,* 538-548.

Berger, W., Quintern, J., & Dietz, V. (1987). Afferent and efferent control of stance and gait: Developmental changes in children. *Electroencephalography and Clinical Neurophysiology, 66* (3), 244-252.

Bergman, J., & Farrell, E. E. (1992). Neurodevelopmental outcome in infants with bronchopulmonary dysplasia. *Clinics in Perinatology, 19,* 673-694.

Berman, B., Vaughan, C. L., & Peacock, W. J. (1989). The effect of rhizotomy on movement in patients with cerebral palsy. *American Journal of Occupational Therapy, 44* (6), 511-516.

Bernstein, N. A. (1996). On dexterity and its development. In M. L. Latash & M. T. Turvey (Eds.), *Dexterity and its development* (pp. 9-244). Mahwah, NJ: Lawrence Erlbaum.

Barry, M. J. (2001, November). Evidence-based practice in pediatric physical therapy. *PT Magazine,* 38-52.

Bertrand, A. M., & Bourbonnais, D. (2001). Effects of upper limb unilateral isometric efforts on postural stabilization in subjects with hemiparesis. *Archives of Physical Medicine and Rehabilitation, 82,* 403-411.

Bierman, J. (1998, September/October). Theoretically speaking. *NDTA Network,* 4-5.

Biguer, B., Jeannerod, M., & Prablanc, C. (1982). The coordination of eye, head, and arm movements during reaching at a single visual target. *Experimental Brain Research, 46,* 301-304.

Bjorklund, A. (1994). Long distance axonal growth in the adult central nervous system. *Journal of Neurology, 241,* S33-35.

Black, F. O., & Nashner, L. M. (1985). Postural control in four classes of vestibular abnormalities. In M. Igarashi & F. O. Black (Eds.), *Vestibular and visual control of posture and locomotor equilibrium* (pp. 271-281). Basel, Switzerland: Karger.

Black, P., Markowitz, R. S., & Cianci, S. N. (1975). Recovery of motor function after lesions in motor cortex of monkeys. *Ciba Foundation Symposium, 34,* 65-83.

Blanche, E. I., Botticelli, T. M., & Hallway, M. K. (1995). *Combining Neuro-Developmental Treatment and sensory integration principles. An approach to pediatric therapy.* Tucson, AZ: Therapy Skill Builders.

Bleck, E. E. (1987). *Orthopedic management in cerebral palsy. Clinics in Developmental Medicine 99/100.* Philadelphia: J. B. Lippincott.

Bly, L. (1999). *Baby treatment based on NDT principles.* San Antonio, TX: Therapy Skill Builders.

Bobath, B. (1948). The importance of the reduction of muscle tone and the control of mass reflex action in the treatment of spasticity. *Occupational Therapy and Rehabilitation, 27* (5), 371-383.

Bobath, B. (1971). Motor development: Its effect on general development and application to the treatment of cerebral palsy. *Physiotherapy, 57,* 526-532.

Bobath, B. (1977). Treatment of adult hemiplegia. *Physiotherapy, 63* (10), 310-313.

Bobath, B. (1985). *Abnormal postural reflex activity caused by brain lesions* (3rd ed.). Rockville, MD: Aspen Systems Corp.

Bobath, B. (1990). *Adult hemiplegia. Evaluation and treatment* (3rd ed.). Boston: Butterworth Heineman.

Bobath, B., & Bobath, K. (1960). Opening address. In G. Beinart (Ed.), Proceedings of a conference on cerebral palsy sponsored by the Cape Province Cerebral Palsy Association, Cape Town, South Africa. *Medical Proceedings, 6* (11), 234-238.

Bobath, B., & Bobath, K. (1975). *Motor development in the different types of cerebral palsy.* London: Heineman.

Bobath, B., & Finnie, N. (1958). Re-education of movement patterns for everyday life in the treatment of cerebral palsy. *British Occupational Therapy Journal, 21,* 1958.

Bobath, K. (1963). The prevention of mental retardation in patients with cerebral palsy. *Acta Paedopsychiatrica, 30* (4), 141-154.

Bobath, K. (1980). *A neurophysiological basis for the treatment of cerebral palsy. Clinics in Developmental Medicine 75.* Philadelphia: J. B. Lippincott.

Bobath, K., & Bobath, B. (1952). A treatment of cerebral palsy based on the analysis of the patient's motor behavior. *British Journal of Physical Medicine, 15,* 107-117.

Bobath, K., & Bobath, B. (1953). Mental activity in infancy. *Lancet,* 598.

Bobath, K., & Bobath, B. (1984). The neuro-developmental treatment. In D. Scrutton (Ed.), *Management of the motor disorders of children with cerebral palsy* (pp. 6-18). *Clinics in Developmental Medicine 90.* Philadelphia: J. B. Lippincott.

Boehme, R. (1998, March/April). When children cry in therapy. *NDTA Network,* 7-10.

Bohannon, R. W. (1989). Is the measurement of muscle strength appropriate in patients with brain lesions? *Physical Therapy, 69,* 225-236.

Bohannon, R. W., & Andrews, A. W. (1990). Shoulder subluxation and pain in stroke patients. *American Journal of Occupational Therapy, 44* (6), 507-509.

Borg, E. (1997). Perinatal asphyxia, hypoxia, ischemia and hearing loss: An overview. *Scandinavian Audiology, 26,* 77-91.

Bourbonnais, D., & Vanden Noven, S. (1989). Weakness in patients with hemiparesis. *American Journal of Occupational Therapy, 43* (5), 319.

Bower, E., & McLellan, D. L. (1992). Effect of increased exposure to physiotherapy on skill acquisition of children with cerebral palsy. *Developmental Medicine and Child Neurology, 34* (1), 25-39.

Bower, E., & McLellan, D. L. (1994). Evaluating therapy in cerebral palsy. *Child: Care, Health and Development, 20* (6), 409-419.

Bower, E., McLellan, D. L., Arney, J., & Campbell, M. J. (1996). A randomized controlled trial of different intensities of physiotherapy and different goal-setting procedures in 44 children with cerebral palsy. *Developmental Medicine and Child Neurology, 38* (3), 226-237.

Bower, E., Mitchell, D., Burnett, M., Campbell, M. J., & McLellan, D. L. (2001). Randomized controlled trial of physiotherapy in 56 children with cerebral palsy followed for 18 months. *Developmental Medicine and Child Neurology, 43* (1), 4-15.

Bradley, N. (2000). Motor control: Developmental aspects of motor control in skill acquisition. In S. K. Campbell (Ed.), *Physical therapy for children* (2nd ed., pp. 45-87). Philadelphia: Churchill Livingstone.

Brogren, E., Hadders-Algra, M., & Forssberg, H. (1998). Postural control in children with spastic diplegia: Muscle activity during perturbations in sitting. *Developmental Medicine and Child Neurology, 38,* 379-388.

Brouwer, B., & Ashby, P. (1991). Altered corticospinal projections to lower limb motorneurons in subjects with cerebral palsy. *Brain, 114,* 1395-1407.

Brown, G. T., & Burns, S. A. (2001). The efficacy of neurodevelopmental treatment in paediatrics: A systematic review. *British Journal of Occupational Therapy, 64,* 235-244.

Buckley, S. L., Sponseller, P. D., & Maged, D. (1991). The acetabulum in congenital and neuromuscular hip instability. *Journal of Pediatric Orthopedics, 11,* 498-501.

Burke, D. (1988). Spasticity as an adaptation to pyramidal tract injury. *Advances in Neurology, 47,* 401-423.

Burkhardt, A. (1998). Edema control. In G. Gillen & A. Burkhard (Eds.), *Stroke rehabilitation. A function-based approach* (pp. 152-160). St. Louis: Mosby.

Burtner, P. A., Woollacott, M. H., & Qualls, C. (1999). Stance balance control with orthoses in a select group of children with and without spasticity. *Developmental Medicine and Child Neurology, 41,* 748-757.

Butler, C. (2001a). Evidence tables and reviews of treatment outcomes. In A. L. Scherzer (Ed.), *Early diagnosis and interventional therapy in cerebral palsy: An interdisciplinary age-focused approach* (3rd ed., pp. 285-330). New York: Marcel Dekker.

Butler, C. (2001b). Research in cerebral palsy. In A. L. Scherzer (Ed.), *Early diagnosis and interventional therapy in cerebral palsy: An interdisciplinary age-focused approach* (3rd ed., pp. 267-283). New York: Marcel Dekker.

Butler, C., & Darrah, J. (2001). Effects of neurodevelopmental treatment (NDT) for cerebral palsy: An AACPDM evidence report. *Developmental Medicine and Child Neurology, 43,* 778-790.

Butterworth, G., & Hicks, L. (1977). Visual proprioception and postural stability in infancy. *Perception, 6,* 255-262.

Byl, N. N., Merzenich, M. M., Cheung, S., Bedenbaugh, P., Nagarajan, S. S., & Jenkins, W. M. (1997). A primate model for studying focal dystonia and repetitive strain injury: Effects on the primary somatosensory cortex. *Physical Therapy, 77* (3), 269-284.

Cahan, L., Adams, J. M., Beeler, L., & Perry, J. (1989). Clinical, electrophysiologic, and kinesiologic observations in selective dorsal rhizotomy in cerebral palsy. In T. S. Park, L. H. Phillips, & W. J. Peacock (Eds.), *Management of spasticity in cerebral palsy and spinal cord injury. Neurosurgery: State of the art reviews* (pp. 477-484). Philadelphia: Hanley and Belfus.

Campbell, S. K. (1991). Framework for the measurement of neurologic impairment and disability. In M. Lister (Ed.), *Contemporary management of motor control problems. Proceedings From II Step Conference. Foundation for Physical Therapy* (pp. 143-154). Alexandria, VA: American Physical Therapy Association.

Campbell, S. K. (1992). Measurement of motor performance in cerebral palsy. In H. Forssberg & H. Hirschfeld (Eds.), *Movement disorders in children* (vol. 36, pp. 264-271). Basel, Switzerland: Medicine and Sport Science/Karger.

Campbell, S. K. (1997). Therapy programs for children that last a lifetime. *Physical and Occupational Therapy in Pediatrics, 17,* 1-15.

Campbell, S. K. (1999a). CNS dysfunction in children. In S. K. Campbell (Ed.), *Pediatric neurologic physical therapy* (2nd ed., pp. 1-18). New York: Churchill Livingstone.

Campbell, S. K. (1999b). Infants at risk for developmental disabilities. In S. K. Campbell (Ed.), *Decision making in pediatric physical therapy* (pp. 260-332). Philadelphia: Churchill Livingstone.

Campbell, S. K. (2000a). The child's development of functional movement. In S. K. Campbell (Ed), *Physical therapy for children* (pp. 3-44). Philadelphia: Churchill Livingstone.

Campbell, S. K. (2000b). Revolution in progress: A conceptual framework for examination and intervention. Part. II. *Neurology Report, 24* (2), 42-46.

Campbell, S. K., Gardner, H. G., & Ramakrishnan, V. (1995). Correlates of physicians' decision to refer children with cerebral palsy to physical therapy. *Developmental Medicine and Child Neurology, 37,* 1062-1074.

Campbell, S. K., Kolobe, T. H. A., Wright, B. D., & Linacre, J. M. (2002). Validity of the Infant Motor Performance for Prediction of 6-, 9- and 12-month scores on the Alberta Infant Motor Scale. *Developmental Medicine and Child Neurology, 44* (4), 263-272.

Carey, L. M. (1995). Somatosensory loss after stroke. *Critical Reviews of Physical Rehabilitation Medicine, 7,* 51-91.

Carey, L. M., Matyas, T. A., & Oke, L. E. (1993). Sensory loss in stroke patients: Effective training of tactile and proprioceptive discrimination. *Archives of Physical Medicine and Rehabilitation, 74,* 602-611.

Carr, J., & Shepherd, R. (2000). A motor learning model for rehabilitation. In J. Carr & R. Shepherd (Eds.), *Movement science. Foundations for physical therapy in rehabilitation* (2nd ed., pp. 33-110). Gaithersburg, MD: Aspen Publishers.

Castle, M. E., Reyman, T. A., & Schneider, M. (1979). Pathology of spastic muscle in cerebral palsy. *Clinical Orthopedics and Related Research, 142,* 223-233.

Chaudhuri, A., & Aruin, A. S. (2000). The effect of shoe lifts on static and dynamic postural control in individuals with hemiparesis. *Archives of Physical Medicine and Rehabilitation, 81* (11), 1498-1503.

Cioni, G., Bertucelli, B., Boldrini, A., Canapicchi, R., Frazzi, B., Guzzetta, A., & Mercuri, E. (2000). Correlation between visual function, neurodevelopmental outcome, and magnetic resonance imaging findings in infants with periventricular leucomalacia. *Archives of Disease in Childhood. Fetal and Neonatal Edition, 82* (2), 134-140.

Cioni, G., Montanaro, D., Tosetti, M., Canapicchi, R., & Ghelarducci, B. (2001). Reorganization of the sensorimotor cortex after early focal brain lesion: A functional MRI study in monozygotic twins. *Neuroreport, 12* (7), 1335-1340.

Cioni, G., Sales, B., Paolicelli, P. B., Petacchi, E., Scusa, M. F., & Canapicchi, R. (1999). MRI and clinical characteristics of children with hemiplegic cerebral palsy. *Neuropediatrics, 30* (5), 249-255.

Cirstea, M. C., & Levin, M. F. (2000). Compensatory strategies for reaching in stroke. *Brain, 123* (Pt. 5), 940-953.

Corso, J. I. (1981). *Aging, sensory systems and perception.* New York: Praeger.

Cote, L., & Crucher, M. D. (1991). The basal ganglia. In E. Kandel, J. Schwartz, & T. Jessell (Eds.), *Principles of neural science* (3rd ed., pp. 647-659). New York: Elsevier.

Craig, C. M., Lee, D. N., Freer, Y. N., & Laing, I. A. (1999). Modulations in breathing patterns during intermittent feeding in term infants and preterm infants with bronchopulmonary dysplasia. *Developmental Medicine and Child Neurology, 41* (9), 616-624.

Craik, R. L. (1991a). Abnormalities of motor behaviour. In M. Lister (Ed.), *Contemporary management of motor control problems. Proceedings From II Step Conference. Foundation for Physical Therapy* (pp. 155-164). Alexandria, VA: American Physical Therapy Association.

Craik, R. L. (1991b). Recovery process: Maximizing function. In M. Lister (Ed.), *Contemporary management of motor control problems. Proceedings From II Step Conference. Foundation for Physical Therapy* (pp. 165-174). Alexandria, VA: American Physical Therapy Association.

Crenna, P., & Inverno, M. (1994). Objective detection of pathophysiological factors contributing to gait disturbance in supraspinal lesions. In E. Fedrizzi, G. Avanzini, & P. Crenna (Eds.), *Motor development in children* (pp. 103-118). New York: John Libbey.

Cusick, B. D. (1990). Progressive casting and splinting for lower extremity deformities in children with neuromotor dysfunction. Tucson, AZ: Therapy Skill Builders.

Damiano, D. L. (1993). Reviewing muscle co-contraction: Is it developmental, pathological or motor control issues? *Physical and Occupational Therapy in Pediatrics, 12* (4), 3-20.

Damiano, D. L., & Abel, M. F. (1998). Functional outcomes of strength training in spastic cerebral palsy. *Archives of Physical Medicine and Rehabilitation, 79,* 119-125.

Damiano, D. L., MacPhail, H. E. A., & Kramer, J. F. (1995). Effect of isokinetic strength-training on functional ability and walking efficiency in adolescents with cerebral palsy. *Developmental Medicine and Child Neurology, 37,* 763-775.

Damiano, D.L., Martellotta, T. L., Sullivan, D. J., Granata, K. P., & Abel, M. F. (2000). Muscle force production and functional performance in spastic cerebral palsy: Relationship of co-contraction. *Archives of Physical Medicine and Rehabilitation, 81* (7), 895-900.

Damiano, D. L., Vaughan, C. L., & Abel, M. F. (1995). Muscle response to heavy resistance exercise in children with spastic cerebral palsy. *Developmental Medicine and Child Neurology, 37,* 731-39.

Darien-Smith, I., Galea, M. P., & Darien-Smith, C. (1996). Manual dexterity: How does the cerebral cortex contribute? *Clinical and Experimental Pharmacology and Physiology, 23,* 948-956.

Davies, P. (1985). *Steps to follow. A guide to treatment of adult hemiplegia.* New York: Springer-Verlag.

DeGangi, G. A., DiPietro, J. A., Greenspan, S. I., & Porges, S. W. (1991). Psychophysiological characteristics of the regulatory disordered infant. *Infant Behavior and Development, 14,* 37-50.

Diamond, M., & Cupps, B. (2002). NDT framework for clinical decision making incorporating a disablement model. In M. Stamer (Ed.), *Progress in Motion.* (pp. 13-29). Laguna Beach, CA. NDTA.

Dickstein, R., Hocherman, S., Pillar, T., & Shaham, R. (1986). Stroke rehabilitation: Three exercise therapy approaches. *Physical Therapy, 66* (8), 1233-1238.

Diener, H. C., Dichgans, J., Guschlbauer, B., & Mau, H. (1984). The significance of proprioception on postural stabilization as assessed by ischemia. *Brain Research, 296,* 103-109.

Diener, H. C., Horak, F. B., & Nashner, L. M. (1988). Influence of stimulus parameters on human postural response. *Journal of Neurophysiology, 59* (6), 1888-1905.

Dietz, V., & Berger, W. (1983). Normal and impaired regulation of muscle stiffness in gait: A new hypothesis about muscle hypertonia. *Experimental Neurology, 79,* 680-687.

Dietz, V., Ketelson, U. P., Berger, S. C., & Quintern, J. (1986). Motor unit involvement in spastic paresis: Relationship between leg muscle activation and histochemistry. *Journal of the Neurological Sciences, 75,* 89-103.

Dietz, V., Quintern, J., & Berger, W. (1981). Electrophysiological studies of gait in spasticity and rigidity: Evidence that altered mechanical properties of muscle contribute to hypertonus. *Brain, 104,* 431-449.

DiFabio, F. P., & Badke, M. B. (1991). Stance duration under sensory conflict conditions in patients with hemiplegia. *Archives of Physical Medicine and Rehabilitation, 72,* 292-295.

Duncan, P., & Badke, M. B. (1987). *Stroke rehabilitation: The recovery of motor control.* Chicago: Year Books.

Edelman, G. M. (1987). *Neural Darwinism. The theory of neuronal group selection.* New York: Basic Books.

Eliasson, A. C., & Gordon, A. M. (2000). Impaired force coordination during object release in children with hemiplegic cerebral palsy. *Developmental Medicine and Child Neurology, 424* (4), 228-234.

Eliasson, A. C., Gordon, A. M., & Forssberg, H. (1992). Impaired anticipatory control of isometric forces during grasping by children with cerebral palsy. *Developmental Medicine and Child Neurology, 34,* 216-225.

Embry, D., Yates, L., & Mott, D. (1990). Effects of neurodevelopmental treatment and orthoses on knee flexion during gait: A single-subject design. *Physical Therapy, 70,* 626-637.

Engardt, M., Knutsson, E., Jonsson, M., & Sternhag, M. (1995). Dynamic muscle strength training in stroke patients: Effects on knee extension torque, electromyographic activity, and motor function. *Archives of Physical Medicine and Rehabilitation, 76* (5), 419-425.

Engberg, J. R., Ross, S. A., & Park, T. S. (1999). Changes in ankle spasticity and strength following selective dorsal rhizotomy and physical therapy for spastic cerebral palsy. *Journal of Neurosurgery, 91,* 727-732.

Erhardt, R. (1994). *Developmental hand dysfunction. Theory, assessment and treatment* (2nd ed.). Tucson, AZ: Therapy Skill Builders.

Erhardt, R. P. (1998, March/April). Improving visual control: Activities for parents and infants. *NDTA Network,* 1, 3.

Esscher, E., Flodmark, O., Hagberg, G., & Hagberg, B. (1996). Non-progressive ataxia: Origins, brain pathology and impairments in 78 Swedish children. *Developmental Medicine and Child Neurology, 38,* 285-296.

Farmer, S. F., Sheean, G. L., Mayston, M. J., Rothwell, J. C., Marsden, C. D., Conway, B. A., Halliday, D. M., Rosenberg, J. R., & Stephens, J. A. (1998). Abnormal motor unit synchronization of antagonist muscles underlies pathological co-contraction in upper limb dystonia. *Brain, 121* (Pt. 5), 801-814.

Farmer, S. F., Swash, M., Ingram, D. A., & Stephens, J. A. (1993). Changes in motor unit synchronization following central nervous lesion in man. *Journal of Physiology (London), 463,* 83-105.

Feldman, R. G., Young, R. R., & Koella, W. P. (1980). *Spasticity: Disordered motor control.* Chicago: Year Book Medical Publications.

Fetters, L. (1991). Cerebral palsy: Contemporary treatment concepts. In M. Lister (Ed.), *Contemporary management of motor control problems. Proceedings From II Step Conference. Foundation for Physical Therapy* (pp. 219-224). Alexandria, VA: American Physical Therapy Association.

Finger, S., & Stein, D. G. (1982). Supersensitivity as a recovery model. In S. Finger & D. G. Stein (Eds.), *Brain damage and recovery: Research and clinical perspectives* (pp. 271-286). New York: Academic Press Inc.

Fisher, A. G., Murray, E., & Bundy, A. (Eds.). (1991). *Sensory integration: Theory and practice.* Philadelphia: F. A. Davis.

Fisher, B., & Woll, S. (1995). Considerations in the restoration of motor control. In J. Montgomery (Ed.), *Clinics in physical therapy: Physical therapy for traumatic brain injury* (pp. 55-78). New York: Churchill Livingstone.

Flick, C. L. (1999). Stroke rehabilitation. 1. Stroke outcome and psychosocial consequences. *Archives of Physical Medicine and Rehabilitation, 80,* 521-526.

Forsstrom, A., & von Hofsten, C. (1982). Visually directed reaching in children with motor impairments. *Developmental Medicine and Child Neurology, 24* (5), 653-661.

Fowler, E. G., Ho, T. W., Nwigwe, A. I., & Dorsey, F. J. (2001). The effect of quadriceps femoris muscle strengthening exercises on spasticity in children with cerebral palsy. *Physical Therapy, 81* (6), 1215-1223.

Frascarelli, M., Mastrogregori, L., & Conforti, L. (1998). Initial motor unit recruitment in patients with spastic hemiplegia. *Electromyography and Clinical Neurophysiology, 38,* 267-271.

Frontera, W. R., Hughes, V. A., Fielding, R. A., Fiatarone, M. A., Evans, W. J., & Roubenoff, R. (2000). Aging of skeletal muscle: A 12-yr longitudinal study. *Journal of Applied Physiology, 88,* 1321-1326.

Gage, J. R. (1991). *Gait analysis in cerebral palsy.* London: Mac Keith Press.

Gage, J. R. (1992). Distal hamstring lengthening, release and rectus femoris transfer. In M. Sussman (Ed.), *The diplegic child* (pp. 317-336). Rosemont, IL: American Academy of Orthopedic Surgeons.

Gajdosik, C. G., & Gajdosik, R. L. (2000). Musculoskeletal development and adaptation. In S. K. Campbell (Ed.), *Physical therapy for children* (2nd ed., pp. 117-197). Philadelphia: W. B. Saunders.

Gardiner, R. (1996). The pathophysiology and clinical implications of neuromuscular changes following cerebrovascular accident. *Australian Physiotherapy, 42* (2), 139-147.

Garland, J. S., Stevenson, T. J., & Ivanova, T. (1997). Postural responses to unilateral arm perturbation in young, elderly, and hemiplegic subjects. *Archives of Physical Medicine and Rehabilitation, 78,* 1072-1077.

Gebler, D. A., Josefczyk, P. B., Herman, D., Good, D. C., & Verhulst, S. J. (1995). Comparison of two therapy approaches in the rehabilitation of the pure motor hemiparetic stroke patient. *Journal of Neurologic Rehabilitation, 9* (4), 191-196.

Ghez, C. (1991). Posture. In E. Kandel, J. Schwartz, & T. Jessell (Eds.), *Principles of neural science* (3rd ed., pp. 596-607). New York: Elsevier.

Gibson, J. J. (1966). *The senses considered as perceptual systems.* Boston: Houghton Mifflin.

Girolami, G., & Campbell, S. K. (1994). Efficacy of a Neuro-Developmental Treatment program to improve motor control of preterm infants. *Pediatric Physical Therapy, 6,* 175-184.

Girolami, G., Ryan, D. F., & Gardner, J. M. (2001). Clinical assessment of the infant. In A. L. Scherzer (Ed.), *Early diagnosis and interventional therapy in cerebral palsy. An interdisciplinary age-focused approach* (3rd ed., pp. 139-184). New York: Marcel Dekker.

Giuliani, C. A. (1991). Dorsal rhizotomy for children with cerebral palsy. Support for concepts of motor control. *Physical Therapy, 71* (3), 248-259.

Giuliani, C. (1997). The relationship of spasticity to movement and considerations for therapeutic interventions. *Neurology Report, 21,* 78-84.

Glassman, R. B., & Smith, A. (1988). Neural spare capacity and the concept of diaschisis: Functional and evolutionary models. In T. E. LeVere, R. B. Almli, & D. G. Stein (Eds.), *Brain injury and recovery: Theoretical and controversial issues* (pp. 45-69). New York: Plenum Press.

Goldman, P. S. (1974). An alternative to developmental plasticity: Heterology of CNS structures in infants and adults. In D. G. Stein, J. J. Rosen, & N. Butters (Eds.), *Plasticity and recovery of function in the central nervous system* (pp. 149-174). New York: Academic Press.

Gonella, C. (1989). Single subject experimental paradigm as a clinical decision tool. *Physical Therapy 69* (7), 91-99.

Gordon, J. (2000). Assumptions underlying physical therapy intervention: Theoretical and historical perspectives. In J. Carr & R. Shepherd (Eds.), *Movement science. Foundations for physical therapy in rehabilitation* (2nd ed., pp. 1-31). Gaithersburg, MD: Aspen Publishers.

Gray, D. B., & Hendershot, G. E. (2000). The ICIDH-2: Developments for a new era of outcomes research. *Archives of Physical Medicine and Rehabilitation, 81,* Suppl. 2, S10-14.

Greenspan, S. (1997). *Growth of the mind.* Reading, MA: Addison-Wesley Publishing Company.

Greiner, B. M., Czerniecki, J. M., & Deitz, J. C. (1993). Gait parameters of children with spastic diplegia: A comparison of effects of posterior and anterior walkers. *Archives of Physical Medicine and Rehabilitation, 74,* 381-385.

Guyton, A. C., & Hall, J. E. (1996). The cerebellum, the basal ganglia and overall motor control. In A. C. Guyton & J. E. Hall (Eds.), *Textbook of medical physiology* (9th ed., pp. 715-730). Philadelphia: W. B. Saunders.

Guzzetta, A., Cioni, G., Cowan, F., & Mercuri, E. (2001). Visual disorders of children with brain lesions: Maturation of visual function in infants with neonatal brain lesions: Correlations with neuroimaging. *European Journal of Paediatric Neurology, 5* (3), 907-914.

Guzzetta, A., Frazzi, B., Mercuri, E., Bertuccelli, B., Carapicchi, R., van Hof-van Duin, J., & Cioni, G. (2001). Visual function in children with hemiplegia in the first year of life. *Developmental Medicine and Child Neurology, 43* (5), 321-329.

Guzzetta, A., Mercuri, E., & Cioni, G. (2001). Visual disorders in children with brain lesions: 2. Visual impairment associated with cerebral palsy. *European Journal of Paediatric Neurology, 5* (3), 115-119.

Hadders-Algra, M. (2000). The neuronal group selection theory: Promising principles for understanding and treating developmental motor disorders. *Developmental Medicine and Child Neurology, 42,* 707-715.

Hadders-Algra, M., Brogren, E., Katz-Salamon, M., & Forssberg, H. (1999). Periventricular leukomalacia and preterm birth have a different detrimental effect on postural adjustments. *Brain, 122,* 727-740.

Hagberg, B., Hagberg, G., Olow, I., & Wendt, L. (1996). The changing panorama of CP in Sweden VII, Prevalence and origin in the birth year period 1987-1990. *Acta Paediatrica Scandinavica, 85,* 954-960.

Hallett, M., & Alverez, N. (1983). Attempted rapid elbow flexion movements in patients with athetosis. *Journal of Neurology, Neurosurgery, and Psychiatry, 46,* 745-750.

Heine, R. G., Jaquiery, A., Lubitz, L., Cameron, D. J., & Catto-Smith, A. G. (1995). Role of gastro-oesophageal reflux in infant irritability. *Archives of the Disabled Child, 73* (2), 121-125.

Heine, R. G., Reddihough, D. S., & Catto-Smith, A. G. (1995). Gastro-oesophageal reflux and feeding problems after gastrostomy in children with severe neurological impairment. *Developmental Medicine and Child Neurology, 37,* 320-329.

Held, J. M. (1998). Environmental enrichment enhances sparing and recovery of function following brain damage. *Neurology Report, 22,* 74-78.

Held, J. M. (2000). Recovery of function after brain damage: Theoretical implications for therapeutic intervention. In J. Carr & R. Shepherd (Eds.), *Movement science. Foundations for physical therapy in rehabilitation* (2nd ed., pp. 189-211). Gaithersburg, MD: Aspen Publishers.

Held, J. M., Gordon, F., & Gentile, A. M. (1985). Environmental influences on locomotor recovery following cortical lesions in rats. *Behavioral Neuroscience, 99,* 678-690.

Henderson, L., Rose, P., & Henderson, S. (1992). Reaction time and movement time in children with a developmental coordination disorder. *Journal of Child Psychology and Psychiatry, 33,* 895-905.

Herbert, R. (1988). The passive mechanical properties of muscle and their adaptations to altered patterns of use. *Australian Journal of Physiotherapy, 34* (3), 141-149.

Heriza, C. (1991a). Implications of a dynamical systems approach to understanding infant kicking behavior. *Physical Therapy, 71* (3), 222-235.

Heriza, C. (1991b). Motor development: Traditional and contemporary theories. In M. Lister (Ed.), *Contemporary management of motor control problems. Proceedings From II Step Conference. Foundation for Physical Therapy* (pp. 99-126). Alexandria, VA: American Physical Therapy Association.

Heuer, H. (1974). Coordination. In H. Heuer & S. W. Keele (Eds.), *Handbook of perception and action* (vol. 2, pp. 121-180). San Diego, CA: Academic Press.

Hirschfeld, H. (1992). Postural control: Acquisition and integration during development. In H. Forssberg & H. Hirschfeld (Eds.), *Movement disorders in children* (vol. 36, pp. 199-208). Basel, Switzerland: Medicine and Sport Science/Karger.

Hodgkinson, I., Jindrich, P., Dubaut, P., Vadot, J. P., Metton, G., & Bernard, C. (2001). Hip pain in 234 non-ambulatory adolescents and young adults with cerebral palsy: A cross-sectional multicenter study. *Developmental Medicine and Child Neurology, 43* (12), 806-808.

Holt, K., Butcher, R., & Fonseca, S. T. (2000). Limb stiffness in active leg swinging of children with spastic hemiplegic cerebral palsy. *Pediatric Physical Therapy, 12,* 50-61.

Holt, K. G., Obusek, J., & Fonseca, S. T. (1996). Constraints on disordered locomotion: A dynamical systems perspective on spastic cerebral palsy. *Human Movement Science, 15,* 177-202.

Horak, F., & Diener, H. C. (1994). Cerebellar control of postural scaling and central set in stance. *Journal of Neurophysiology, 72,* 479-493.

Horak, F. B., Esselman, P., Anderson, M. E., & Lynch, M. K. (1984). The effects of movement velocity, mass displaced and task certainty on associated postural adjustments made by normal and hemiplegic individuals. *Journal of Neurology, Neurosurgery, and Psychiatry, 47,* 1020-1028.

Horak, F. B., Nashner, L. M., & Diener, H. C. (1990). Postural strategies associated with somatosensory and vestibular loss. *Experimental Brain Research, 82,* 167-177.

Horak, F. B., Nutt, J. G., & Nashner, L. M. (1992). Postural inflexibility in Parkinsonian subjects. *Journal of Neurology and Science, 111* (1), 46-58.

Horvat, M. (1987). Effects of a progressive resistance training program on an individual with spastic cerebral palsy. *American Corrective Therapy Journal, 41,* 7-10.

Howle, J. (1999a). Cerebral palsy. In S. K. Campbell (Ed.), *Decision making in pediatric neurologic physical therapy* (pp. 23-83). Philadelphia: Churchill Livingstone.

Howle, J. (1999b). Description, assessment and treatment progression of a child with ataxic cerebral palsy: A single subject case study: Part I, *NDT Network,* March/April, 1, 3, 4, 19; Part II, *NDT Network,* May/June, 1, 3, 12, 19.

Humphrey, D. R., & Reed, D. J. (1983). Separate cortical systems for control of joint movement. In J. E. Desmedt (Ed.), *Motor control mechanisms in health and disease. Advances in Neurology,* #39. New York: Raven Press.

Ibrahim, I. K., Berger, W., Trippel, M., & Dietz, V. (1993). Stretch-induced electromyographic activity and torque in spastic elbow muscles. *Brain, 116,* 971-989.

Indredavik, B., Bakke, F., Slordahl, S. A., Rokseth, R., & Haheim, L. L. (1999). Stroke unit treatment. 10-year follow-up. *Stroke, 30* (8), 1524-1527.

Ito, J., Araki, A., Tanaka, H., Tasaki, T., Cho, K., & Yamazaki, R. (1996). Muscle histopathology in spastic cerebral palsy. *Brain and Development, 18,* 299-303.

Jeannerod, M. (1990). *The neural and behavioral organization of goal-directed movements.* New York: Clarendon Press.

Jensen, J. L., Schneider, K., Ulrich, B. D., Zernicke, R. F., & Thelen, E. (1994). Adaptive dynamics of the leg movement patterns of human infants: I. The effect of posture on spontaneous kicking. *Journal of Motor Behavior, 26* (4), 303-312.

Josefczyk, P. B., & Gebler, D. (1995). Stroke rehabilitation outcome: A prospective comparison of traditional functional rehabilitation versus neurodevelopmental technique in the moderately impaired stroke patient. *Journal of Neurologic Rehabilitation, 9* (4), 127-128.

Jouen, F. (1990). Early visual-vestibular interactions and postural development. In H. Block & B. I. Bertenthal (Eds.), *Sensory-motor organization and development in infancy and early childhood* (pp. 190-205). Dordrecht, Holland: Kluwer.

Kahn-D'Angelo, L., & Unanue, R. A. (2000). The special care nursery. In S. K. Campbell (Ed.), *Physical therapy for children* (2nd ed., pp. 840-880). Philadelphia: W. B. Saunders.

Kalar, L. (1994). The influence of stroke unit rehabilitation on functional recovery from stroke. *Stroke, 25,* 821-825.

Karnath, H. O., Ferber, S., & Dichgans, J. (2000a). The neural representation of postural control in humans. *Proceedings of the National Academy of Sciences of the United States of America, 97* (25), 13931-13936.

Karnath, H. O., Ferber, S., & Dichgans, J. (2000b). The origin of contraversive pushing: Evidence for a second graviceptive system in humans. *Neurology, 55* (9), 1298-1304.

Katz, R., & Rymer, Z. (1989). Spastic hypertonia: Mechanisms and measurements. *Archives of Physical Medicine and Rehabilitation, 70,* 114-155.

Kelly, M. K. (2000). Children with ventilator dependence. In S. K. Campbell (Ed.), *Physical therapy for children* (pp. 633-685). Philadelphia: W. B. Saunders.

Kelso, J. A., & Tuller, B. (1984). Converging evidence in support of common dynamical principles for speech and movement coordination. *American Journal of Physiology, 246,* 928-935.

Kennard, M. A. (1940). Relation of age to motor impairment in man and in sub-human primates. *Archives of Neurology and Psychiatry, 44,* 377-398.

Kennard, M. A. (1942). Cortical reorganization of motor function: Studies on a series of monkeys of various ages from infancy to maturity. *Archives of Neurology and Psychiatry, 48,* 227-240.

Kent-Braun, J. A., Ng, A. V., & Young, K. (2000). Skeletal muscle contractile and noncontractile components in young and older women and men. *Journal of Applied Physiology, 88,* 662-668.

Kershner, E. A. (1991). How theoretical framework biases evaluation and treatment. In M. Lister (Ed.), *Contemporary management of motor control problems. Proceedings From II Step Conference. Foundation for Physical Therapy* (pp. 37-48). Alexandria, VA: American Physical Therapy Association.

Ketellaar, M., Vermeer, A. (1998). Functional motor abilities of children with cerebral palsy: a systematic literature review of assessment measures. *Clinical Rehabilitation, 12, 369-380.*

Knickerbocker, B. (1980). *A holistic approach to learning disabilities.* Thorofare, NJ: Slack Publishers.

Knox, V., Evans A.L. (2002) Evaluation of the functional effects of a course of Bobath therapy in children with cerebral palsy: a preliminary study. *Developmental Medicine and Child Neurology, 44, 447-460.*

Knutsson, E. (1994). Can gait analysis improve gait training in stroke patients? *Scandinavian Journal of Rehabilitation Medicine Suppl., 30,* 73-80.

Knutsson, E., & Martensson, A. (1980). Dynamic motor capacity in spastic paresis and its relation to prime mover dysfunction, spastic reflexes and antagonist co-activation. *Scandinavian Journal of Rehabilitation Medicine, 12,* 93-106.

Knutsson, E., & Richards, C. (1979). Different types of disturbed motor control in gait of hemiparetic patients. *Brain, 102,* 405-430.

Koop, S. E., J. L. Stout, W. H. Drinken, & R. C. Starr. (1989). Energy cost of walking in children with cerebral palsy (abstract). *Physical Therapy, 69,* 386.

Krageloh-Mann, I., Hagberg, G., Meisner, C., Schelp, B., Haas, G., Eeg-Olofsson, K. E., Selbmann, H. K., Hagberg, B., & Michaelis, R. (1993). Bilateral spastic cerebral palsy. A comparative study between south-west Germany and western Sweden I: Clinical patterns and disabilities. *Developmental Medicine and Child Neurology, 35,* 1037-1047.

Kundi, M., Cahan, L. D., & Starr, A. (1988). Somatosensory evoked potentials in cerebral palsied subjects with spastic diplegia before and after partial selective dorsal root rhizotomy. *Archives of Neurology, 46,* 524-527.

Kusoffsky, A., Apel, I., & Hirschfeld, H. (2001). Reaching-lifting-placing task during standing after stroke: Coordination among ground forces, ankle muscle activity and hand movement. *Archives of Physical Medicine and Rehabilitation, 82,* 650-660.

Lance, J. W. (1980). Symposium synopsis. In F. G. Feldman, R. R. Young, & W. P. Koella (Eds.), *Spasticity: Disordered motor control* (pp. 485-500). Chicago: Year Book Medical Publications.

Law, M., Russell, D., Pollock, N., Rosenbaum, P., Walter, S., & King, G. (1997). A comparison of intensive neurodevelopmental therapy plus casting and a regular occupational therapy program for children with cerebral palsy. *Developmental Medicine and Child Neurology, 39* (10), 664-670.

Lee, D. N. (1978). The functions of vision. In H. Pick & E. Saltzman (Eds.), *Modes of perceiving and processing information.* Hillsdale, NJ: Erlbaum.

Lee, D. N., & Aronson, E. (1974). Visual proprioceptive control of standing in human infants. *Perception and Psychophysics, 15,* 529-532.

Lee, D. N., Georgopoulos, A. P., Clark, M. J., Craig, C. M., & Port, N. L. (2001). Guiding contact by coupling the taus of gaps. *Experimental Brain Research, 139* (2), 151-159.

Lee, W. (1983). Neuromotor synergies as a basis for coordinated intentional action. *Journal of Motor Behavior, 16* (2), 135-170.

Lee, W. A. (1988). A control systems framework for understanding normal and abnormal posture. *American Journal of Occupational Therapy, 43* (5), 291-301.

Leonard, C. T., Hirschfeld, H., Moritani, T., & Forssberg, H. (1991). Myostatic reflex development in normal children and in children with cerebral palsy. *Experimental Neurology, 111,* 329-382.

Leonard, C. T., Moritani, T., Hirschfeld, H., & Forssberg, H. (1990). Deficits in reciprocal inhibition of children with cerebral palsy as revealed by H reflex testing. *Developmental Medicine and Child Neurology, 32,* 974-984.

Lesny, I. A. (1979). Follow-up study of hypotonic forms of cerebral palsy. *Brain and Development, 1,* 87-90.

Levangie, P. K., Guihan, M. F., Meyer, P., & Stuhr, K. (1989). Effect of altering handle position of a rolling walker on gait in children with cerebral palsy. *Physical Therapy, 69* (2), 130-134.

LeVeau, B. F., & Bernhardt, D. B. (1984). Effects of forces on the growth, development and maintenance of the human body. *Physical Therapy, 64,* 1874-1882.

Levin, M. F. (1996). Interjoint coordination during pointing movements is disrupted in spastic hemiparesis. *Brain, 119,* 281-293.

Levin, M. F., & Hui-Chan, C. (1993). Are H and stretch reflexes in hemiparesis reproducible and correlated with spasticity? *Journal of Neurology, 240* (2), 63-71.

Levin, M. F., Michaelsen, S. M., Cirstea, C. M., & Roby-Brami, A. (2002). Use of the trunk for reaching targets placed within and beyond the reach in adult hemiparesis. *Experimental Brain Research, 143* (2), 171-180.

Lewis, C., & Bottomley, J. (1990). Musculoskeletal changes with age. In C. Lewis (Ed.), *Aging: Health care's challenge* (2nd ed., pp. 145-164). Philadelphia: F. A. Davis.

Liepert, J., Bauder, H., Wolfgang, H. R., Miltner, W. H. R., Taub, E., & Weiller, C. (2000). Treatment-induced cortical reorganization after stroke in humans. *Stroke, 31,* 1210-1216.

Lin, J. P., Brown, J. K., & Brotherstone, R. (1994a). Assessment of spasticity in hemiplegic cerebral palsy. I: Proximal lower-limb reflex excitability. *Developmental Medicine and Child Neurology, 36,* 116-129.

Lin, J. P., Brown, J. K., & Brotherstone, R. (1994b). Assessment of spasticity in hemiplegic cerebral palsy. II. Distal lower-limb reflex excitability and function. *Developmental Medicine and Child Neurology, 36,* 290-303.

Lipsitz, L. A., Jonsson, P. V., Kelley, M. M., & Koestner, J. S. (1991). Causes and correlates of recurrent falls in ambulatory frail elderly. *Journal of Gerontology, 46,* M114-122.

Logan, L., Byers-Hinley, K., & Ciccone, C. (1990). Anterior vs. posterior walkers for children with cerebral palsy: A gait analysis study. *Developmental Medicine and Child Neurology, 32,* 1044-1048.

Lundberg, A., Ovenfors, C. O., & Saltin, B. (1967). The effect of physical training on school children with cerebral palsy. *Acta Paediatrica Scandinavica, 56,* 182-188.

Luria, A. R., Naydin, V. L., Tsvetkova, L. S., & Vinarskaya, E. N. (1969). Restoration of higher cortical function following local brain damage. In R. J. Vinken & G. W. Bruyn (Eds.), *Handbook of clinical neurology* (vol. 3, pp. 368-433). Amsterdam: North Holland Publishers.

Magill-Evans, J. E., & Restall, G. (1991). Self-esteem of persons with CP: From adolescence to adulthood. *South African Journal of Occupational Therapy, 45* (9), 819-825.

Manheim, C. J. (1994). *The myofascial release manual* (2nd ed.). Thorofare, NJ: Slack, Inc.

Massery, M., & Moerchen, V. (1996, November/December). Coordinating transitional movements and breathing in patients with neuromotor dysfunction. *NDTA Network,* 3-7.

Mayer, N. H., Esquenazi, A., & Childers, M. K. (1997). Common patterns of clinical motor dysfunction. *Muscle and Nerve, 6,* S21-35.

McAuliffe, C. A., Wenger, R. E., Schneider, J. W., & Gaebler-Spira, D. J. (1998). Usefulness of the Wee-Functional Independence Measure to detect functional change in children with cerebral palsy. *Pediatric Physical Therapy, 10* (1), 23-28.

McComas, A. J., Sica, R. E. P., Upton, A. R., & Aguilera, N. (1973). Functional changes in motorneurons of hemiparetic patients. *Journal of Neurology, Neurosurgery, and Psychiatry, 36,* 183-193.

Michaelsen, S. M., Luta, A., Roby-Brami, A., & Levin, M. F. (2001). Effect of trunk restraint on the recovery of reaching movements in hemiparetic patients. *Stroke, 32* (8), 1875-1883.

Milla, P. T., & Jackson, A. D. M. (1977). A controlled treatment of baclofen in children with cerebral palsy. *Journal of International Medical Research, 5,* 398-401.

Miller, L. J., & Lane, S. J. (2000). Toward a consensus in terminology in sensory integration theory and practice: Part I: Taxonomy of neurophysiological processes. *Sensory Integration Special Interest Section Quarterly 23* (1), 1-13. Part II, Sensory integration patterns of function and dysfunction, *23* (2), 1-3. Part III, Observable behaviors: Sensory integration dysfunction, *23* (3), 1-3.

Milner, B. (1974). Sparing of language functions after early unilateral brain damage. *Neurosciences Research Program Bulletin, 12,* 213-217.

Milner-Brown, H. S., & Penn, R. D. (1979). Pathophysiological mechanisms in cerebral palsy. *Journal of Neurology, Neurosurgery, and Psychiatry, 42,* 606-618.

Montgomery, P. C. (1991). Perceptual issues in motor control. In M. Lister (Ed.), *Contemporary management of motor control problems. Proceedings From II Step Conference. Foundation for Physical Therapy* (pp. 175-184). Alexandria, VA: American Physical Therapy Association.

Montgomery, P. C. (2000). Achievement of gross motor skills in two children with cerebellar hypoplasia: Longitudinal case reports. *Pediatric Physical Therapy, 12,* 68-76.

Moore, J. (1984, May). The neuroanatomy and pathology of cerebral palsy. In *Selected Proceedings from the Barbro Salek Memorial Symposium,* 3–60.

Morris, S. E., & Dunn, M. K. (2000). *Pre-feeding skills. A comprehensive resource for feeding development* (2nd ed.). Austin, TX: Therapy Skill Builders.

Muir, R. B., & Lemon, R. N. (1983). Corticospinal neurons with a special role in precision grip. *Brain Research, 261* (2), 312-316.

Murphy, K. P., Molnar, G., & Lankasky, K. (1995). Medical and functional status of adults with cerebral palsy. *Developmental Medicine and Child Neurology, 37,* 1075-1084.

Mutch, L., Alberman, E., Hagberg, B., Kodama, K., & Perat, M. V. (1992). Cerebral palsy epidemiology: Where we are now, and where we are going? *Developmental Medicine and Child Neurology, 34,* 547-555.

Mullens, P. A. (2001, January/February). AACPDM evidence reports–Defined. *NDT Network,* 8-9.

Nakayama, H., Jorgensen, H. S., Raaschon, H. O., & Olsen, T. S. (1994). Recovery of upper extremity function in stroke patients: The Copenhagen stroke study. *Archives of Physical Medicine and Rehabilitation, 75,* 394-398.

Horak, J. B., Nutt, J. G., & Nashner, L. M. (1992). Postural inflexibility in parkinsonian subjects. *Journal of Neurological Science, 111* (1), 46-58.

Nashner, L. M., Black, F. O., & Wall, C., III. (1982) Adaptation to altered support and visual conditions during stance: Patients with vestibular deficits. *Journal of Neuroscience, 2 (5),* 536-544.

Nashner, L. M., Shumway-Cook, A., & Marin, O. (1983). Stance posture control in select groups of children with cerebral palsy: Deficits in sensory organization and muscular coordination. *Experimental Brain Research, 49,* 393-409.

Nashner, L., & Woollacott, M. (1979). The organization of rapid postural adjustments of standing humans: An experimental-conceptual model. In R. E. Talbott & D. R. Humphrey (Eds.), *Posture and movement* (pp. 243-257). New York: Raven.

Neilson, P. D., & McCaughey, J. (1982). Self-regulation of spasm and spasticity in cerebral palsy. *Journal of Neurology, Neurosurgery, and Psychiatry, 45,* 320-330.

Nelson, C. (2001, July/August). The effect of visual dysfunction on motor development. *NDTA Network, 8* (4), 1, 4, 6.

Nicolaides, P., & Appleton, R. E. (1996). Stroke in children. *Developmental Medicine and Child Neurology, 38,* 172-180.

Noth, J. (1991). Trends in the pathophysiology and pharmacotherapy of spasticity. *Journal of Neurology, 238,* 131-139.

Nudo, R. J. (1998). Role of cortical plasticity in motor recovery after stroke. *Neurology Report, 22* (2), 61-67.

O'Dwyer, N. J., Ada, L., & Neilson, P. D. (1996). Spasticity and muscle contracture following stroke. *Brain, 119,* 1737-1749.

Olney, S. J. (1985). Quantitative evaluation of contraction of knee and ankle muscles during walking. In D. A. Winter, R. W. Norman, R. P. Wells, K. C. Hayes, & A. E. Potla (Eds.), *Biomechanics IX-A* (pp. 431-435). Champaign, IL: Human Kinetics.

Olney, S. J., & Wright, M. J. (2000). Cerebral palsy. In S. K. Campbell (Ed.), *Physical therapy for children* (2nd ed., pp. 533-570). Philadelphia: W. B. Saunders.

O'Shea, T. M., Goldstein, D. J., deRegnier, R. A., Shaeffer, C. I., Roberts, D. D., & Dillard, R. G. (1996). Outcome at 4 to 5 years in children recovered from neonatal chronic lung disease. *Developmental Medicine and Child Neurology, 38,* 830-839.

O'Sullivan, M. C., Miller, S., Ramesh, V., Conway, E., Gilfillan, K., McDonough, S., & Eyre, J. A. (1998). Abnormal development of the biceps brachii phasic stretch reflex and persistence of short latency heteronymous reflexes from the biceps brachii in spastic cerebral palsy. *Brain, 121,* 2381-2395.

Ottenbacher, K., Biocca, Z., DeCremer, G., Gevelinger, M., Jedlovec, K., & Johnson, M. (1986). Quantitative analysis of the effectiveness of pediatric therapy. *Physical Therapy, 66,* 1095-1101.

Ottenbacher, K. J., & Hinderer, S. R. (2001). Evidence-based practice: Methods to evaluate individual patient improvement. *American Journal of Physical Medicine and Rehabilitation, 80* (10), 786-796.

Pai, Y. C., Rogers, M. W., Hedman, L. D., & Hanke, T. A. (1994). Alterations in weight-transfer capabilities in adults with hemiparesis. *Physical Therapy, 74,* 647-657.

Palisano, R., Rosenbaum, P., Walter, S., Russell, D., Wood, E., & Galuppi, B. (1997). The development and reliability of a system to classify gross motor function in children with CP. *Developmental Medicine and Child Neurology, 39,* 214-223.

Palmer, F. B., Shapiro, B. K., Wachtel, R. C., Allen, M. C., Hiller, J. E., Harryman, S. E., Mosher, B. S., Meinert, C. L., & Capute, A. J. (1988). The effects of physical therapy on cerebral palsy. A controlled trial in infants with spastic diplegia. *New England Journal of Medicine, 318,* 803-808.

Palta, A. E., & Shumway-Cook, A. (1999). Dimensions of mobility defining the complexity and difficulties associated with community mobility. *Journal of Aging and Physical Activity, 1,* 7-19.

Perry, J. (1992). *Gait analysis: Normal and pathological function.* Thorofare, NJ: Slack, Inc.

Perry, J., & Newsam, C. (1992). Function of the hamstrings in cerebral palsy. In M. D. Sussman (Ed.), *The diplegic child* (pp. 299-307). Rosemont, IL: American Academy of Orthopedic Surgeons.

Post-Stroke Rehabilitation Guideline Panel. (1995). *Post-stroke rehabilitation: Clinical practice guidelines.* AHCPR Pub. No. 95-0662. Rockville, MD: U. S. Department of Health and Human Services. Public Health Service.

Powell, J. (2001, July/August). Vision contributes to the "why?" *NDTA Network, 8* (4), 10.

Prechtl, H. F. R. (1990). Qualitative changes of spontaneous movements in fetus and preterm infants are a marker of neurological dysfunction. *Early Human Development 23,* 151-158.

Prechtl, H. F. R. (2001). General movement assessment as a method of developmental neurology: New paradigms and their consequences. *Developmental Medicine and Child Neurology, 43,* 836-842.

Prechtl, H. F. R., Einspieler, C., Cioni, G., Bos, A. F., Ferrari, F., & Sontheimer, D. (1997). An early marker for neurological deficits after perinatal brain lesions. *Lancet, 349,* 1361-3197.

Quintana, L. A. (1995). Evaluation of perception and cognition. In C. A. Trombly (Ed.), *Occupational therapy for physical dysfunction* (pp. 201-223). Baltimore: Williams and Wilkins.

Reeves, G. R. (1998). From cells to systems. The neural regulatory emotions and behavior. *Sensory Integration Special Interest Section Quarterly, 21* (3), 1-3.

Rempel, G. R., Colwell, S. O., & Nelson, R. P. (1988). Growth in children with cerebral palsy via gastrostomy. *Pediatrics, 82* (6), 857-862.

Rosblad, B., & von Hofsten, C. (1994). Repetitive goal directed arm movements in children with developmental coordination disorders: Role of visual information. *Adapted Physical Activities Quarterly, 11,* 190-202.

Rose, J., Haskell, W. L., Gamble, J. G., Hamilton, R. L., Brown, D. A., & Rinsky, L. (1994). Muscle pathology and clinical measures of disability in children with cerebral palsy. *Journal of Orthopaedic Research, 12,* 758-768.

Rose, S. J., & Rothstein, J. M. (1982). Muscle mutability: Part 1. General concepts and adaptation to altered patterns of use. *Physical Therapy, 62,* 1773-1784.

Rosenflack, A., & Andreasson, S. (1980). Impaired regulation of force and firing patterns of single motor units in patients with spasticity. *Journal of Neurology, Neurosurgery, and Psychiatry, 43,* 907-916.

Ryerson, S., & Levit, K. (1997). *Functional movement reeducation.* New York: Churchill Livingstone.

Sackett, D. L., Strauss, S., Richardson, W. S., Rosenberg, W., & Haynes, R. B. (2000). *Evidence-based medicine: How to practice and teach EBM* (2nd ed.). New York: Churchill Livingstone.

Sackett, D. L., Rosenberg, W. M., & Gray, J. A. (1996). Evidence-based medicine: What it is and what it isn't. *British Medical Journal, 312,* 71-72.

Sahrmann, S., & Norton, S. A. (1977). The relationship of voluntary movement to spasticity in upper motor neuron syndrome. *Annals of Neurology, 2* (6), 460-465.

Saint-Anne Dargassies, S. (1977). *Neurological development in the full-term and premature neonate.* New York: Excerpta Medica.

Sanders, H. N. (1990). Feeding dependent eaters among geriatric patients. *Journal of Nutrition for the Elderly, 9* (3), 69-74.

Sanders, K. D., Cox, K., Cannon, R., Blanchard, D., Pitcher, J., Papthakis, P., Varella, L., & Maughan, R. (1990). Growth response to enteral feeding by children with cerebral palsy. *JPEN. Journal of Parenteral and Enteral Nutrition, 14* (1), 23-26.

Scalzitti, D. A. (2001). Evidence-based guidelines: Application to clinical practice. *Physical Therapy, 81* (10), 1622-1628.

Schenkman, M. (1989). Interrelationship of neurological and mechanical factors in balance control. In P. Duncan (Ed.), *Balance: Proceedings of the APTA Forum* (pp. 29-41). Alexandria, VA: American Physical Therapy Association.

Schenkman, M., & Butler, R. B. (1992). "Automatic postural tone" in posture, movement, and function. *Forum on physical therapy issues related to cerebrovascular accident* (pp. 16-21). Alexandria, VA: American Physical Therapy Association.

Scherzer, A. L. (2001). *Early diagnosis and interventional therapy in CP* (3rd ed.). New York: Marcel Dekker.

Scrutton, D., Baird, G., & Smeeton, N. (2001). Hip dysplasia in CP: Incidence and natural history in children aged 18 months to 5 years. *Developmental Medicine and Child Neurology, 43,* 586-600.

Sears, T. A., & Newsom-Davis, J. (1968). The control of respiratory muscles during voluntary breathing. *Annals of the New York Academy of Sciences, 155,* 183-190.

Sharkey, M. A. (1996, January/February). Age of referral to enter intervention as a dependent factor in the acquisition of gross motor skills. *NDTA Network,* 1, 3, 5, 6-9, 10.

Sharkey, M. A., Banaitis, D. A., Giuffrida, C., Mullens, P., & Rast, M. (2002). *Neuro-Developmental Treatment for cerebral palsy–Is it effective? Developmental Medicine and Child Neurology, 44* (6), 430-431.

Shea, C. H., Guadagnoli, M. A., & Dean, M. (1995). Response biases: Tonic neck response and aftercontraction phenomenon. *Journal of Motor Behavior, 27* (1), 41-51.

Shumway-Cook, A., & Woollacott, M. (2000). Attentional demands and postural control: The effect of sensory context. *Journal of Gerontology A. Biological Science and Medical Science, 55* (1), M10-16.

Shumway-Cook, A., & Woollacott, M. H. (2001). *Motor control. Theory and practical applications* (2nd ed.). Philadelphia: J. B. Lippincott.

Silver, L. (1988). *The misunderstood child: A guide for parents of learning disabled children.* New York: McGraw-Hill.

Sinkjaer, T., & Magnussen, I. (1994). Passive, intrinsic and reflex-mediated stiffness in the ankle extensors of hemiparetic muscles. *Brain, 117,* 355-363.

Sporns, O., & Edelman, G. M. (1993). Solving Bernstein's problem: A proposal for the development of coordinated movement by selection. *Child Development, 64,* 960-981.

Stallings, V. A., Charney, E. B., Davies, J. C., & Cronk, C. E. (1993). Nutritional status and growth of children with diplegic or hemiplegic cerebral palsy. *Developmental Medicine and Child Neurology, 35* (11), 997-1006.

Stamer, M. (2000). *Posture and movement of the child with cerebral palsy.* San Antonio, TX: Therapy Skill Builders.

Steenbergen, B., Hulstijn, W., Lemmens, I. H. L., & Meulenbroek, R. G. J. (1998). The timing of prehensile movements in subjects with cerebral palsy. *Developmental Medicine and Child Neurology, 40,* 108-114.

Stein, D. G. (1998). Brain injury and theories of recovery. In L. B. Goldstein (Ed.), *Restorative neurology: Advances in pharmacotherapy for recovery after stroke* (pp. 2-66). Armonk, NY: Futura Publishing.

Stein, D. G., Brailowsky, S., & Will, B. (1995). *Brain repair.* New York: Oxford University Press.

Steinlin, M., Zangger, B., & Boltshauser, E. (1998). Non-progressive congenital ataxia with or without cerebellar hypoplasia: A review of 34 subjects. *Developmental Medicine and Child Neurology, 40,* 148-154.

Sterba, J. A., Rogers, B. T., France, A. P., & Vokes, D. A. (2002). Horseback riding in children with cerebral palsy: Effect on gross motor function. *Developmental Medicine and Child Neurology, 44* (5), 301-307.

Steward, O. (1989). Reorganization of neuronal connections following CNS trauma: Principles and experimental paradigms. *Journal of Neurotrauma, 6,* 99-151.

Stewart, D. G. (1999). Stroke rehabilitation. 1. Epidemologic aspects and acute management. *Archives of Physical Medicine and Rehabilitation, 80,* S4-6.

Stineman, M. G., A. Jette, R. Fiedler, & C. Granger. (1997). Impairment-specific dimensions within the Functional Independence Measure. *Archives of Physical Medicine and Rehabilitation, 78,* 6636-6643.

Stockmeyer, S. (2000, May). *What about tone?* Paper presented at the meeting of the Neuro-Developmental Treatment Association, Cincinnati, OH.

Stout, J. (2000a). Gait: Development and analysis. In S. K. Campbell (Ed.), *Physical therapy for children* (2nd ed., pp. 99-126). Philadelphia: Churchill Livingstone.

Stout, J. (2000b). Physical fitness during childhood and adolescence. In S. K. Campbell (Ed.), *Physical therapy for children* (2nd ed., pp. 141-169). Philadelphia: Churchill Livingstone.

Subramanian, N., Vaughan, C. L., Peter, J. C., & Arnes, L. J. (1998). Gait before and 10 years after rhizotomy in children with cerebral palsy spasticity. *Journal of Neurosurgery, 88,* 1014-1019.

Sutton, G. J., & Rowe, S. J. (1997). Risk factors for childhood sensorineural hearing loss in the Oxford region. *British Journal of Audiology, 31,* 39-54.

Sweeney, J. K., & Chandler, L. S. (1990). Neonatal physical therapy: Medical risks and professional education. *Infants and Young Children, 2* (3), 59-68.

Sweeney, J. K., & Swanson, M. W. (1995). Neonatal care and follow-up for infants at neuromotor risk. In D. A. Umphred (Ed.), *Neurological rehabilitation* (3rd ed., pp. 203-262). St. Louis, MO: Mosby.

Tang, A., & Rymer, W. (1981). Abnormal force-EMG relations in paretic limbs of hemiparetic human subjects. *Journal of Neurology, Neurosurgery, and Psychiatry, 44,* 690-698.

Tangeman, P. T., Banaitis, D. A., & Williams, A. K. (1990). Rehabilitation of chronic stroke patients: Changes in functional performance. *Archives of Physical Medicine and Rehabilitation, 71* (11), 876-880.

Tardieu, C., de al Tour, E. H., Bret, M. D., & Tardieu, G. (1982). Muscle hypoextensibility in children with cerebral palsy: I. Clinical and experimental observations. *Archives of Physical Medicine and Rehabilitation,* 63, 97-102.

Taub, E. (1980). Somatosensory deafferentation research with monkeys. In L. P. Ince (Ed.), *Behavioral psychology and rehabilitation medicine* (pp. 371-401). Baltimore: Williams and Wilkins.

Thelen, E., & Fisher, D. M. (1982). Newborn stepping: An explanation for a "disappearing" reflex. *Developmental Psychology, 18,* 760-775.

Thillmann, A. F. D., Fellows, S. J., & Garms, E. (1990). Pathological stretch reflexes on the "good" side of hemiparetic patients. *Journal of Neurology, Neurosurgery, and Psychiatry, 53,* 208-214.

Thillmann, A. F., Fellows, S. J., & Garms, E. (1991). The mechanism of spastic muscle hypertonus. *Brain, 114,* 233-244.

Thomas, S. S., Aiona, M. D., Buckon, C. E., & Piatt, J. H. (1997). Does gait continue to improve 2 years after selective dorsal rhizotomy? *Journal of Pediatric Orthopaedics, 17,* 387-391.

Trahan, J., & Malouin, F. (1999). Changes in the gross motor function measure in children with different types of cerebral palsy: An eight-month follow-up study. *Pediatric Physical Therapy, 11* (1), 12-17.

Trahan, J., & Malouin, F. (2002). Intermittent intensive physiotherapy in children with cerebral palsy: A pilot study. *Developmental Medicine and Child Neurology, 44* (4), 233-239.

Trombly, C. A., & Wu, C. Y. (1999). Effect of rehabilitation tasks on organization of movement after stroke. *American Journal of Occupational Therapy, 53* (4), 333-344.

Tscharnuter, I. (1993). A new therapy approach to movement organization. *Physical and Occupational Therapy in Pediatrics, 13* (2), 19-40.

Tscharnuter, I. (2002). Clinical application of dynamic theory concepts according to Tscharnuter Akademie for Movement Organization (TAMO) Therapy. *Pediatric Physical Therapy, 14,* 29-37.

Tuller, B., Turvey, M. T., & Fitch, H. (1976). The Bernstein perspective II. The concept of muscle linkage or coordinative structure. In G. E. Stelmach (Ed.), *Motor control: Issues and trends* (pp. 253-270). New York: Academic Press.

Turvey, M. T., Fitch, H., & Tuller, B. (1976). The Bernstein perspective I. The problem of degrees of freedom and context-conditioned variability. In G. E. Stelmach (Ed.), *Motor control: Issues and trends* (pp. 239-252). New York: Academic Press.

Valvano, J., & Newell, K. M. (1998). Practice of a precision isometric grip-force task by children with spastic CP. *Developmental Medicine and Child Neurology, 4* (7), 464-473.

Van den Berg-Emons, R. J. G., van Baak, M. A., de Barbanson, D. C., Speth, L., & Saris, W. H. M. (1996). Reliability of tests to determine peak aerobic power, anaerobic power and isokinetic muscle strength in children with spastic cerebral palsy. *Developmental Medicine and Child Neurology, 38,* 1117-1125.

van der Meer, A. L., van der Weel, F. R., & Lee, D. N. (1996). Lifting weights in neonates: Developing visual control of reaching. *Scandinavian Journal of Psychology, 37* (4), 424-436.

Van Deusen, J., & Brunt, D. (Eds.). (1997). *Assessment in occupational therapy and physical therapy.* Philadelphia: W. B. Saunders.

Van Heest, A., House, J., & Putnam, M. (1993). Sensibility deficiencies in the hands of children with spastic hemiplegia. *Journal of Hand Surgery, 18,* 278.

Van Vliet, P., Sheridan, M., Kerwin, D. G., & Fentem, P. (1995). The influence of functional goals on the kinematics of reaching following stroke. *Neurology Report, 19* (1), 11-16.

Vicari, S., Albertoni, A., Chilosi, A. M., Cipriani, P., Cioni, G., & Bates, E. (2000). Plasticity and reorganization during language development in children with early brain injury. *Cortex, 336* (1), 31-46.

von Hofsten, C., & Ronnqvist, L. (1993). The structuring of neonatal arm movements. *Child Development, 64,* 1046-1057.

von Koch, C. S., Park, T. S., Steinbok, P., Smyth, M., & Peacock, W. J. (2001). Selective posterior rhizotomy and intrathecal baclofen for the treatment of spasticity. *Pediatric Neurosurgery, 35* (2), 57-65.

Wade, D. T., & Hewer, R. L. (1987). Functional abilities after stroke: Measurement, natural history and prognosis. *Journal of Neurology, Neurosurgery and Psychiatry, 50* (2), 177-182.

Wagenaar, R. C., Meijer, O. G., van Wieringen, P. C. W., Kuik, D., Hazenberg, G. J., Lindeboom, J., Wichers, F., & Rijswijk, H. (1990). The functional recovery of stroke: A comparison between Neuro-Developmental Treatment and the Brunstrom method. *Scandinavian Journal of Rehabilitation Medicine, 22,* 1-8.

Wall, J. C., & Turnbull, G. I. (1986). Gait asymmetries in residual hemiplegia. *Archives of Physical Medicine and Rehabilitation, 67,* 550-553.

Wannstedt, G. T., & Herman, R. M. (1978). Use of augmented sensory feed-back to achieve symmetrical standing. *Physical Therapy, 58,* 553-559.

Warburg, C. L. (1994). Assessment and treatment planning strategies for perceptual deficits. In S. O'Sullivan & T. Schmitz (Eds.), *Physical rehabilitation: Assessment and treatment* (2nd ed., pp. 603-632). Philadelphia: F. A. Davis.

Wiklund, L., & Uvebrant, P. (1991). Hemiplegic cerebral palsy: Correlation between CT morphology and clinical findings. *Developmental Medicine and Child Neurology, 33* (6), 512-523.

Wilbarger, J. (1998). The emerging concept of sensory modulation disorders. *Sensory Integration Special Interest Section Quarterly, 21* (3), 3-4.

Wiley, M. E., & Damiano, D. L. (1998). Lower extremity strength profiles in spastic cerebral palsy. *Developmental Medicine and Child Neurology, 40,* 100-107.

Williams, G. N., Higgins, M. J., & Lewek, M. D. (2002). Aging skeletal muscle: Physiologic changes and effects of training. *Physical Therapy, 82* (1), 62-68.

Wilson, J. M. (1989). Outpatient-based physical therapy program for children with cerebral palsy undergoing selective dorsal rhizotomy. In T. S. Park, L. H. Phillips, & W. J. Peacock (Eds.), *Management of spasticity in cerebral palsy and spinal cord injury* (pp. 417-429). Philadelphia: Hanley and Belfus.

Wing, A. M., & Frazer, C. (1983). The contribution of the thumb to reaching movements. *Quarterly Journal of Experimental Psychology, 35A,* 297-309.

Winstein, C. J., Merians, A. S., & Sullivan, K. J. (1999). Motor learning after unilateral brain damage. *Neuropsychologia, 37* (8), 975-987.

Wolf, L. S., & Glass, R. P. (1992). *Feeding and swallowing disorders in infancy.* Tucson, AZ: Therapy Skill Builders.

Woll, S. P., & Utley, J. (2001, January/February). Forced use–A handling strategy. *NDTA Network,* 1, 4-6.

Woods, B. T. (1980). The restricted effects of right hemispheric lesions after age one: Wechsler test data. *Neuropsychologia, 18,* 65-70.

Woollacott, M. (1989). Aging, posture control and movement preparation. In M. H. Woollacott & A. Shumway-Cook (Eds.), *Development of posture and gait across the life span* (pp. 155-175). Columbia, SC: University of South Carolina Press.

Woollacott, M., Burtner, P., Jensen, J., Jasiewicz, J., Roncesvalles, N., & Sveistrup, H. (1998). Development of postural responses during standing in healthy children and in children with spastic diplegia. *Neuroscience and Biobehavioral Reviews, 22,* 583-589.

World Health Organization. (1999). *ICIDH-2: International classification of functioning and disability. Beta-2 draft, full version.* Geneva, Switzerland: Author.

World Health Organization. (2001). ICF: International classification of functioning, disability and health. Geneva, Switzerland: Author.

Yan, K., Fang, J., & Shahani, B. T. (1998a). An assessment of motor unit discharge patterns in stroke patients using surface electromyographic technique. *Muscle and Nerve, 21,* 946-947.

Yan, K., Fang, J., & Shahani, B. T. (1998b). Motor unit discharge behavior in stroke patients. *Muscle and Nerve, 21,* 1502-1506.

Zacharewicz, L. (2002). Stretch and strengthen: Use of NDT to improve functional outcomes of a patient with chronic hemiplegia. *NDT Network*, 9 (4). 1, 7-10.

Zhan, S., & Ottenbacher, K. J. (2001). Single-subject research designs for disability research. *Disability and Rehabilitation, 23* (1), 1-8.

Chapter 3

Principles and Process of Examination

"The assessment should enable the therapist to make a systematic treatment plan related to the individual patient's main difficulties and needs." (K. Bobath & B. Bobath, 1979, p. 4)

Introduction

The NDT problem-solving model guides clinicians from examination through goal setting and evaluation of intervention implementation. Because NDT focuses on the management of the posture and movement problems that limit motor functions, physical therapy (PT), occupational therapy (OT), and speech-language pathology (SLP) are always core professions in the examination and intervention process. Other professions (such as medicine, psychology, nursing, nutrition, ophthalmology, social service, and education, among others) are added depending on the client's needs, level of development or recovery, the physical setting, and the system of service delivery. This chapter describes the principles underlying the process that form the basis of assessment (examination and evaluation), goal development, and plan of care (including recommendations for intervention). Two written examples demonstrate the application of this process to the assessment of an adult with hemiplegia following stroke and a child with cerebral palsy (CP) following traumatic brain injury (TBI).

> ***NDT Focus: The problem-solving examination process is fundamental to the NDT approach and begins with the examination of the client's abilities and limitations in various contexts.***

The NDT assessment and treatment-planning process is modeled on Mrs. Bobath's teachings and writings, with changes in terminology adapted from the *APTA Guide to Physical Therapist Practice* (2nd ed., American Physical Therapy Association, 2001). Assessment consists of examination and evaluation, reflects the NDT model of enablement described in Chapter 2, and includes the information that Mrs. Bobath described in her original assessment protocol (see Chapter 5).

Figure 3.1 (which was introduced in Chapter 2) illustrates the dynamic relationships among the various parameters that NDT's clinical problem-solving model considers. The triangle represents the person with competencies and limitations; the square depicts events and contexts external but meaningful to the person. In this chapter, the circle is added to represent the global view that NDT clinicians use when assessing and planning treatment. Throughout the chapter, this illustration will help focus the reader on the importance of the interactions of the dynamic parameters, either when considering the principles or applying the process of examination and intervention.

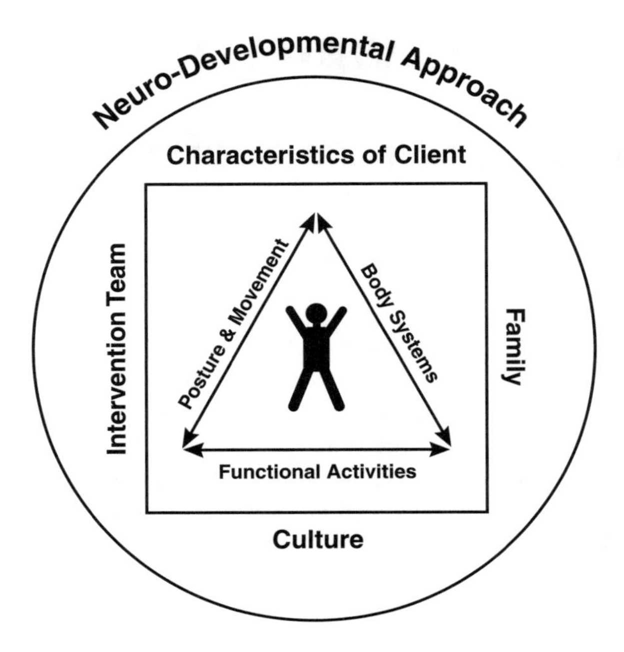

Figure 3.1. Dynamics in NDT examination and intervention.
(Illustration by Claire Wenstrom.)

Principles of Examination and Evaluation

1. △ **The NDT examination process evaluates each client as a unique person with multiple competencies and limitations.** This perspective comes directly from Mrs. Bobath (1990), who asserted that the way in which the medical/therapeutic team views the client determines the therapeutic approach to the treatment of that individual. For example, a 3-year-old child with athetoid CP who is unable to speak, but who has created and uses an informal "sign language" that his family understands, is quite competent in getting his basic needs met in his home. In this setting, at this age, he is perceived as "clever" and lack of speech is not a limitation in participating in expected family roles (Pennington & McConachie, 2001). The child's competency in developing gesture language secures his place in the family. On the other hand, a 65-year-old man who, because of a stroke, cannot speak and who has lost the spontaneity of gesture language, will be limited in communicating his needs with medical personnel in the hospital setting. In addition, he might be embarrassed to attempt alternative communication methods and, as a result could appear incompetent to his family or to medical personnel in ways that are only remotely related to the lack of speech. Neither of these individuals has speech, yet one is viewed as competent and the other as incompetent. These examples clearly demonstrate that each function or its limitation must be considered as only one part of each individual's overall competency as a person at a particular time and in a specific context.

The clinician using an NDT framework recognizes that each client is part of a family unit and has personal interests, preferences, values, and goals. This information is part of the initial data the clinician collects on the client's history and background, as well as the individual's current standing as a family and community member within his or her subculture (e.g., working-class, Italian-American family) that exists within a larger culture (e.g., northeast, urban-American culture). For an adult with stroke, his or her standing in the family and community undergoes an unexpected change after the onset of stroke. For example, a man who had been head of a household, primary financial provider, and decision maker might find himself (at least initially) to be a dependent, care-receiving family member. However, with time, he might become a more attentive grandparent, appreciative of the time he can spend with his loved ones, and develop a new and equally satisfying role in the family. In another example, a first-born child with severe CP does not fulfill the expected role of "big sister" who is able to guide and direct younger siblings, but this child can still "teach" younger siblings compassion and patience.

Various studies have shown that there is a great diversity of effects on families who have a member with a chronic disability. Lonsdale (1978) found that more than half of the families he interviewed reported marriage difficulties resulting from the birth of a child with a handicap. High rates of stress, negative feelings, and physical and mental ill health among parents of children with disabilities have been reported as well (Burden, 1980; Butler, Gill, & Pomeroy, 1978; Floyd & Zmich, 1991; McMichaels, 1971). On the other hand, the majority of the studies reviewed by Dunlap and Hollingsworth (1977) did not support the perception that having a family member with a disability has a substantial negative effect on family life. Some studies have shown that siblings of children with disabilities can actually benefit from their experience and are often well-adjusted (Grossmann, 1972; Shankoff & Hausen-Cram, 1987). In this author's personal experience, interviews with siblings of children with severe disabilities have indicated that at different times during their development, siblings expressed anger, resentment, dislike, compassion, sympathy, and understanding toward their parents and their sibling. Although it is impossible to know what might stress a particular family at any given time, the presence of a child with a disability in the family does not dictate any one effect on family life (Peterson & Wikoff, 1987). The NDT therapist does not presume that the presence of a family member with a disability disturbs the structure or function of a strong family unit. Clinicians view each family uniquely without making judgments, and support the client and the family by providing education, resources, networking with other families, and intervention accordingly.

The NDT examination process establishes an individualized care plan by gathering information that allows the clinician to get to know the client as a complete person, with likes and dislikes, abilities and limitations, and personal priorities in lifestyle. The initial data collection includes:

* Personality: motivation, cooperation, temperament, self-regulation, emotional stability, desires, and dreams

* Social and family data: education; profession; job or school experiences; social support systems; current participation in family's daily routine, educational, work, and social settings

* Personal data: the individual's level of understanding and acceptance of his or her diagnosis, learning styles, preferences, adaptability, coping strategies, attention, and self-esteem; and physical characteristics, including weight and height (age-appropriate), general strength, and endurance

* Activity data: level of and interest in activities and motor skills prior to disability (athletic, sedentary, flexible, active, or inactive in general lifestyle); current activity level, interest, and energy available for participation in family, educational, and work environments

2. △ **NDT examines each client in a life-cycle framework.** An initial examination clarifies the problems and functions of the individual at some *point in time* and therefore must consider the client's prior experiences, medical and developmental history, and projections for future changes based on age, growth, development, and the aging processes. A number of well-designed tests for adults and children can help to establish the level of function at a specific period in time and provide a basis for understanding the changes that occur with development, maturation, aging, and intervention. This chapter's section on the Examination Process describes these tests.

In addition, the life-cycle framework assumes that goals and therapeutic strategies must change over the life span to continue to meet the client's changing needs. Changes in the family and environment are a normal part of the life cycle. These contextual factors can act as facilitators of, or barriers to, the client's recovery or developmental processes. For example, divorce in a family, birth of a sibling, or moving from one community to another can have either positive or negative effects on a child with CP. A spouse's failing health can alter a significant support system for a client with stroke. In a lesser way, change of school or teacher or alteration in a family member's visitation schedule can also have an impact on motor performance. NDT intervention cannot change the family or society, but knowledge of external events enables the clinician to anticipate performance fluctuations and focus on ways to help the client adapt and make the best of a situation that cannot be altered.

For example, on a particular day during OT, Mrs. J. was not performing well in a series of activities designed to accomplish the outcomes of independence in bathing, toileting, and personal grooming in preparation for her discharge to her own home. On this day, not only was she having difficulty with the physical activities, she was unusually distracted and irritable. Finally, after several unsuccessful attempts, she burst forth with an emotional response, saying that the social worker had just informed her that her insurance would no longer pay for additional days in the stroke unit and that she was to be discharged to an extended-care facility because she did not yet have the independence to live at home with her aging husband. Later that week, she learned that her oldest granddaughter would live with her and her husband while attending a local college. During a subsequent OT session, her now-positive outlook was reflected in high energy and determination, increasing her willingness to attempt difficult activities to reach her aim of personal independence in anticipation of her discharge home. In summary, the clinician needs to evaluate "who the client is" on any given day.

> ***NDT Focus: The need to look at the impact of contextual facilitators and barriers on the individual's daily performance is an important focus of the NDT life-cycle framework.***

3. △ **The NDT examination process incorporates an interdisciplinary therapeutic management team that includes and respects the client and the family as primary and active participants in decision making.** The therapeutic management team consists of the client, family members and caregivers, therapy specialists, and other relevant professions (medical, social work, nutrition, education, etc.) as part of the team for establishing outcome goals and treatment strategies. The family is the constant in the client's life. Each family's resources and priorities define the professional's role (Kolobe, Sparling, & Daniels, 2000). The therapeutic management team is a flexible unit with core members who use input from other professionals and paraprofessionals, community resources and agencies as needed to meet the client's and family's needs. Because not all problems are identified at the same time and because secondary problems can arise later, the composition of the team–both service providers and family members–can change to reflect alterations in the client's needs. The following examples illustrate this. A child with spastic diplegia who has just had a dorsal rhizotomy needs intensive PT, but the added appointments might dictate temporarily discontinuing OT for a few months following surgery as the family commits their time to the postsurgical PT appointments. A young adult with CP now living outside the family might need a group home supervisor added as part of her team. A woman with a stroke might need a personal care assistant to help her live at home as safely and independently as possible. At all stages in the life cycle, the interdisciplinary team understands and respects the multidimensional aspects of contemporary family structures, the capabilities and limitations of the client and family members, and the availability of, or access to, other support services in the community.

In some situations, a family might not have enough information to participate fully as an advocate for their family member; thus, family education would be a top priority. In addition to knowledge about the diagnosis and expected progression of recovery or development, the family must be educated about community resources and family member's rights to access those services (Blaskey & Jennings, 1999). The initial collaboration between the family and the therapist begins a pattern of establishing the importance of the family's opinions and concerns as part of ongoing interactions between the family and professionals. As the family and client are empowered with an increase in knowledge, they become responsible for identifying and synthesizing the information they receive and can make appropriate decisions for their family unit. The collaboration between professionals and the family is mandated in the United States by public laws (Individuals with Disabilities Education Act of 1990, PL 102-119; Individuals with Disabilities Education Act [IDEA] of 1997, PL 105-17). Other countries may have parallel laws that support collaboration. More important, the trust and credibility between the family and the clinician set into motion patterns of thought and behavior that will last for years (Howle, 1999).

For example, when a child with athetoid CP is referred for SLP at age 3 or 4, the family is familiar with the diagnosis of CP and is usually able to describe the child's speech production and language comprehension, as well as oral-motor skills, and can state reasons for their desire to seek an SLP referral. However, when a pediatrician refers a child to an SLP at 2 or 3 months of age, with no clearly defined diagnosis or prognostic indicator but only a history of prematurity and failure to thrive, the family might not know what to expect of any infant at that age. They almost certainly do not understand what a SLP has to offer their irritable, difficult-to-feed, underweight infant. In another situation, the husband of a woman who has had a stroke might not know that respite care is available through home health services in the community so that he can resume his golf day, or that he can request that the OT make a home visit, prior to discharge, to assess the home so as to ensure a safe and accessible environment. Education of the family is a priority so that the family can seek the overall best care for their family member and themselves.

4. ❍ **The NDT examination begins the problem-solving process that enables the clinician to make sound clinical decisions that combine evidence from clinical research with experience and judgment**. Clinical decision making begins at the initial examination and requires the clinician to interpret clinical findings within an enablement framework, with the knowledge of clinical research results, and best standards of practice of the profession (Diamond & Schenkman, 1996). This process encompasses a complex set of tasks that moves beyond experience, learning, intuition, and judgment. At the time of this writing, the available evidence supporting various aspects of NDT offers inconsistent findings, making it impossible to objectively relate clinical decisions to expected outcomes (Barry, 2001). However, systematically gathering data in an enablement model balances the clinician's judgment with objective data. NDT uses a systematic, individualized

approach to understanding the effects of the health condition on the level of function and prognosis for each client. The NDT approach provides a flexible framework with general guidelines, but without specific prescriptions for intervention strategies, which places responsibility on the therapist to be clear about the observations of functions and their limitations and to analyze the possible system or motor impairments that can affect the client's functional abilities. During the examination and development of the care plan, the clinician analyzes the impact of each system's integrity (or impairment) on performance, the environmental demands of the selected task, and the client's capacity for performing the task (Adler, 2002). The clinician repeatedly ponders, "How do the functional activity limitations relate to the client's and family's desired outcomes?", "Is there evidence in the clinical research that I can share with the family that could help them make informed decisions?" and, "Is it possible to change functions by addressing the underlying impairments?" The NDT clinician has the responsibility to consider the individual client's values and expectations, his or her own level of expertise, and the available evidence when making decisions regarding intervention and care (Sackett, Rosenberg, & Gray, 1996).

NDT Focus: Mary Quinton initially used an analogy to describe the process of clinical reasoning: first train the "outer eye" to observe and record, then look with the "inner eye" to analyze the probable causes for what the outer eye sees. This remains a guiding principle for the process of assessing the client's problems (Bly, 2001).

5. ❍ **NDT examination and intervention incorporate principles from the study of motor control, motor learning, and motor development.** Chapter 1 covers the principles of motor control, motor learning, and motor development in detail. The following list highlights the main ideas from each area as they apply to examination and intervention.

* NDT recognizes that efficient motor control is organized around task demands and requires the interaction and interdependency of the task components, the environment, and the internal systems of the individual.

* Motor learning is an active process. The role of the clinician is to guide the client through the stages from preparation to skilled movement, focusing on strategies to optimize performance and functional outcomes.

* NDT therapists use the knowledge of motor development across the life span to respect individual differences and recognizes common and typical patterns in the developmental process that prepare and enhance skill performance commensurate with age and current ability.

6. △ **The distinguishing feature of the NDT examination is the emphasis on components of posture and movement that are efficient or inefficient in persons with stroke or CP.** This focus strengthens the problem-solving process by adding another level of analysis connecting function and individual systems. NDT recognizes that the client's ineffective postures and movements link functional limitations with system impairments. The use of atypical strategies to perform functional tasks can create ineffective posture and movement, which produce secondary system impairments; alternatively, system impairments (primary or secondary) can create problems in posture and movement, which in turn produce functional limitations. In this part of the examination, the clinician analyzes the quality of posture and movement, specifically effective or ineffective alignment, weight bearing, coordination, balance, tone, and movement combinations that are observable symptoms of motor function or dysfunction but are not in themselves either functions or system impairments.

Examination Process

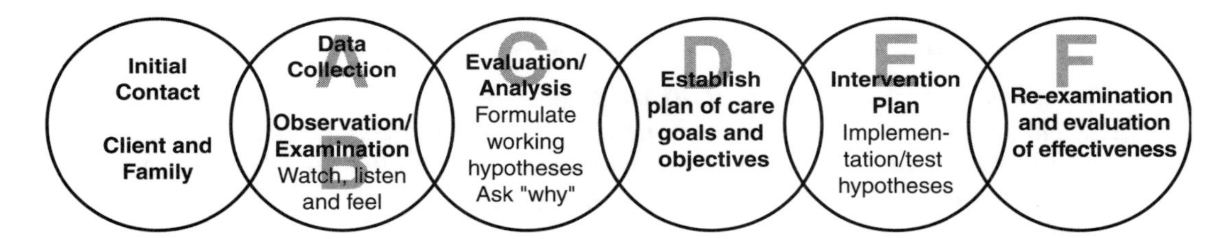

Figure 3.2.The NDT examination and treatment-planning process progresses through overlapping phases, from initial contact with the client and family through the examination, evaluation, development of plan of care, and treatment implementation. (Schematic developed by the NDT Theory Committee.)

NDT Focus: The purpose of the NDT examination is to identify the client's abilities and limitations. Identifying what the client can and cannot do leads to an optimal, individualized intervention plan and provides a basis for comparing the client's abilities at a later point in time.

Data Collection

The first part of the examination process is data collection, during which the clinician defines the scope of the problem(s) and determines the relevant procedures for examination. The initial data collection sets up the "big picture" based on the clinician's impressions of the client and family regarding *their* goals, *their* level of understanding of the diagnosis and prognosis, and *their* understanding and knowledge of the current problem. The clinician accesses this data by reviewing medical records and previous examinations, treatment plans, and educational or employment records; by interviewing the family about their questions and reasons for seeking intervention services; and by directly interviewing and observing the client. The initial data collection provides the historical and current information necessary for the therapist to hypothesize about the existence and origin of impairments or functional limitations that are commonly related to medical conditions, socio-demographic factors, or personal characteristics (American Physical Therapy Association, 2001). The information obtained in this initial stage of examination includes the following:

* **Reason for referral:** The client, family, or person making the referral generates a statement of why the client or family is seeking examination and intervention services and what is their desired outcome. For example, an adult with hemiplegia might say, "I want to regain the use of my right hand so that I can resume taking care of myself and enjoy networking on my computer." A teenager with CP heading to college might say, "I want to learn ways to maintain my flexibility and strength so I won't get tired walking on campus." A mother might say, "I want Luke to gain more strength in his hands to be able to keep up with the written work he must do in second grade and remain in his community school." Another parent might say, "I want my baby to eat and drink without choking and spitting."

* **Medical history:** For children with CP, the medical history consists of a prenatal, perinatal, and developmental history. In the case of adults with stroke, the medical history covers prior and current medical conditions, their impact on the current status of the client, and the period of time since the onset of the stroke (in intensive care unit, acute-care hospital, or inpatient stroke unit). The medical history will explain, or at least contribute to an understanding of the current health condition and chief complaints. The medical history can also provide information about coexisting health problems (e.g., the child with CP also has asthma, or the man with stroke has congestive heart disease). Such coexisting conditions often have implications for intervention.

* **General level of function:** The clinician generates a concise description of the client by summarizing observable functions in just a few sentences, such as, "Mr. Stern walks slowly with a cane and is reported to do most of his daily living skills with moderate physical assistance. He wears glasses and hearing aids and prefers familiar routines. He understands, but his speech is limited to naming objects or persons." Or, "At 7 months of age, Alexia is curious about her environment, recognizes familiar persons, communicates with sounds and facial and body gestures. She becomes frustrated when she is unable to use her hands to play with age-appropriate toys or feed finger foods. She sits when supported around the trunk, rolls from stomach to back. She has no means of independent mobility." The purpose of this summary statement is to create a brief characterization of the client so that any other health professionals, or the clinician on subsequent appointments, will be able to review the chart quickly, develop an image of the individual, and respond appropriately when meeting the person.

* **Family and environmental characteristics:** Factors such as the size of the family and household; the stability of the family's relationships and physical environment; general daily routines; cultural standards; the family's understanding of the disability and expectations for change or improvements; their concerns; and their availability and support systems, including financial, emotional, and intellectual resources.

Examination

> ***NDT Focus: During the examination phase of the assessment, the NDT therapist searches for constraints that limit the client's ability to perform functional activities.***

After organizing the available data (both the past and present) relating to why the client and family are seeking the services of therapists, the clinician begins observation and standardized testing. The examination, therefore, involves more than collecting and recording information, and includes prioritizing the client's functional problems, simultaneous analysis of the relationship to posture and movement, and generation of hypotheses about the underlying system impairments. The goal of this depth of examination is that ultimately the treatment sessions can be designed to address the client's most significant problems efficiently. The more subjective and flexible component of the examination relies on the therapist's training, skill, intuition, and knowledge, and includes:

1. Examination of the client's functional skills or limitation of skills and their impact on participation in life roles, at the present time and in anticipation of the future.
2. An in-depth look at the control of posture and movement components (e.g., alignment, relationship of base of support (BOS) and center of mass (COM), anticipatory control and weight shift, symmetry and asymmetry, movement strategies for manipulation, oral-motor functions and gait, postural tone, compensatory strategies, and the relationship of this motor dimension to function.
3. Individual systems review, which includes a brief examination of the anatomical and physiological status of those critical systems and subsystems (sensory, respiratory, gastrointestinal, cardiovascular, integumentary, musculoskeletal, neuromuscular, perceptual/cognitive, and regulatory) that contribute to functional limitations.

The following section describes the examination procedure as a linear relationship for clarity and comprehensiveness. In reality, as the examination proceeds, the therapist's methods of collecting and evaluating this data can change (often intuitively rather than deliberately), moving among the various components of examination of functions, analysis of posture and movement, and individual systems review, being led by the client's responses in the test situation.

The examination section also incorporates structured test results from norm-referenced tests, criterion-referenced tests, and/or self-referenced tests of functional abilities. This data must be collected according to the test procedures.

Functional Skills

Examination of functional skills gathers objective information about functional activities or limitations in functional activities. Functional activities consist of an individual's observable tasks or actions (World Health Organization, 2001).

The clinician observes and identifies:

* Functional abilities that can be used as a foundation for interventions that relate to the problems and goals identified by the client and family and address the question, "How can the client's positive attributes contribute to achieving functional outcomes?" For example, the client wants to be able to eat with the family, but cannot use the arms and hands independently from each other to reach for and manipulate silverware and food. The OT first identifies those sitting postures (including the support surface and special seating) that provide stability and support the client's ability to chew and swallow various liquids and solids, the individual's food preferences, and the client's desire to be part of the family during mealtime. These positive characteristics will be useful when working on the motor components needed to reach in space and manipulate silverware and food.

* Functional activity limitations. In another example, the SLP identifies activities that the client is unable to do and in what contexts. "This 75-year-old woman is unable to move food around with her tongue and cheeks so that she cannot adequately chew or clear her mouth of food when she swallows." The SLP then asks him or herself while observing, "Is this true with all textures and foods? Does this occur under all eating or mealtime conditions? Are there conditions that make this problem better or worse? Under what conditions is this activity most limited?"

NDT Focus: Assessing the capacity for change is a critical component of an NDT client examination.

* Potential to change function. Once the clinician determines what a client can do without assistance, an NDT examination *requires* the clinician to place his or her hands on the client to determine the difference between performance (what the individual does) and capacity (what the individual can do). The clinician's hands can (a) offer postural support or stability, (b) provide physical guidance for the initiation or completion of a movement sequence, (c) model the task goal, (d) constrain the temporal or spatial characteristics of the action, (e) ease the effort required during the task, (f) direct the client's attention to a particular part of the action to be carried out, and/or (g) provide the feeling of the component or sequence of posture or movements to complete the task most efficiently.

With hands on, the clinician might wonder, "Can Mrs. K get up to standing from her chair with less effort if I assist her weight shift forward? If I give her the feeling of pushing into the support, can she then do it without my assistance? If I prevent her from hyperextending her knee when she initially stands up, can she maintain this postural alignment?" Or, "Will the baby increase the amount of time he reaches forward with both hands if I provide proximal support at the shoulder girdle or guide the direction of his arms or if I set boundaries for scapular adduction and shoulder retraction? If I add toys with strong visual and auditory stimulation, will he maintain his hands on the toy and explore it?" Adding or changing various components of posture and movement through handling allows the clinician to discern the client's ability to adapt movement responses in controlled situations.

Examination of the capacity for changing function begins the process of identifying what NDT intervention methods will contribute toward achieving this client's goals. For example, "If a child with athetoid CP can reach out and take a small item when the forearm is pronated, what effect does my repositioning the object have? If I change the relationship of the child's body to the object? If I facilitate supination? If an adult can walk with a cane, what happens to postural stability and gait pattern when I facilitate weight shift and pelvic rotation at the trunk?" Evaluating the difference between performance and capacity requires that the therapist identify functional activities the client can do with the assistance of therapeutic handling, modification of the environment, or restructuring of the learning situation, and compare this to the quality and quantity of skills that the person can do unassisted.

* Clusters of critical functional activities and activity limitations with common motor or system impairments. For example, an adult with stroke sits with her head forward and back rounded during mealtime, is unable to stabilize her right arm when manipulating utensils, and makes requests for food with such a low volume that the staff cannot hear her requests for assistance. All these activities require thoracic extension, which is a critical component for stable posture, upper extremity (UE) control, and respiratory support. Clustering activities with similar movement components helps to answer the question, "What are the intermediate posture or movement goals (in this case, generating isometric thoracic extension) that need to be addressed in order to reach broad functional outcomes and improve the efficiency of therapeutic intervention?" While each therapist is working on discipline-specific functional outcomes (where, for example, the OT outcome is improved reaching during mealtime, the SLP outcome is improved speech volume when asking for food or engaging in social conversation at mealtime, and the PT outcome is improved sitting posture at the table, yet all develop strategies to improve thoracic extension), they can address a number of functions simultaneously that are related to this postural control impairment. The work of each discipline directly supports the goals and outcomes of the other disciplines.

* The relationship between the client's participation and functional activity level. For example, an adult with stroke cannot resume shopping at the mall because she tires and does not have the endurance to walk long distances. Walking, even with a cane, is functional only around the house. To increase participation, the therapist might prescribe an electric scooter for use outside the home while developing treatment methods to increase walking endurance.

Functional activities and their limitations are observed and measured by a single professional discipline or multiple disciplines. Functional activities and limitations are usually grouped into the following performance categories:

Gross Motor Control: posture and movement of the body in and through space for functional mobility (e.g., transitions, crawling, general mobility within a position, gait characteristics).

Communications: speaking, reading, facial expressions and body gesturing, signing, comprehending, and oral-motor abilities. *Note:* Clients with neuropathology often have significant oral-motor dysfunction. In such cases, oral-motor function becomes a separate category under functional skills, as described in the case-study examinations in this chapter.

Fine Motor Control or task-directed functions: reaching, manipulating and exploring objects, eating and drinking, dexterity for play, self-care skills, work, school and leisure activities.

Control of Behavior and Emotions: alertness, attention span, cooperation, tolerance for change, adaptability, perseverance, motivation, learning style, interpersonal interactions, ability to follow social rules.

Contextual Factors: Conditions and Constraints on Function. Each function is examined within the conditions and context that are most commonly linked with the action. NDT therapists understand that the environment is critical in eliciting the type of action that is functional for the client and that quality of function can vary within different environmental contexts. Altering the context allows the therapist to determine whether the client can adapt behavior and motor performance in novel situations (Girolami, Ryan, & Gardner, 2001). Depending on the setting for the examination, the clinician might initially be able to obtain this information by questioning the client, family, teacher, or other caregivers who observe the function under the most normal or frequently occurring conditions. For example, does the function of walking change outside? On grass? On concrete? On uneven terrain? In crowds? With time constraints? With changes in speed? Or, in another example, can the child wash his own hands in the bathroom at home? At school? In a public restroom? When unsupervised? With or without external support for standing?

Assistive Technology Devices. Examination of assistive technology (AT) devices is part of the examination of functional abilities. Inclusion of AT services that are mandated in the Individuals with Disabilities Education Act (Public Law 102-119, 1990) and the Technology-Related Assistance for Individuals with Disabilities Act (Public Law 100-407, 1998) presents AT as part of the contextual facilitators and barriers in the NDT enablement model. This gives credibility to the importance of this aspect of examination and intervention. Considering AT as an "adjunct to therapy" is no longer appropriate; rather, in NDT, AT is an integral part of the functional examination and treatment strategies. AT includes those items that assist the client to actively perform tasks that would otherwise be difficult or impossible, due to the underlying system impairments (Seelman, 1999). AT encompasses any useful device, such as high-tech computer-generated communication devices, adaptive seating and positioning equipment, daily and personal care items, ambulation aids, and automated learning devices (Carlson & Ramsey, 2000, Cook & Hassey 2002, De Ruyter 2002).

Various investigators have shown that appropriate selection and use of AT allows individuals with disabilities to participate in and contribute more fully to activities in their home, school, work, and community (Lunnen, 1999; Mann, Ottenbacher, Fraas, Tomita, & Granger, 1999; Miedaner, 1990; Persperin, 1990). Persperin reported a direct correlation between seating/positioning equipment and the prevention of pressure sores, orthopedic deformities, and muscle contractures; and qualitative improvement of respiration, digestion, heart rate, and functional skills. Gudjondottir and Mercer (2002) demonstrated increases in measures of bonemineral density in children who participated in an 8-week standing program using prone standers. Miedaner (1990) correlated improved speech intelligibility and vocalization, head control, self-feeding, and drinking to the use of adaptive seating and positioning devices. Various investigators have reported on the impact of walker design on the mobility of children with CP. Three different studies found that posterior walkers improved gait characteristics and produced a more upright posture during walking than anterior walkers (Greiner, Czerniecki, & Dietz, 1993; Levangie, Chimera, Johnson, Robinson, & Wobeskya, 1989; Logan, Byers-Hinley, & Ciccone, 1990).

The clinician must identify the use of the AT equipment as it relates to the client's motor functions or limitations. The range of choices of AT, the complexity of options, the availability of sophisticated technology, and the attitudes of the client and family toward the inclusion of AT in their daily life challenge the clinician as he or she determines whether AT actually has a positive affect on function.

Splinting and Orthotics. Splints and orthotics are common in the management of adults and children with neuropathology. The goal in using such devices is to improve hand function, facilitate balance in sitting and standing, change gait characteristics, or prevent the development of muscle contractures and structural deformities that affect functional skills (Girolami et al., 2001; Ryerson & Levit, 1997, De Ruyter, 2002). The NDT examination describes (a) the splint or orthotic device, (b) the structural and functional rationale for its use, and (c) the change in function (positive or negative) that results from inclusion of orthotics in the plan of care. The therapist needs to evaluate the specific need for an orthotic device and to determine its effectiveness with the same attention to functional goals as any other aspect of the plan of care (Howle, 1999). The clinician observes the client with and without the device to determine whether the device enhances the functional goal. Because slings, splints, and orthotics restrict motion at one joint in order to benefit movement at other joints, the clinician must pay attention to the overall goal, the duration of use of the device, and the potential for contributions to muscle shortening, stiffness, and weakness resulting from non-use of the splinted part (Carr & Shepherd, 2000; Howle, 1999).

Observation of Posture and Movement

Determining the posture and movement components that facilitate performance of functional activities, as well as those components that are significantly atypical during performance, is essential to the NDT problem-solving process. During the examination of functional activities, the NDT therapist searches for constraints that limit the ability of the client to perform various functions or tasks. Posture and movement functions and dysfunctions are detailed in Chapter 2 and include atypical alignment and abnormal patterns of weight bearing, abnormal muscle and postural tone, postural control and balance problems, kinesiological and biomechanical components of movement, and coordination. This part of the examination includes the following five steps.

* **The clinician notes the effectiveness of spontaneous posture and movement during functional activities within an appropriate time and place context and the frequency with which specific postural and movement components occur.** The client must have adequate time to initiate and complete tasks while the therapist analyzes the person's ability to organize and perform age-appropriate actions. The therapist identifies these components and correlates them with the overall function. For example, what interferes with independent eating? Ineffective postural stability to support the arm and hand moving through space? Limited patterns of grasp that prevent holding a fork or knife? Inability to rotate the shoulder, to supinate the forearm to bring the utensil smoothly to the mouth? Inability to coordinate chewing and swallowing with lip closure? Ineffective intralimb coordination to stop smoothly and change direction of the movement? Ineffective distal co-activation combined with reciprocal activation patterns to flex and extend the elbow? Inability to quickly adapt grasp for different utensils or to use a utensil for different purposes? Limitations in interlimb coordination that hinder cutting or managing two utensils at the same time?
* **The therapist observes the variability of posture and movement, both typical and atypical, that exists during functional activities.** Normal variation in task performance reflects both the stability of the body systems and adaptability for flexible performance. In an NDT examination, it is important to observe the client in as many positions as possible and to encourage the client to change from one position to another, noting changes in the base of support, alignment, and shifts in COM within positions and during transitions. A rich variation in posture and movement allows the selection of the most appropriate response pattern for the function that can then be softly assembled and adapted to the task-specific constraints (Hadders-Algra, 2001; Thelen, 1994). Limited postures and movements reduce fluency and can lead to secondary impairments. For example, a client with hemiplegia might be able to initiate movement only with the less-involved side, which restricts the availability of this side for postural tasks. If the client uses the left hand to reach, he cannot also use this hand to stabilize his posture. Or if this individual needs to use the less-involved side for support when rising to stand, he cannot rise to stand while holding an article in this hand. In another example, in order to look at an object or person, a child with athetoid CP moves the head and eyes together. Upward gaze is limited so that looking upward induces thrusting of the trunk and head backward into extension. Visual orientation and attending are accompanied by inappropriate changes in alignment and weight bearing (B. Bobath, 1975). These stereotypic, inflexible movement synergies are characteristic of individuals with CNS pathology. It is important for the therapist to observe variability (or lack of it) in posture and movement

during the examination because changes can be made only when the individual has sufficient flexibility to explore and select new solutions. If movements are stereotypic and limited, intervention begins with increasing movement options and variability.

* **The therapist analyzes postures and movements to determine significant missing and atypical components and the resulting compensatory movement strategies.** For example, a woman with hemiplegia cannot turn around to sit down in a chair. The therapist asks, "Why not?" Possible problems in posture and movement might be that (a) she lacks head and trunk rotation to follow visual orientation, (b) her balance is too precarious to adapt to the weight shifts needed while turning, (c) her movements are slow and laborious and require too much energy, (d) she may have rotation but does not use it because she fears falling, or (e) she is unable to scale the muscle forces appropriately to the degree of instability during the task. Other constraints on this function might include (f) the client's inability to interpret visual perception of spatial relationships and (g) an inability to allocate attention to the task when engaged in multiple activities. Any one (or many) of these components contributes to the inability to turn and sit down. The therapist's role during the examination is to consider *all* possible posture and movement components and system constraints on the functional limitation.

* **Therapeutic handling during examination gives the clinician insights into alignment, weight bearing, balance, coordination, muscle and postural tone, and movement components and can influence the client's muscle execution patterns.** A therapist can *feel* as well as see if the postural alignment is appropriate for the task and wonder, "If I reposition the client, will functional improvement follow? If I increase the BOS, will the client spontaneously demonstrate increased freedom of movement of the extremities? Is the UE paucity of movement compensatory for decreased proximal stability so that, if I support the trunk, the variety and of arm movements will increase? Do the extremities feel stiff before or during active movement? Does moving increase or decrease the stiffness? If I set limits for scapular retraction, will the client select more appropriate activation patterns for reaching? Will spontaneous use of the hands follow?" Therapeutic handling allows the therapist to *feel* the client's response to many options for changing movement strategies and provides critical information about the underlying impairments that are not fully-apparent by observation alone.

* **The therapist analyzes those components of posture and movement that constrain energy-efficient actions in settings in which the individual must function effectively**. For example, a child with ataxic CP can maintain stability in standing only by standing with excessive lumbar extension and compensating with thoracic and cervical flexion and arms and hands clasped in front to prevent losing balance backward. Because of unpredictability of force production and timing of the muscles supporting one leg, the child keeps both feet on the floor at all times and keeps the BOS wide. These children do not use rotation of the body for transitions because they cannot overcome the priority for steady-state balance that they need to maintain stability. At best they combine flexion and extension, but in only very limited patterns. Movement of the extremities or head independent of whole-body movement is almost impossible (B. Bobath,

1975; Montgomery, 2000). The energy requirements for stable posture are so high that energy is not available for tasks in a standing position.

> ***NDT Focus: The hallmark of the NDT examination is observing and feeling the way the individual executes components of posture and movement during functional skills.***

Individual System Review Related to Function

This section highlights how the individual systems affect overall motor behavior and additionally might require referral to other health professionals.

* Neuromuscular system: examination of coordinated movement for oral-motor, fine motor, and gross motor skills, including the positive and negative impairments discussed in Chapter 2; spasticity; impaired inter- and intralimb selective control; impaired synergies; insufficient force generation; timing impairments; hypokenesia; and loss of fractionated movement
* Musculoskeletal system: biomechanics, active range of motion (ROM), muscle extensibility, joint and soft tissue flexibility, strength and endurance, skeletal abnormalities, measures of physical characteristics (height, weight, bony structure, limb circumference and symmetry)
* Respiratory system: patterns of respiration, rate, breath control, capacity, endurance, rhythm of respiration and phonation, respiratory diseases, allergies, asthma, emphysema
* Cardiovascular system: heart rate, blood pressure, edema, aerobic power and endurance, measures of fitness and conditioning
* Integumentary system: skin integrity, color, mobility, scarring
* Gastrointestinal system: motility, reflux, constipation, control of bladder and bowel, peptic ulcer disease, food sensitivities or allergies
* Sensory systems: vision, hearing, gustatory, somatosensory, vestibular functions, responsiveness to sensory input and feedback
* Perceptual/Cognitive system: intelligence, memory, ability to make needs known, orientation to sensory information, executive functions, judgment, safety, adaptability to persons and places
* Regulatory system: threshold for arousal, state regulation, emotions, pain, fear, orientation and modulation of attention and interest, interpersonal interactions, appropriateness of emotional/behavioral responses
* Limbic system: emotions, pain, fear

Objective Test Results

Norm-referenced tests. NDT emphasizes the need for informal, ongoing examinations as part of treatment to identify the success of treatment strategies. However, norm- or criterion-referenced tests are used to gauge changes that occur with development, maturation, aging, and intervention. Norm-referenced tests compare an individual's performance with the performance of peers without disability, using a standard format. VanDeusen and Brunt (1997) describe many of the tests commonly used with infants, children, and adults.

* The Bayley II is a test for children from birth to 42 months. The scales contain norm-referenced motor and mental scales and a criterion-referenced behavior scale for examining affect, attention, and exploration (Bayley, 1993).
* The Test of Infant Motor Performance (TIMP) is a test for infants younger than 4 months of age. This scale defines function as the postural and selective control needed for functional movements in early infancy, including head and trunk control in supine, prone, and vertical positions (Campbell, Ostern, Kolobe, & Fisher, 1993; Campbell, Ostern, Kolobe, Lenke, & Girolami, 1995; Campbell, Wright, & Linacre, 2002).
* The Alberta Infant Motor Scale (AIMS) is an observational scale for assessing gross motor milestones in infants from birth through the stage of independent walking. This test defines function as spontaneous motor behaviors performed with a specified level of postural control (Piper & Darrah, 1994).
* The Rosetti Infant-Toddler Language Scales examine functions of parent-child attachment, play, gestures, and pragmatics as well as receptive and expressive language (Rosetti, 1990).
* The Preschool Language Scale (3rd ed.) contains norm-referenced receptive and expressive language items for children 6 months to 6 years (Zimmerman, Steiner, & Pond, 1991).
* The Pediatric Evaluation of Disability Inventory (PEDI) is standardized for children 6 months to 7.5 years and detects functional limitations and disability in age-appropriate independence. This evaluation defines function as the ability to perform activities of daily living (ADL), mobility, and social skills, which include communication (Haley, Coster, Ludlow, Haltiwanger, & Andrellos, 1992).
* The Functional Independence Measure for Children (WeeFIM) is a discipline-free test of disability for assessing functions in self-care, mobility, locomotion, communication, and social cognition. It is standardized for children 6 months to 7 years. This measure defines function as the amount of caregiver assistance needed to accomplish daily tasks. This test documents change in functional abilities in children with developmental disabilities (Granger, Hamilton, & Kayton, 1989; Ottenbacher et al., 2000).

The following are tests for school-aged children:

* The Bruininks-Oseretsky Test of Motor Proficiency evaluates gross, fine, and visual-motor control in school-aged children (Bruininks, 1978; Duger, Bumin, Uyanik, Aki, & Kayihan, 1999; Wilson, Polatajko, Kaplan, & Faris, 1995).

* The School Functional Assessment identifies strengths and limitations related to performance of school-related functional tasks (Coster, Deeney, Haltiwanger, & Haley, 1998).

* The Jebsen-Taylor Test of Hand Function simulates hand functions common to many ADL tasks and has established norms for adults and children. The original norm data included individuals with hemiplegia. This tool assesses handwriting skills and contains items that test both hands in picking up and handling large and small items (Jebsen, Taylor, Trieschmann, Trotter, & Howard, 1969; Taylor, Sand, & Jebsen, 1973).

There are numerous tests for adults addressing self-care, mobility, and fine motor skills (Zacharewicz, 2001):

* The Barthel Index evaluates function during rehabilitation. It is not particularly useful for high-functioning clients with stroke (Hsuch, Lee, & Hsish, 2001; Mahoney & Barthel, 1965).

* The Fugl-Meyer assessment of sensorimotor functions gauges upper and lower extremity functions, sensation, ROM, and balance and has been rigorously analyzed for reliability and validity (Duncan, Propst, & Nelson, 1983; Fugl-Meyer, Jaasko, Leyman, Olsson, & Steglind, 1975; Malouin, Pichard, Bonneau, Durand, & Corriveau, 1994).

* The Functional Independent Measure (FIM) was developed using the ICIDIH-2 classification of impairments, disabilities, and handicaps (now called ICF, International Classification of Functioning, disability and health) (World Health Organization, 2001). Like the WeeFIM, it measures function in areas of self-care, mobility control, locomotion, sphincter control, communication, and social cognition (Granger, Hamilton, Linacre, Heinemann, & Wright, 1993).

* The Motor Assessment Scale (MAS) measures motor and functional abilities including balance, transitions, arm and hand functions, and general tone (Carr, Shepherd, Nordholm, & Lynne, 1985; Loewn & Anderson, 1988, 1990; Poole & Whitney, 1988).

* The Porch Index of Communicative Ability assesses auditory and visual comprehension, written and verbal expression, and pantomime. This tool is valid and reliable; standardization included individuals with left and right hemiplegia (Porch, 1981).

Numerous other tests, such as the Berg Balance Scale (Berg, Wood-Dauphinee, & Williams, 1995; Berg, Wood-Dauphinee, Williams, & Gayton, 1992) and the Rivermead Mobility Index (Adams, 1993; Lincoln & Leadbitter, 1979; Wade, 1992) evaluate specific motor functions.

Criterion-referenced Tests. Criterion-referenced tests compare a client's performance to a predetermined behavioral criterion and report performance in terms of what the individual can do. Many of these tests have been designed specifically to evaluate skills in children or adults with physical handicaps and are more sensitive to changes than norm-referenced tests that are normed with typical populations (Jain, Turner, & Worrell, 1994). Although criterion-referenced tests are not normed, they do provide a way to track a client's progress over time. Mrs. Bobath taught that it was very useful to have a basis against which to compare the client's condition at later stages (B. Bobath, 1990). Examples of criterion-referenced tests for children are:

* The Gross Motor Function Measure (GMFM) gauges change over time in gross motor function in children with CP. This measure defines function as the child's degree of achievement of a motor behavior regardless of quality (Bjornson, Grauber, Buford, & McLaughlin, 1998; Bjornson, Grauber, McLaughlin, Kerfeld, & Clark, 1990; Russell et al., 1989; Russell et al., 1990).

* The Carolina Curriculum for Handicapped Infants at Risk and its companion for older children, the Carolina Curriculum for Preschoolers with Special Needs, evaluate functions in gross motor mobility, fine motor skills, social skills, communication, and self-help skills (Johnson-Martin, Attermeier, & Hacker, 1990; Johnson-Martin, Jens, & Attermeier, 1986).

* The Vulpe Assessment Battery for the Atypical Child is designed for children 0-6 years and provides information on the child's manner and degree of independence in task performance in gross motor, fine motor, communication, self-care, and educational readiness skills (Vulpe, 1979).

* The Erhardt Developmental Prehension Assessment describes hand functions in children who are delayed or atypical (Erhardt, 1994).

The following are criterion-referenced tests for adults:

* The Canadian Occupational Therapy Measure evaluates changes in the client's perception of performance and his or her satisfaction with performance in self-care, productivity, and leisure. The tool also measures client satisfaction with outcomes (Law et al., 1990; Law et al., 1994).

* The Get Up and Go test is a quick screening tool for detecting balance problems affecting daily mobility skills (Mathias, Nayak, & Isaacs, 1986).

* The Functional Reach Test examines the limits of stability when reaching forward from a standing position and is a quick screen for balance problems in older adults (Duncan, Weiner, Chandler, & Studenski, 1990).

Nonstandardized self-referenced tests. NDT clinicians test a client at the beginning and end of a single treatment session to evaluate the treatment's effectiveness in producing change in the client's posture, movement, or functional activities. This practice allows the clinician to collect and record information about changes (or lack of change) in the client's functional skills in a systematic and objective manner. It also gives a baseline measure of function at a given time, and serves as an aid to evaluating change resulting from applying a specific intervention over a specific period of time, using the client as his or her own comparison (Howle, 1999). At the beginning and end of a therapy session, for example, a clinician might note how long it takes a client to climb a set of stairs, how far a client can reach out in various directions while seated, how quickly a client can dress, how many coins a client can put in a coin purse, how long or how far the individual can walk on a treadmill, or how many words or how long a sentence a client can speak with one breath or while maintaining appropriate volume. Self-referenced testing can easily be incorporated into a single treatment session, is noninvasive, and takes very little additional time because the targeted goals or anticipated outcomes are part of the treatment. The client and the family can participate in deciding whether the goals or outcomes have been met and whether they see targeted changes. Using this approach to evaluate a single treatment session helps the clinician decide which activities to continue and which to discard for the next treatment session, depending on whether the client is making progress toward the goal or functional outcome. This informal testing is motivating to the client, the family, and the therapist by providing immediate feedback on the results of treatment. However, self-referenced tests do not provide data that directly compare outcome to intervention and are not truly objective because the tester and the client have a vested interest in the outcome. The therapist must be cautious when interpreting findings based on self-referenced tests.

Evaluation

It is essential for the NDT therapist to *observe* functions and the contributions of the body systems, efficient posture and movement, and environmental contexts, however, these observations alone do not provide sufficient information from which to form a plan of care. A clinician must be able to *describe* the relationships among various dimensions, *analyze* these relationships as they relate to the specific client's problems, and *form hypotheses* linking treatment planning and outcomes. A clinician's evaluation skills depend on appropriate blending of experience, clinical and theoretical knowledge, problem-solving skills, and insight and intuition regarding the dimensions affecting motor behavior.

Although presented here as two separate steps, examination and evaluation occur simultaneously during contact with a client. The therapist observes, listening to and watching the client; places his or her hands on the client to feel the tone of muscles at rest, their readiness to move, and their responsiveness to change; analyzes "why" the client does or does not meet task goals; watches for change in responsiveness to this therapeutic input; develops working hypotheses; explores and tests the hypotheses through handling; and continues to observe. Mrs. Bobath initially taught that this dynamic, problem-solving process occurs throughout the initial assessment, as well as during each treatment session. This process continues to provide the framework for the examination, as well as the NDT treatment approach.

> ***NDT Focus: One of the unique contributions of the NDT approach is the depth of the analysis of effective and ineffective postures and movements that link functions and their limitations to systems and their impairments.***

The evaluation consists of:

* **Statements that accentuate the client's competencies in participation in society, functional activities, effective posture and movement, and system integrity.** The list of strengths includes information regarding internal and contextual resources. Internal resources consist of all personal attributes (intelligence, interest, attention, motivation, cooperation, and self-concept), as well as posture, movement, and other body systems. External or contextual facilitators include; the family size and physical presence, interest, level of understanding of the client's abilities, family goals, energy available for interaction and therapy, and financial resources for care. Building on competencies can facilitate progress toward specific functional outcomes and movement goals.

* **Identifying and prioritizing functional limitations and participation restrictions.** For example, a teenager with CP who walks efficiently with forearm crutches is unable to attend the sporting events at his high school because even though the sports field and gymnasium are accessible, he is unable to move sideways into the bleachers and sit securely without back support to watch a game. Although this teen walks quickly and safely with his crutches, his inability to move sideways and sit securely on a narrow seat restricts his participation in age-appropriate activities.

* **Relating the critical components of posture and movement to underlying system integrity/impairments and hypothesizing how these dimensions affect functional activities and limitations and participation or restrictions in society.** This step goes deeper than observing the constraints on function and includes an analysis of the primary or secondary system impairments that are discussed in Chapter 2. The clinician asks, "Which posture and movements components appear to constrain the client's functional limitations, and which specific system impairments are the most probable cause of these motor problems?"

* **Prioritizing the structural and functional impairments of the multiple systems as they affect activity limitation.** For example, a man with right hemiplegia cannot put on his jacket because he does not have the ROM in the right UE, lacks proactive and reactive balance while sitting, has motor planning and visual (hemianopsia) problems, and cannot time and coordinate muscle activation patterns of dexterity needed to change his grip patterns while moving his arms through space and through the sleeves. All of these are important impairments, but this individual cannot change the timing and coordination of muscle synergies if ROM is not first available and he does not have a stable posture to permit him to safely lift his arms from a support and move them through space.

* **Analyzing the potential for change.** The clinician assesses the client's ability to alter posture and movement, which the clinician determines through therapeutic handling and by changing elements in the environment during the examination. The clinician also evaluates structural constraints, such as effects of surgery, contractures, or deformities that prevent change. For example, Robert had a triple arthrodesis of his right ankle at age 14, which limits mobility in all motions of this ankle. This affects his ability to push

off during gait. The therapist must also anticipate the development of further impairments, additional problems in posture and movement, and functional limitations based on the typical recovery process and progression of the disorder with growth, development, and aging. This appraisal includes the primary neuromuscular and musculoskeletal impairments, as well as secondary behavioral, cognitive, perceptual, and biomechanical components of the musculoskeletal system and social and environmental barriers. Is it possible to reduce impairments through intervention? Is it possible to prevent secondary impairments or deterioration in function? Will changing impairments result in improved function?

The process of first enumerating strengths and then describing problems enables the therapist to focus on the unique qualities of this individual, even in the face of obvious limitations, and to utilize the individual's strengths when selecting intervention strategies.

> ***NDT Focus: NDT examination has always focused on what the patient can or cannot do, the quality (accuracy, coordination, efficiency, quickness, and effectiveness) of the performance, and the potential for change. In Mrs. Bobath's words, the clinician must "find, obtain and develop any potential . . . which is being neglected." (B. Bobath, 1990, p. 24).***

Plan of Care

The plan of care consists of statements that specify the anticipated goals and expected outcomes, predicted level of optimal improvement, specific interventions to be used, and proposed duration and frequency of the interventions that are required to reach the anticipated goals and expected outcomes (American Physical Therapy Association, 2001). The plan of care is the culmination of the data collection, examination, and evaluation process. The clinician interprets the results of the examination and evaluation in collaboration with the client and the caregivers (family, teachers, and others), then determines outcomes and goals that are meaningful to the client, based on typical and age-appropriate movement function, and the impact on future development.

The following items are the elements of an NDT plan of care:

1. Recommendations for intervention in a care plan follow each discipline's best standard of practice. The plan of care identifies and prioritizes critical impairments and functions that can be addressed in NDT treatment and includes measurable outcomes and goals of the intervention. The recommendations for intervention include the frequency and duration. The treatment plan incorporates client and family education along with the development or modification of client-centered programs based on the individual's lifestyle.
2. The team sets functional outcomes and goals. The client (when appropriate) and family, along with all the therapy disciplines involved in the examination, write

functional outcomes and goals based on the identified functional abilities and limitations. *Outcomes* refer to the functional activities that the team, including the family and client, anticipates that the client will achieve. *Goals* refer to changes in individual systems or system interactions (Diamond & Cupps, 2002). For example, when the anticipated functional outcomes are determined in the care plan, it is important to know what systems, posture, and movements contribute to achieving these outcomes. For a client to accomplish the *outcome* of getting out of bed without assistance, the individual must meet *goals* of adequate muscle strength, postural control, weight shift, and movement synergies that combine flexion and extension with rotation, as well goals of other systems, including motivation and attention to the task to safely achieve this outcome. It is important to set specific and measurable goals as well as outcomes. The therapists can then set the frequency and duration of intervention that will be optimal to achieve these goals and outcomes.

3. The clinician identifies strategies the client is currently using to accomplish functions, as well as broad strategies that might be more energy-efficient or successful in preventing the development of additional impairments. Girolami et al. (2001) and Kolobe (1992) suggested that the clinician develop recommendations for therapeutic management of a given client, then present this list of alternatives to the family. The recommendations would cover all appropriate options, including the use of adaptive equipment, assistive technology, orthoses, medication, and surgery, as well as various service models, such as clinic-based individual or group therapy, consultative, or home-based models that would allow the family to select the program and methods to achieve the "best" outcome that works for the individual situation. For example, a child currently gets around at school with a posture walker, however, this is slow, energy- and time-consuming, and limits the distance the child can go with classmates. The teacher and family want to consider a wheelchair for long distances and playground use, but at the same time, the family does not want to compromise on the long-term goal of ambulation. The therapist believes that walking is an important consideration for maintaining flexibility, reducing the potential for contractures, and maintaining physical fitness and self-image; and the child wants to be with friends. The physical or occupational therapist is consulted in the process of selecting appropriate equipment that can meet all these needs. This process considers availability, materials and construction, source of funding, portability, stability, ease of adjustment, ease of modification, and aesthetics (Wilson, 1993, Cook & Hussey 2002). Other considerations include the available space in the environment to store the equipment, the client's and caregivers' ability to manage and maintain the equipment, type of vehicle to transport it, lifestyle of the family, and typical activities and settings in which the equipment will be used (Lunnen, 1999). The therapist lists the options and discusses these with the client and family. Together they decide if a manual or power chair will provide the most energy-efficient mobility for the child in these various settings without limiting the child's potential for ambulation.

4. The care plan identifies measures to promote health, wellness, and fitness and provides means to prevent functional decline, secondary impairments, and need for additional services. This often addresses the issue of pain, mobility, and strength that limit the participation of adults with physical disabilities in society and affect the quality of life (Campbell, 1997; Jones, Molloy, Chamberlain, & Tennant, 2001).
5. The care plan describes the role of family and other medical and educational professionals involved in the care. The plan of care states specifically who is responsible for various parts of the program. The various family members might be responsible for transporting the client for the intervention program and/or directly involved in carrying out specific treatment strategies and providing practice opportunities. Classroom teachers might be responsible for opportunities for practice in the school setting and scheduling time in the school day for a specific therapy program. Although these roles are described in the plan of care, the therapist must make certain that the care plan is updated as roles and responsibilities change. For example, a mother cannot provide the same intensity of support when a second child is born; a spouse can become more directly involved when he retires from full-time employment; and a sibling can become responsible for transportation at the time he or she obtains a driver's license. Although it is ideal for each family to participate actively in carrying out specific activities with the client and thus expand the settings for practice, not all families are capable in this role, and therapists cannot expect any one family to be capable of actively carrying out specific therapeutic activities throughout the entire life span of the client.
6. Re-examination is an ongoing part of the plan of care, and the schedule is stated as part of the care plan. This could consist of formal standardized examination determined by the model of service within a designated time (e.g., all babies in the special infant care program will be reexamined on the TIMS at 2 and 4 months of age) or informal (e.g., the speed and distance of walking, including use of equipment and orthoses, of all clients with stroke will be recorded when they enter the rehabilitation unit and again when they are discharged). Additionally, NDT clinicians continually evaluate the effect of treatment throughout a session. At the end of each session and after a series of sessions, therapists also re-evaluate to answer the questions: Have the functional outcomes been achieved? Have impairment-related goals been met? Are treatment strategies optimal? These questions lead to additional questions: Is there a need to re-evaluate the relationships among impairments, functional activity limitations, and the client's and family's desired outcomes? Do the hypotheses formulated at the evaluation level need to be revised? Do functional outcomes and/or impairment-related goals need to be revised? If the client has achieved the outcomes, therapy can be discontinued, or new outcomes can be added. If the client has not achieved them, do treatment strategies need to be altered? Is there evidence that the client cannot meet the outcome objectives? Is there a need for referral to other professionals?

Writing up anticipated outcomes and goals provides an opportunity for objective communication between the family and the therapeutic team. All outcomes are written up to assist in demonstrating measurable, observable changes in functions as a result of the treatment intervention, even when the testing is self-referenced. Goals state changes in system or motor impairments. Frequently goals and anticipated outcomes are described together. For example, "During treatment today, while seated on a small bench so that her feet were planted on the floor, Becky was able to maintain her balance and successfully pull her T-shirt off over her head. Two weeks ago, she lost her balance as soon as her vision was occluded by the T-shirt and she could not complete the task." Such statements encourage the child and present the family with realistic expectations for progress. The expected functional outcome is consistent with the client's age, developmental status, and family concerns. Any outcome or goal, whether long-term, short-term, or single treatment, is stated in terms of a specific activity or function that the client will accomplish and defines the circumstances and environment in which the outcomes and goals will be evaluated. The inclusion of specific performance conditions (time, duration, speed, environmental conditions, etc.) allows objective assessment of the outcome and goals by the treating therapist or any other person. Words such as *better, worse,* or *improved* are not acceptable in written goals and objectives.

Third-party payers and the model of service delivery often define short- and long-term outcomes and goals, as well as frequency and duration of treatment. For the client in an acute-care hospital following stroke, the short-term outcomes will include functions that the person can accomplish before discharge to home or a rehabilitation setting, however, the length of stay might be determined by the person's health-care plan. For a child in school, the short-term outcome might be determined by the individual educational plan (IEP) with times for re-examination built in, whereas the frequency and duration of treatment might be determined by the availability of a therapist. Short-term outcomes and goals are particularly useful to make certain that the intervention is on target, and if not, to prevent the loss of valuable treatment time by helping the clinician to revise outcome goals or change treatment strategies (Palisano, 2000).

Case Studies:
Examination, Evaluation, Plan of Care

This section uses case studies to illustrate the application of NDT theory and principles to the process of NDT multidisciplinary examination and care-plan development. These case studies give examples of the NDT problem-solving process, which begins with client examination. Notes in *italics* allow the reader to follow the decision-making process that the clinicians used during the examination. The first case is a child with CP following TBI at 1 year of age; the second case is a 75-year-old man, 5 weeks post stroke on admission to an outpatient rehabilitation program.

Case 1: Child With Cerebral Palsy

Name: Megan

Date of Birth: 5/12/95

Date of Examination: 12/3/01

Diagnosis: Right hemiplegic, level III, CP secondary to TBI

Examiners: Loren Arnaboldi, M.A., CCC; Judith Bierman, PT; Gail Ritchie, OTR/L

Data Collection

Reason for referral: The family sought an evaluation by this NDT multidisciplinary team to gain a realistic understanding of Megan's performance and capabilities. In addition, they asked the team to make recommendations for future therapies.

Medical history and background: Megan was born following a full-term, uncomplicated pregnancy. Her development followed a typical progression until age 1 year, at which time she received a traumatic brain injury. Since that time, she has been involved in intensive rehabilitation, including occupational, physical, and speech and language intervention, as well as special education, music therapy, hippotherapy, and aquatic therapy. At age 2 1/2 years she began attending a therapeutic preschool with typically and atypically developing children. She will continue to attend this program for half days for the remainder of the school year. Results of a hearing test indicate that her hearing is normal. Vision has also been evaluated and at this time glasses are not recommended.

Overview of Function: Megan is a happy, social child who interacts readily with adults. She reportedly enjoys music, singing, and watching Barney and Sesame Street. She is able to attend to a program for 30 minutes. Megan demonstrates good receptive language skills, although not at an age-appropriate level, and is able to communicate by pointing, gesturing, or bringing an object to an adult or vice versa. She can walk using her quad cane, but requires assistance to get to a standing position with it. She often scoots on the floor to move around a room. She can cruise next to furniture.

Megan's typical day begins at 6:00 a.m. after sleeping well through the night. Her morning routine includes assisting in toileting, hygiene, and dressing. She reportedly is able to self-feed with a fork once her plate is set up, and she drinks from a cup. She takes a bus to school at 7:45 and is in school until 2:30. At school, a one-on-one aide provides physical assistance for motor activities and helps her focus attention to the critical aspects of motor and cognitive tasks. After school she attends outpatient therapy or adjunct after-school activities.

Family and home routine: Megan lives at home with her parents, younger sister, and older brother. Her grandmother is nearby and serves as a resource for the family on a regular basis. Her father owns and operates a small business. Her mother was a special education teacher, but has stopped working to better provide Megan with the services that she needs to reach her potential. Both parents are knowledgeable about the extent of Megan's limitations and prognosis. They are particularly hopeful that she will gain understandable speech, and they recognize this as a major problem as she gets older and needs to interact with persons outside the family and preschool.

At this time, Megan wears bilateral dynamic ankle-foot orthoses (DAFO). One is an ankle-foot orthosis (AFO) style and one a supramalleolar orthosis (SMO) style. They fit well. She has a resting/positioning UE splint for the right that she wears at night. She does not have a wheelchair and is transported in a double stroller with her younger sister. She utilizes a quad cane that her grandfather fabricated from PVC piping. She has no other adaptive equipment or assistive devices.

When asked her desired outcome from this examination, Megan's mother indicated she wanted a realistic assessment of Megan's capabilities. She and Megan's father are particularly interested in discovering ways in which Megan can improve her attention, articulation, and comprehension skills; increase the use of her right hand for self-care and school skills; and become more independent in mobility, particularly getting up to standing and when walking.

The PT, OT, and SLP were present during the entire examination. Megan was engaging and interacted comfortably with all the team members. Her parents described the motor and social behaviors she exhibited as typical of daily performance.

Note: *During the initial data collection, it was apparent that Megan's comfort level was the result of previous intervention and positive interactions with various therapists. This contributed to the ease with which this team was able to gather information. Although the NDT team might not agree with all aspects of previous or ongoing intervention, it is important not to undermine the confidence that the family has placed in previous therapists and to focus on the current status of the client and how NDT intervention might contribute at this point to additional improvements in function.*

Examination

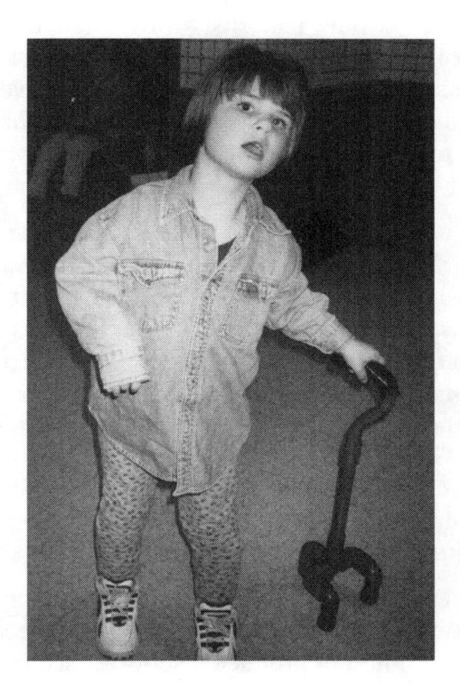

Figure 3.3. Six-year-old Megan ambulates cautiously with a quad cane, given predictable surfaces, few distractions, and familiar environments.

Morphology

Megan is an attractive, well-proportioned 6-year-old girl. Height and weight measurements were not taken today. Her legs are symmetrical in length at 21 inches. The circumferences of her arms and legs are symmetrical. Examination of the peripheral oral mechanism revealed that her maxillary arch is not fully developed, but her bite is characterized by normal alignment of her molars.

Functional Tasks

Gross motor/control of the body in and through space. Megan moves independently from prone and supine to sitting on the floor. She typically sits in a modified long-sit position and moves around the floor by scooting in a sitting position using her left arm and leg. With effort, she can pull up to a bench and, with the physical assistance of the PT during the exam, she was able to turn and seat herself. She is unable to pull to standing independently; however, once standing she can balance without her cane for a few seconds. She can take steps with her quad cane for support, but is unable to negotiate obstacles in her pathway. She does not routinely move up and down off the floor independently or initiate walking.

Fine motor/task-related skills. Megan participated in all presented play activities utilizing age-appropriate reaching and grasping patterns with the left UE only. Object exploration included raking, patting, poking, tilting, and shaking. She turned the pages of a book and attempted to imitate crayon strokes and spoon-fed a doll. Given verbal or physical cues, she engaged the right hand to assist the left and brought the right hand to midline to transfer objects from her right hand to the left when a toy was placed in her right hand. She was able to release a variety of small toys accurately and demonstrated various pinches with the left hand only.

Activities of daily living. Megan willingly assisted in donning and doffing clothing to the best of her ability. She was able to remove her jacket and shirt after the fasteners were detached and her right UE was removed from the sleeve. She was able to doff her socks and her pants once they were pulled down over her knees. Megan completed the last phase of shoe and brace removal. She assisted with donning her clothing by pushing her left UE through the sleeves of her shirt and jacket. Megan reportedly participates in a toileting program at home and school. She remains dependent in hygiene and doffing her pants. She requires assistance to engage the right hand to wash her hands. She is dependent in bathing. She is able to self-feed using a spoon and fork, once set up. She needs supervision during mealtime because she frequently overstuffs her mouth and is at risk for choking.

Oral-motor skills. Megan eats most food consistencies and drinks regular liquids from a cup and through a small straw. She demonstrated no difficulty coordinating the suck/swallow with her breathing, but she did not produce a series of sequential suck/swallows while drinking.

Communication. Megan's receptive communication skills are characterized by alerting and attempting to localize both non-speech and speech sounds. She appears easily distracted by extraneous environmental noises and maintains focused attention to an activity for less than a minute. The examiners were frequently successful in redirecting Megan to activities with simple verbal prompts. Megan demonstrated recognition of several body parts and familiar objects when named by the examiner. Megan responded to simple verbal commands involving familiar routines, but when presented with less familiar actions or novel objects, she required additional visual or physical prompts to respond appropriately. She did not respond to commands involving more than one step.

Megan's expressive skills are vocalizations and gestures to gain attention, indicate pleasure or distress, and request objects. Her vocalizations exhibit changes in pitch and intensity. She produces vowel sounds requiring either a low or posterior tongue position (i.e., "o," "uh," "aw," "ah"). The consonants require either lip closure (i.e., "b," "m"), posterior tongue placement (i.e., "k," "g"), or limited tongue elevation (i.e., "y" as in "yuh"). Megan appeared to enjoy vocal play and repeated her utterances when a clinician imitated her vocalizations. The only identifiable words were "yeah" and "baby." Although Megan frequently shook her head when excited, on several occasions she appeared to be shaking her head to indicate "no." Other communicative gestures included pointing, offering objects, and waving. No symbolic gesturing (i.e., sign language) was observed, and no other non-vocal communication strategies were explored during this examination.

Social/Behavior. Megan presented as a happy, social child who readily engaged with the therapists during the examination. She maintained attention to play for a short time, but demonstrated frustration when activities did not go well for her.

Tests and Measures

Test results. The PEDI, GMFM, and Preschool Language Scale-3 were administered. The standard scores on the PEDI were all below 4 standard deviations, indicating that Megan was performing significantly below expectations for her age in self-care, mobility, and social functions, which includes speech and language. Her scaled scores showed a distribution consistent for a child with a significant physical disability and additional systems impairments, resulting from widespread neuropathology. The scaled scores are more appropriate than the standard scores for charting progress during therapy because her standard scores were so low that they are not likely to be sensitive to changes that can be expected in a reasonable time frame.

Domain	Raw Score	Normative Standard Score	Scaled Score
Self-Care	34	<10	51.7
Mobility	22	<10	44.3
Social Function	13	<10	37.0

Table 3.1. Pediatric Evaluation of Disability Inventory (PEDI) Composite Scores

By exploring Megan's movement capabilities in a variety of positions, the GMFM added information regarding ineffective posture and movements that underlie Megan's functional limitations. This test clearly indicated that she has significant problems in antigravity activities that require postural control, various aspects of balance, and integration of movements of the two sides of her body.

Dimension	Score %
A. Lying and rolling	86
B. Sitting	90
C. Crawling and kneeling	50
D. Standing	23
E. Walking, running, jumping	20
Total Score	54
Goal total score (C, D, E)	31

Table 3.2. Gross Motor Function Measure (GMFM) Summary Scores

The Preschool Language Scale-3 provides specific information regarding engagement in structured tasks, processing auditory/visual information for responding to verbal directions, comprehension of language concepts, and the production of words and phrases for functional communication. Megan's results clearly indicated significant functional limitations in communication skills, both receptively and expressively, and were consistent with the global impairments identified by the PEDI.

Communication Skills	Raw Score	Standard Score	Percentile Rank	Age Equivalent
Auditory Comprehension	16	50	1	1 yr. 7 mos.
Expressive Communication	15	50	1	1 yr. 7 mos.
Total Language Score	31	50	1	1 yr. 7 mos.

Table 3.3. Preschool Language Scale-3

Note: *Because the family was seeking a second opinion regarding realistic prognosis for change, the therapists felt it was particularly important to include objective examination data.*

Examination of Posture and Movement During Functional Tasks

Note: *To gain information about posture and movement, the therapists use direct handling to combine observations of functions with the information gained by feeling the weight shifts in anticipation of movement and effort and initiation of muscle activity as the client attempts various activities. This handling provides critical information about the underlying impairments that is not fully apparent from observation alone. The therapists' correlations between what they see and what they feel are the foundation from which they begin to hypothesize about the underlying causes for the client's posture and movement difficulties.*

Relationship of COM and BOS: Megan tended to keep a wide base of support and position her COM somewhat lower to the BOS and slightly to the left side when sitting or standing.

Alignment: Megan did not align herself equally over her base of support. This was particularly apparent in the frontal plane. She typically held her head tilted to the left. She had pelvic obliquity with the pelvis retracted on the right side, contributing to LE asymmetry. She held the right UE in humeral adduction or horizontal abduction, internal rotation, elbow flexion, wrist flexion, and ulnar deviation, with the hand fisted. Her movement was very asymmetrical, using the left side for movement and the right side to compensate for the lack of proximal stability. She did not spontaneously engage her right UE in functional activity. This deficit appeared to be related to her asymmetric neural lesion rather than a secondary problem developing with growth and changes in body mass because muscle atrophy and bone shortening were not evident.

Anticipatory control and weight shift: Megan did not demonstrate any ability to anticipate the need for postural adjustment prior to a task that involved changing her COM relative to her BOS. She was often unable to initiate movement with the appropriate body part for the task, frequently initiating movement through space with a lateral shift of her head.

Movement components: Megan confined most of her movements to small, unvaried excursions of flexion and extension without axial rotation. When the therapist facilitated these movement combinations as Megan seated herself on a bench or moved into a sitting position on the floor, Megan was able to change her movement patterns, demonstrating the potential for change under these conditions.

Muscle tone: Hypertonus in the flexor muscles of her arm and hand contributed to abnormal positioning of her UE, with internal shoulder rotation, elbow flexion, pronation, and wrist and hand flexion. This stiffness increased with activity and the effort to balance and move in standing. Right LE stiffness resulted in excessive co-activation at the knee and ankle, limiting her stride length and speed of swing phase of gait. Excessive stiffness added to the inability to adapt muscles in preparation of movement.

Spasticity could be elicited in the ankle plantar flexors, hip adductors, and elbow and wrist flexors, but this did not account for much of the stiffness in the extremities, which was evident without changes in velocity.

Movement synergies and compensations: Megan's movements were limited in variety, more so on the right side than the left, but this limitation was also evident on the left side. The shoulder girdle remained strongly linked to postural control, with the scapula and humerus moving as a single unit. Her feet were held in postures of plantar flexion and eversion, which were linked to extensor posture of the LEs. In standing, she compensated for lack of steady-state balance and postural control with genu recurvatum. She had a habitual open-mouth posture with slight lip/jaw retraction and her tongue spread to press against her upper molars in attempts to compensate for instability (see figure 3.3). She was able to adjust the tension in her lips and cheeks to move food over her teeth for chewing and demonstrated tongue spreading and tilting to both sides, but did not exhibit more mature lateral movements of her tongue, including discrete movements of her tongue tip. It was apparent that encouraging Megan to actively alternate between positions combining movements in all three planes has been a focus in therapy and for her family because she was comfortable and cooperative when the therapists facilitated changes in her habitual movement strategies or inhibited her compensation patterns. Although she did not combine movements spontaneously, she did not have any muscle contractures or skeletal deformities that might result from such limited movement options.

Gait analysis: This examination did not include a comprehensive gait analysis. However, the team noted that she had marked asymmetry in step length and stance time. There was short stance on the right, as well as short stride so that the right foot never stepped in front of the left. The right hip was held in a position of retraction. The right foot then was in a position of external rotation compared to the line of progression. She was not able to make accommodations in her gait for even small obstacles in her path. She was unable to make quick changes in direction or speed. She was insecure because balance and reliable visual information were unavailable during progression. The use of a quad cane shifted her BOS to the left.

Note: *The PT made the decision not to include a comprehensive gait analysis at this time because Megan was not walking in functional settings and the characteristics of her gait pattern were very inconsistent. The only way she would walk for the examiners was with her quad cane, and that added an artifact that did not seem consistent with her other patterns of movement. The PT decided to wait until Megan was comfortable with walking without the quad cane to see if her COM would be more appropriately placed within her BOS. Although the inconsistencies in her walking pattern indicate that she is capable of change, and therefore changing her gait is an appropriate goal for PT, the data available for examination purposes is not reliable.*

Examination of Individual Systems

Neuromuscular system. Major impairments were noted in the neuromuscular system, directly related to her TBI. These impairments in motor execution constrained functional skills.

Ineffective postural control and balance: Megan demonstrated difficulty anticipating the postural forces necessary for controlling her body's position in space to achieve orientation and stability against the force of gravity. Inefficient balance affected movement in all positions. She sought additional postural stability by adding flexion of the UE, excessive use of the scapular muscles and quadratus lumborum and even tongue spreading instead of depending on proximal dynamic stabilization of the trunk muscles. She was resistant to moving outside her BOS and confined most of her spontaneous movements to small, unvaried excursions of flexion and extension without axial rotation. This strategy limited movements available for transitions, balance, and skilled UE movements. Generally, she was unable to activate balance in advance of a potentially destabilizing movement in order to avoid instability, and was unable to recover from an unexpected perturbation. She was not able to generate the muscle forces appropriate to the degree of instability to control her position in space.

Note: *The therapists decided to include the examination of postural control under the neuromuscular system rather than as a component of posture and movement because Megan's lack of control of posture and dynamic balance appeared to be directly related to cerebellar damage secondary to her TBI.*

Impaired movement strategies: Megan had restricted variability in movement strategies and limited movement repertoires that further restricted the information she could obtain about her body and her environment. She initiated most movement with her left side. Any movement on her right side was limited to predictable synergies with limited active joint excursion during the movement. Her right arm was consistently held with flexion of the elbow and wrist. Effort decreased the range, speed, and variability of movement options. Because she was unable to adapt her movement strategies to the task, she frequently used strategies that were inefficient and energy-consuming.

Atypical inter- and intralimb control: Megan was unable to move the joints of the LEs independent of each other, and movements of one LE were strongly linked to movements of the other so that flexion of one hip was coupled with flexion of the other. Effort to move the LEs produced a flexion synergy of the right UE, particularly when standing and walking. Within one LE, knee flexion was coupled with dorsiflexion and knee extension with plantar flexion. Similarly, she evidenced decreased ability to isolate movements of the eyes from the head and the head from the trunk. Movement of the left UE produced flexion of the fingers and wrist of the right UE. This overflow of activity in multiple muscles interfered with normal reciprocal relationships during purposeful movement and prevented the ability to stabilize with one body segment while moving another.

Lack of dissociated or fractionated movements: Lack of dissociated movement of the fingers and thumb of the left hand prevented refined coordination of grasp and manipulation. She had no ability to use the digits of the right hand independent from one another or without associated movements of the left hand. Loss of fractionated movements of the oral-motor structures limited her ability to accurately produce discrete sounds for speech.

Abnormal co-activation: Agonist and antagonist muscles activated simultaneously during eccentric and concentric contractions in the extremities, which prevented normal synergies needed for quick, accurate movement. Megan used this increased joint stiffness to assist with stability in standing, but this strategy hindered normal amounts of knee flexion during swing phase of gait. Excessive co-activation prohibited midrange control, particularly with respect to axial rotation. She had great difficulty in eccentric control of muscles, relying instead on excessive isometric holding. Decreased co-activation of the trunk muscles for postural control resulted in excessive use of muscles of the scapula and pelvis to stabilize against the force of gravity.

Abnormal Timing: Megan had limited ability to initiate, sustain, or terminate movement to adapt self-initiated movements to the requirements of the tasks. Increased reaction time resulted in her inability to initiate movement quickly once she desired to move, and increased movement time affected her ability to recruit the appropriate muscles or to execute a movement within the time appropriate for a task. These timing problems affected acceleration and deceleration of movement as well as the spatial components of movements of the right UE and both LEs.

Extraneous movements: Extraneous movements interfered with functional abilities. Megan had small lateral oscillations of her jaw paralleled with a lateral oscillation of her eyes. In addition, she frequently demonstrated a slight proximal tremor, which increased with postural challenges.

Note: *Extraneous movements, including tremor and nystagmus are frequent findings in clients with TBI. For this reason, a separate section discussing these issues is included in Megan's examination.*

Musculoskeletal system

Range of motion:

1. Passive ROM at all LE joints measured within normal limits except for right ankle dorsiflexion with knee extension, which was limited to 5°.
2. Limitations in end range in shoulder flexion, elbow extension, and forearm supination were noted but not measured.
3. Active ROM was limited in all attempts to produce movements in the right UE. It was increasingly difficult for Megan to obtain the end range of active movement when she exerted excessive effort. Slow active ROM produced increases in active range in the fingers and wrist of the right UE.

Strength: Muscle strength was not measured because there are many factors that interfered with spontaneous or directed use of individual muscles. Marked weakness in the right UE was evident when Megan attempted any active movement. Decreased force production, combined with stiffness in her right hand, limited all spontaneous or directed use of this hand. On the left, she could not easily alter the power of grasp or release adapted for the task, but this was also related to neuromuscular impairments. She could not sustain power to maintain hip control in the LEs for gait. She had poor endurance and could not repeat movement without deterioration in the quality. There was no muscle atrophy.

Muscle stiffness: During functional activities, the therapist felt dynamic stiffness in all muscles of the right UE when Megan initiated movement or when the joints were moved passively. Spasticity could be elicited with rapid passive movements of the ankles and hip adductors, but this did not account for most of the muscle stiffness that interfered with active ROM. Stiffness appeared to involve muscles but not the joints, as indicated by normal range of passive movement in the left UE and LE with no joint contractures. However, this excessive stiffness appeared to interfere with Megan's active ROM in all right UE movements and gross active movement of the right LE. In addition, stiffness was apparent in the oral mechanism, with increases in stiffness related to the effort to speak or move or with laughter or other emotions relative to the task presented.

Note: *The examiners felt that stiffness, rather than spasticity, interfered with Megan's postures and movements. According to her mother, the stiffness Megan exhibited on examination was more than the stiffness she experienced when doing these same activities at home. The examiners felt that Megan's desire to perform well and her insecurity in this unfamiliar setting with new examiners contributed to the excessive stiffness seen on this day. The therapists will continue to assess stiffness as Megan becomes familiar with the team who work with her on a regular basis.*

Sensory systems

Somatosensory: Megan was unable to register or discriminate somatosensory information throughout her right UE and LE, as noted by her under-responsiveness to input, the inability to perceive light and deep touch, and to use somatosensory information to alter posture, most notably her head-trunk alignment. Megan demonstrated an overall neglect of her right UE. She also did not respond to light tactile stimuli in and around her mouth. She often required strong input to her trunk to obtain a change in alignment.

Vestibular: Megan's vestibular system appeared compromised by her inability to stabilize her head and eyes and her decreased midline control and balance. However, by report, she does enjoy vestibular input and does not demonstrate any adverse reaction to play on a swing or merry-go-round on the playground.

Vision: Testing indicated normal visual acuity. Her gaze was compromised by her inability to stabilize her eyes when moving her head. Given external stability at her head and neck, she was able to track objects horizontally from the periphery across the midline. Megan also exhibited a midline eye jerk and blink during this activity. Diagonal and circular tracking were difficult. She was able to converge and diverge between near and midspace, but had difficulty organizing her vision for far space. She tilted her head toward the left to gain stability for visual tracking. Changes in the environment were distracting for Megan, and she appeared unable to pick up or prioritize the important visual cues for functional skills.

Auditory: Megan's hearing had been tested previously, and today Megan demonstrated auditory thresholds within normal levels. She alerted to and localized sounds of interest, particularly familiar people talking. She tended to be easily distracted by environmental sounds, but she was able to respond to auditory cues to bring her back to task.

Sensory modulation: Megan's arousal state fluctuated between high and low levels of alertness. At times she required increases in input to respond, while at other times only minimal input was necessary. She was visually and auditorially distractible, which caused difficulty in maintaining her attention to complete a task.

Cardiovascular system. Megan showed signs of poor distal supply. Her feet were cool to the touch, and both feet and her right UE were slightly red in comparison to the rest of her body color. The exam did not include specific measures of heart rate with postural changes and activity. These tests should be done to establish a base for cardiovascular fitness and endurance. Megan's mother expressed concern about Megan's easy fatigability and low endurance.

Respiratory system. Megan used primarily a belly-breathing pattern. She was able to shift into a thoracic breathing pattern required by activity. Resting breathing rate was 15 breaths per minute. Breathing rate during activity was not measured. She had more active mobility of the rib cage on the left than on the right. She demonstrated breath holding to achieve postural stability. Although most of Megan's vocalizations were short, she demonstrated several examples of extended vocalizations without any unusual effort and consistently exhibited easy onset of voicing.

Perceptual/Cognitive system. Megan had been tested for intelligence and the results indicated that she functions below age level in all areas tested. Cognition impairments were complicated by Megan's limited attention, speech, and language problems described in this examination. She was unable to allocate attention appropriately when engaged in multiple activities. She could solve simple tasks, but had difficulties interpreting information from her environment and the task that would permit generalization and application to more complex situations. These problems were evident in general motor tasks and oral-motor tasks. She demonstrated memory based on repetition and practice. She exhibited real difficulties in executive functions, such as the ability to set goals, anticipate and plan safe movements, and inhibit unwanted behaviors based on anticipated consequences.

Note: *Even at this point in the examination, the therapists felt that progress in motor skills would be limited by her attention and cognitive abilities. The interdependency and interactions between the motor and cognitive systems would be included in the discussion with her family to assist them in understanding the rate of change in functional skills they could expect.*

Evaluation

Client Strengths

1. Visual and auditory acuity that support interactions with people, tasks, and varying contexts
2. Adequate passive and active ROM for all age-appropriate functions
3. Functional strength for standing and play
4. Ability to move through environment independently, which supports exploration and experimentation
5. Capacity to engage briefly in play independently and with adults
6. Ability to communicate with gestures and pointing and initiate interactions with others
7. General curiosity and motivation within her physical and cognitive abilities
8. Social child, eager to cooperate and please adults; high frustration tolerance

Contextual Facilitators

1. Supportive, realistic parents who understand Megan's successes, challenges, and progress and who place a high priority on continued intervention
2. Older brother and younger sister who enjoy Megan for who she is
3. Extended family that supports parents and Megan
4. Financial resources to provide services and equipment for Megan
5. General family lifestyle that includes Megan's therapeutic appointments and schedule

Areas of Concern

Functional Limitations

1. Short attention span for teaching/learning situations
2. Inability to communicate with speech
3. Dependent in all areas of self-help
4. No functional household or community ambulation
5. Inability to assume standing from chair sitting
6. Inability to use hands to engage in age-appropriate play, especially with age-matched peers

Posture and Movement Problems

1. Asymmetry in alignment and inability to anticipate and adapt her body alignment necessary to support movement execution
2. Decreased use of LEs as an adaptable BOS
3. Inability to spontaneously reposition her COM within a moving BOS
4. Inability to shift weight to the right in anticipation of movement synergies for effective movement
5. Poor coordination of movements, including efficiency, accuracy, reliability, adaptability, and quickness
6. Limitations in motor planning
7. Abnormalities in postural and muscle tone, including hypertonus, hypotonus, and spasticity

Impairments

Neuromuscular system: Abnormal co-activation, impaired movement strategies, impaired selective control of patterns of muscle activation with loss of inter- and intralimb isolated control, loss of dissociated movements, extraneous movements, ineffective postural control, abnormal timing of muscle activation

Musculoskeletal system: Muscle stiffness, decreased active ROM, weakness

Sensory system: Decreased somatosensory awareness on the right side, unreliable visual attention and perception, increased auditory distractibility, inconsistent sensory modulation

Regulatory system: Inconsistent arousal and attention states, labile emotions

Respiratory system: Atypical respiratory patterns, breath holding

Perceptual/Cognitive system: Decreased executive functions; inability to set goals, solve complex problems, and adapt behavior based on consequences

Contextual Barriers

1. Megan's distractibility
2. Lack of aid in classroom

Summary

Megan is a 6-year-old girl with multiple and complex impairments that significantly limit her functional abilities. She has definite asymmetries in all postures and with all movements. She is motivated to play and explore her environments and has a very knowledgeable and supportive family. Consequently, she is likely to make consistent progress with a coordinated intervention plan. At this time, she probably will require PT, OT, and SLT services on a weekly basis. The intervention will most likely need to continue periodically throughout her life span. Such therapies will support her ability to gain independence in ambulation, greater communication with a wide variety of individuals, and increased independence in activities of daily living, as well as help decrease the likelihood of developing secondary impairments such as scoliosis, hip dislocation, or UE contractures. She is an excellent candidate for therapeutic intervention.

Note: *The therapists noted that Megan and her family were not new to the intervention process and acknowledged the need to intensify therapy now because commitment to a therapy program would become increasingly difficult as she got older and the demands of her educational program increased. The family decided to dedicate this next year to making improvements in the motor areas, which they (and the therapists) felt would directly affect her functional independence and the choice of learning environments.*

Expected Functional Outcomes (discipline-specific)

Physical Therapy

Long-term outcomes: 1 year

1. Megan will ambulate independently without an assistive device for distances of 10-20 feet in familiar surroundings.
2. Megan will move from the floor to standing with her quad cane, independent of additional physical assistance.
3. Megan will ascend and descend at least 15 steps with her left hand on the rail and close stand-by guarding.
4. Megan will ambulate 200 feet outdoors with her quad cane.
5. Megan will be able to get in and out of the family vehicle with assistance, but without lifting by the caregiver.

Short-term outcomes: 3 months

1. Megan will get up from bench sitting to standing with her quad cane with only verbal prompts.
2. Megan will step up a 1-inch rise with assistance from her quad cane.
3. Megan will walk with her quad cane between rooms, making turns of 90° to either direction to follow her mom or caregiver.

Speech and Language Therapy

Long-term outcomes: 1 year

1. In a structured setting, Megan will produce tongue-tip sounds (t, d, s) in individual words 80% of the time, given models, visual cues, and tactile prompts.
2. Megan will spontaneously produce three, two-word utterances during engagement in a one-on-one play interaction while sitting quietly, pairing expressive communication with activities.
3. Megan will produce simple signs involving the left hand moving in relation to the right, given postural support for sitting and visual/tactile cues for the signs, 20 times per session.
4. Megan will complete a three-step play sequence involving the combination of at least two objects, given postural support for sitting and visual/tactile cues for the steps, 10 times per session.

Short-term outcomes: 3 months

1. Megan will accurately imitate a vocalization containing pitch and vowel change during reciprocal play to link sounds with objects and events, given tactile/visual cues that facilitate alignment and independent head movement, 60% of the time.
2. Megan will produce a tongue click, given postural support for sitting and visual/tactile cues for tongue placement, 10 times per session.
3. Megan will produce a two-handed gesture to request an object or activity, given somatosensory cues to the right arm and hand at least once in each session.
4. Megan will complete a two-step play sequence involving the combination of two objects, 10 times per session.

Occupational Therapy

Long-term outcomes: 1 year

1. Megan will carry a light-weighted basket of toys to her play area without loss of the bilateral grasp, walking at least 15 feet.

2. Megan will place her jacket over her right UE and pull the jacket on, requiring assistance with the fasteners only.
3. Megan will doff her pants over her hips and seat herself on the toilet with stand-by assistance only.
4. Megan will complete a six-dot-to-dot picture using her right UE as a stabilizer.

Short-term outcomes: 3 months

1. Megan will pull her jacket over her right UE once her hand is through the sleeve.
2. Megan will complete a four-dot picture using her right UE as a stabilizer with visual cueing to perceive the sequence of the dots.
3. Megan will push her pants down from her hips, once started, and seat herself on a regular toilet using a small step.
4. Megan will fasten her pants/jacket using anterior hook-and-pile fasteners independently.

Impairment-Related Posture and Movement Goals (all disciplines)

1. Megan will demonstrate increased symmetry in weight bearing in sitting and standing postures.
2. Megan will align her head relative to her body, grading her head movements in all planes appropriately for the task.
3. Megan will demonstrate typical, effective co-activation of the head, neck, and trunk for central control of posture.
4. Megan will demonstrate increased awareness of the posture and movement of her right UE during all structured activities.
5. Megan will demonstrate increased variety of spontaneous movements as she moves in sitting and between postures, leading with either the left or the right side, as appropriate.
6. Megan will demonstrate increased isolated movements between her UEs, using swiping and batting movements of the right UE while keeping the left UE quiet, and increased precision and dexterity of patterns of grasp, manipulation, and release of the left UE while keeping the right UE quiet.
7. Megan will demonstrate effective, discrete oral movements with graded control of her head movements in all planes.
8. Megan will incorporate axial rotation when moving in sitting and upright postures.

Plan of Care

1. The family has decided to pursue private, clinic-based therapeutic intervention in addition to Megan's school program. The caregiver who brings her will attend and participate in each session, as appropriate. Activities in all disciplines will pair posture and movement with age-appropriate functional skills, including play. Strategies to increase Megan's attention to and organization of her behavior will be stressed in all therapeutic settings to increase the application of her repertoire of posture and movement to many settings. At the end of each session, the therapist will discuss with the family how to incorporate into daily life at home those activities that have been successful and to set up practice opportunities. The clinician will provide the family with activities they can do at home that fit into their lifestyle and daily routines. Services among educators, therapists, and medical management will be coordinated to ensure that all areas of need are being addressed with a similar approach, but not duplicated.

2. Megan will receive PT one or two times a week for 60-minute sessions. Intervention will be provided in a one-on-one format, in a contained space with limited environmental distraction. Sessions will stress gait training as well as independent transitions from the floor to standing. The PT will monitor equipment such as AFOs and assistive devices for fit and use.

3. Megan will receive OT two times a week for 60-minute sessions. Treatment will focus on increasing use of both UEs for refinement of fine motor and adaptive skills. The clinician will address the use of a right UE splint.

4. Megan will receive SLP two times a week for 45-minute sessions. Treatment will focus on accurate imitation of an increasing variety of sound combinations, discrete oral movements, and demonstrating understanding of two-step directions during play.

5. Megan will be informally re-examined in 3 months to determine if the therapeutic strategies are appropriate for realizing the short-term posture and movement goals and functional objectives described here. The team will re-examine her using standardized measures in 9 months.

Case 2: Adult With Stroke

Name: Mr. Ron Winkler

Date of Birth: 11/25/1925

Date of Examination: 10/27/01

Diagnosis: Right hemiplegia, dysphasia secondary to CVA, onset 9/16/01

Examiners: Monica Diamond, M.S., PT; Laura Gaudynski, OTR; Heidi Ruedinger, M.S./CCC-SLP

Data Collection

Reason for referral: The inpatient rehabilitation team at the time of discharge recommended that Ron continue with a program to develop right UE function and independent ambulation. Speech was also recommended. Ron and his wife, Lorraine, pursued this recommendation. Ron reported that he was most interested in regaining use of his right arm and hand, improving his speech, and walking.

Note: *It is the policy of this program that all staff initially address each adult client as "Mr.," "Mrs.," "Ms.," or "Dr.," as they introduce themselves, and then ask each client how he or she wants to be addressed. This procedure makes certain that clinicians do not offend clients or family members by assuming any particular level of informality. The Winklers had asked the staff to use their first names when Ron was hospitalized following his stroke. This examination continued that practice.*

Medical history and background: Prior to the CVA, Ron was a relatively healthy, 75-year-old retired man living with his wife. At the onset of his stroke, Ron was admitted to an acute-care hospital and received medical management for the ischemic infarct with right hemiparesis and dysphasia, his primary pathophysiology at that time. Additional pathophysiologies included chronic atrial fibrillation, Type II diabetes, and cardiomegaly. Ron also had a history of problems with his left eye over many years (strabismus, glaucoma, and retinal detachment) and had little vision in that eye since birth. Ron's acute hospital stay was 3 days, followed by admission to an inpatient rehabilitation unit. On admission to that unit, he was medically stable and was taking medication for diabetes and high cholesterol as well as digoxin, coumadin, and a diuretic for his blood pressure. He remained in the rehabilitation unit for 4 weeks.

At discharge from the rehabilitation unit, he performed bed mobility with verbal cues and stand-by assistance, basic transfers with minimal to moderate physical assistance, and car transfers with a sliding board and moderate assistance from his wife. He could propel his wheelchair on level surfaces. He had begun walking with a quad cane in the protected setting of the rehab therapy department, but required moderate physical assistance for balance and right LE advancement.

In ADL, Ron performed upper-body bathing with verbal cues and use of a long-handled bath sponge. Lower-body bathing required physical assistance. Shaving and teeth brushing required only set-up. He required physical assistance with toileting and tub transfers.

Ron's dysphasia demonstrated rapid and relatively functional recovery during his rehab stay. He had begun demonstrating more independent use of strategies to increase volume and intelligibility while speaking; however, he continued to speak using residual air and demonstrated difficulties with timing and sequencing of breathing and voicing, as well as oral-motor weakness. His diet had no restrictions.

Overview of function: Upon admission to this outpatient program, Ron is alert but socially reserved, a characteristic reported by his wife to be his general makeup. He is interested in regaining the movements and skills necessary for independent function. He demonstrates functional receptive language and cognitive skills. Although his voicing is often inaudible, he tries hard to be understood and is not hesitant to repeat if not understood. He cannot move his right arm or hand independently against the force of gravity. He is unable to walk unassisted, but propels his wheelchair with his left extremities.

Contextual factors/family and home routines: Ron and Lorraine provided the information about his progress at home. They live in their ranch-style home with adult children and friends nearby. Prior to retirement, he had worked as a manufacturing supervisor and since retirement had increased the time he spent with hobbies such as woodcarving. Ron enjoyed yard work, wood carving, ushering at church, and travel to their cabin in the north. His wife was primarily responsible for cooking and indoor homemaking activities. In general, they report that Ron is doing well since discharge and, although he is not independent in any area, they both feel he needs less assistance as he practices new ways to function at home. Although he seems to be mildly depressed, he is always willing to participate in therapy and, with the assistance and encouragement of his wife, follows through with exercises and activities at home as instructed. He is on a general diet, but needs his food prepared and cut up in order to manage with his left hand. Lorraine reports that she can usually understand him, although she frequently has to ask him to repeat what he said, partly because of his low volume and her mild hearing loss. She is willing and able to assist in transfers from bed to wheelchair and to his recliner, so he seldom spends time in his wheelchair except for ADLs in the morning and to get from place to place in his home. He gets dressed every day and spends most of his time in the den because the living room is "sunken" and he cannot negotiate the step. He eats his meals at the dining room table, because he is unable to sit at the breakfast bar as he had prior to the stroke. Fortunately the bathroom is wheelchair-accessible, and he can sit for grooming functions. At this time, Ron and Lorraine find the daily routine to be quite time consuming for both of them. They are still adjusting to the change in their lifestyle. Friends, two adult children, and three grandchildren, all who live in the area, have visited several times and are willing to help transport him for additional outpatient therapy. They have discussed going to a restaurant, but have not done so because Ron needs help with car transfers and needs the wheelchair to get from the house to the car and into the restaurant and because he is embarrassed when his wife must cut up his food in public. They will wait until transfers are easier and Ron and Lorraine are more comfortable with them before they attempt to go anywhere that is not a required outing. To aid his independence at home, the rehab hospital has provided a raised toilet seat with arms, bathroom grab bars, tub transfer bench, sliding board, prefabricated right AFO, wheelchair, right wrist splint, rocker knife, elastic shoelaces, and a long-handled bath sponge.

Note: *Even as the therapists collected this data regarding participation and participation restrictions, they began to prioritize the various functions that would allow Ron to participate in activities that were important to him and his wife. It was apparent that intervention needed to address his motor impairments in order to develop functional skills. The therapists pondered these questions: "Are there ways that Ron can become more active even with such limited motor control? What is his potential for motor recovery? What positive characteristics can be used to develop the motor components? What will be motivating to the client? Are there ways to vary the task and the environment to enhance his function at home in ways that are consistent with Ron's and Lorraine's goals and priorities?"*

Ron and Lorraine are concerned with the amount and speed of recovery that they can expect over the next few months. Although both are optimistic, his wife is concerned that he might become depressed if progress is slow. Antidepressants had been considered during his rehab stay, but with all the medications he is taking for other system impairments, Ron and his wife decided not to add another drug at this time. They expressed interest in finding ways to decrease his dependence on his wife. Lorraine, who had not done much driving before Ron's stroke, hopes he will be able to drive again, but more important to them is gaining independence in his home, specifically using his right arm and hand and walking around the house in order to participate in various aspects of the daily routine and the activities he enjoys.

Examination

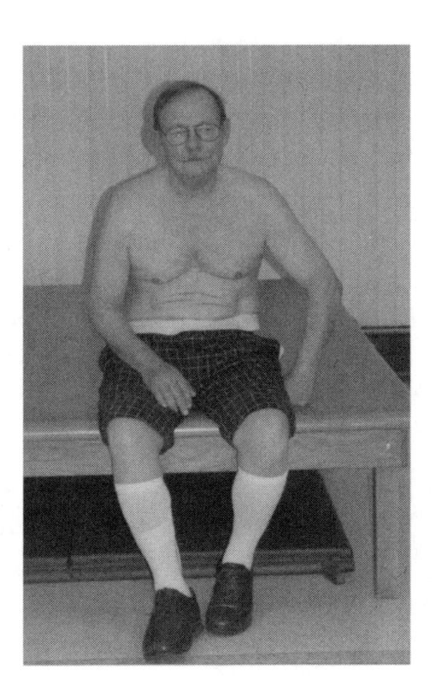

Figure 3.4. At the time of admission to the outpatient program, Ron's postural muscles remained inactive and movement was initiated through his left side.

Morphology

Ron has an average build, is not overweight, and was generally active before his stroke. He has kyphosis of the thoracic spine with abduction of the scapulas, but this is typical of his age. The appearance of asymmetry is due to the lack of tone and movement since his stroke. There is no muscle atrophy nor are there joint contractures.

Examination of Functional Skills

Gross motor/control of the body in and through space. This is a significant problem area for Ron. He moved to the side of the mat and sat up with supervision but no physical assistance. This was very energy consuming, however. He propelled his wheelchair on level surfaces and maneuvered it to position himself at a table. He could not get up from his wheelchair to stand, transfer from one surface to another, or walk unaided. He required physical assistance when moving his entire body against gravity, but could move his left extremities and partially lift his right leg. He rarely adjusted his position unless a task demanded a postural adjustment.

Fine motor/task-related skills. Ron was unable to do any function with the right arm and hand. It was noted, via interview and observation in the clinic, that Ron used his left UE for stabilization and manipulation of objects and did not incorporate the right UE for any task. He was right-handed before his stroke, and attempting to do all functions with the left hand produced awkward, inefficient, and energy-consuming effort. When presented with forms to sign or items of clothing during the examination, Ron attempted to stabilize the material and manipulate the object with his left hand, including signing his name slowly with his left hand. He seldom spontaneously incorporated the right side for any task. When asked to assist with the right, he initiated the movement by hiking his shoulder or leaning to the left, which were the only options he had. If he needed to move the right arm for safety reasons, or as part of a gross motor function, such as moving from supine to sit, he did so by lifting his right arm with his left.

Activities of daily living. During the examination, Ron assisted with dressing and grooming using his left arm and hand if the clothing and articles were set up for him and he was in a seated position. He needed physical assistance for toileting. Additional daily activities were reported by Ron and Lorraine and are described in the section detailing his home routines.

Oral-motor skills. Ron is on a general diet and by report can eat most foods that he enjoyed before his stroke. He demonstrated some problem with swallowing thin liquids and tended to cough, but these problems were mostly resolved by the time of his discharge from the inpatient rehab program. Breath support for speech was limited, and volume was low. Asymmetry in the face muscles was apparent, and he was observed to chew foods with the teeth on the left side. Tongue protrusion showed asymmetry.

Communication. Ron spoke in short phrases. He had occasional word-finding problems. His voice was often inaudible, and articulation was sometimes unclear. Length of verbalization was limited by inadequate breath support.

Social/Behavior. Ron interacts appropriately with the therapeutic team. He maintains attention and attempts all tasks. He persists even when tasks were difficult. Affect is somewhat flat, but he appears to be invested in the therapeutic activities. Problem-solving skills appears appropriate at the intermediate and advanced level when observed in a structured setting.

Note: *As the therapists examined functional skills, it became clear that communication and cognitive skills were strengths that could be used to develop the sensorimotor areas. The therapists began to note relationships among functions that could be the basis for intervention.*

Tests and Measures

Test results. The Functional Independent Measure Profile (FIM™) was completed when Ron was admitted to the inpatient rehabilitation unit and again at discharge, just prior to his admission to the outpatient rehabilitation program. The results indicate the need for assistance in all functional skills in the motor areas, with greater independence in communication and social/cognition areas. This confirms the findings during the informal, systematic examination.

FIM PROFILE

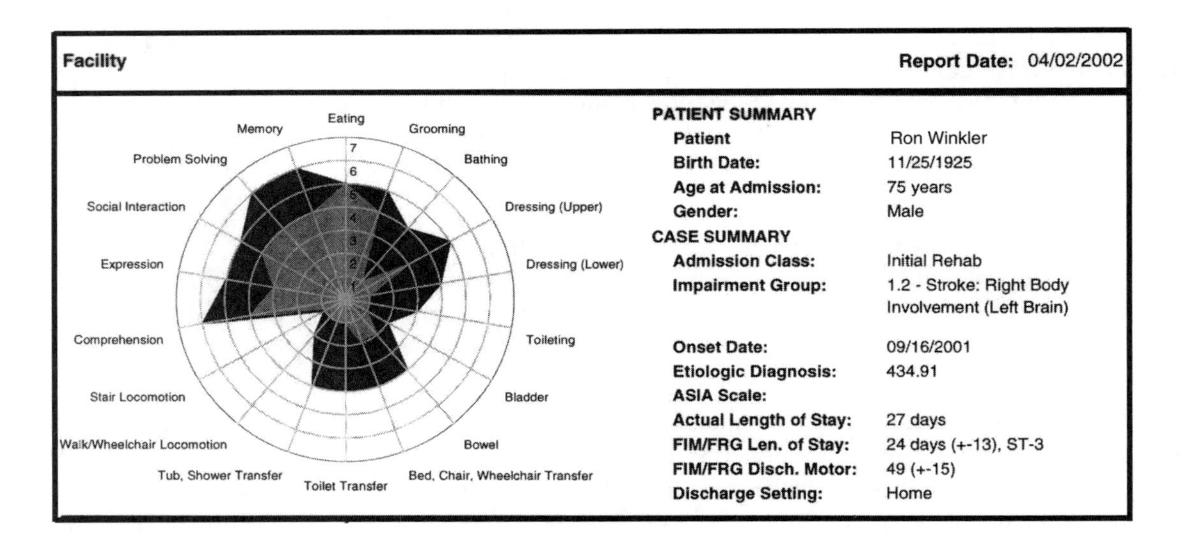

Facility **Report Date:** 04/02/2002

PATIENT SUMMARY

Patient	Ron Winkler
Birth Date:	11/25/1925
Age at Admission:	75 years
Gender:	Male

CASE SUMMARY

Admission Class:	Initial Rehab
Impairment Group:	1.2 - Stroke: Right Body Involvement (Left Brain)
Onset Date:	09/16/2001
Etiologic Diagnosis:	434.91
ASIA Scale:	
Actual Length of Stay:	27 days
FIM/FRG Len. of Stay:	24 days (+-13), ST-3
FIM/FRG Disch. Motor:	49 (+-15)
Discharge Setting:	Home

FIM Levels

No Helper

7 Complete Independence (Timely, safely)

6 Modified Independence (Device)

Helper - Modified Dependence

5 Supervision (Subject = 100%)

4 Minimal Assistance (Subject = 75% or more)

3 Moderate Assistance (Subject = 50% or more)

Helper - Complete Dependence

2 Maximal Assistance (Subject = 25% or more)

1 Total Assistance or not testable (Subject = less than 25%)

FIM is a service mark of the Uniform Data System for Medical Rehabilitation

FIM Assessment:	1	2
Legend:		
Encounter:	Inpatient	Inpatient
Type:	Admission	Discharge
Date:	09/19/2001	10/16/2001
Self Care		
A. Eating	5	5
B. Grooming	4	5
C. Bathing	1	4
D. Dressing - Upper Body	3	5
E. Dressing - Lower Body	1	4
F. Toileting	1	3
Sphincter Control		
G. Bladder Management	1	2
H. Bowel Management	2	4
Mobility		
I. Bed, Chair, Wheelchair	2	4
J. Toilet	1	4
K. Tub, Shower	1	4
Locomotion		
L. Walk/Wheelchair	1	2
M. Stairs	1	1
Motor Skills Subtotal	**24**	**47**
Motor Skills Average	**1.8**	**3.6**
Communication		
N. Comprehension	4	6
O. Expression	3	5
Social Cognition		
P. Social Interaction	4	5
Q. Problem Solving	4	6
R. Memory	4	6
Cognitive Skills Subtotal	**19**	**28**
Cognitive Skills Average	**3.8**	**5.6**
FIM Total	**43**	**75**
FIM Average	**2.4**	**4.2**

Table 3.4. FIM™ profile for Ron Winkler. (Reprinted with permission from the Uniform Data System for Medical Rehabilitation, Buffalo, NY, 14214: State University of New York at Buffalo; 1997.)

Examination of Posture and Movement During Functional Tasks

Note: *As in Megan's examination, the therapists used direct handling to combine observations of functions with the information gained by feeling alignment, initiation, and effort required to move in order to hypothesize causes for the client's posture and movement impairments.*

Abnormal tone/spasticity. There was little evidence of spasticity except in the flexors of the elbow and unsustained clonus at the ankle. Clonus was evident in the ankle when the ankle was passively dorsiflexed. Weight bearing did not activate clonus. The postural tone in the right LE was not adequate to support normal weight distribution over his two feet when standing. Inadequate postural tone in the trunk and the right LE interfered with attempts to bear weight fully on the right LE, resulting in malalignment throughout the trunk, shifting of his trunk to the left due to the inadequate support from the right LE, and inability to maintain right knee extension during stance.

Relationship of COM to BOS. Ron was stable in sitting, although his alignment was asymmetrical and he was unable to change the relationship of his COM to his BOS to orient for various tasks such as reaching while sitting. In order to achieve postural control in standing, he widened his base of support, shifting his COM over his more stable left side (see Figure 3.5). This strategy limits movements available for activities such as balancing to perform ADL tasks, or stepping to perform transfers.

Anticipatory balance (proactive) and weight shift. Ron did not demonstrate an ability to anticipate the need for postural adjustment prior to tasks that involved changing his COM relative to his BOS. He initiated movement from the head and upper trunk or with the left UE from an initial posture with his weight shifted to the left side, instead of using finely graded movements within the trunk in anticipation of weight shift. He sometimes substituted momentum rather than active control to bring his COM over his BOS when changing positions (as in moving from sit to stand).

Alignment. In sitting or standing, Ron did not align himself equally over his BOS in the frontal or sagittal planes. When he attempted to come to stand from sitting, he did not realign his COM over his feet, but instead kept his weight behind his feet and therefore was unable to complete this task without assistance or requiring several attempts and the use of momentum.

Equilibrium (reactive-balance). Ron was able to recover balance if his weight was displaced slowly and for short distances to the left. With further displacement, he was able to use a protective response of the left UE, but was unable to produce an effective equilibrium response through the trunk due to difficulty activating and shortening the right lateral trunk flexors. He could not recover balance if displaced rapidly or with wide excursions to the right. He did not have independent balance in standing and did not use stepping or in-place equilibrium strategies while standing.

Movement strategies. Ron had a variety of movement strategies available with the left extremities. He spontaneously used various strategies to get himself from supine to sitting or to move in supine. Although he used his left arm and leg actively to assist with all tasks, inadequate postural control limited the effectiveness of the left side as well as the right. Active movement was limited on the right side (arm movements were more limited than leg movements), and Ron frequently used strategies that were not effective in combining postural control with movement execution of the right side, particularly the right UE. However, when the therapist facilitated strategies that were not his usual patterns, he followed manual and verbal cues, varying his posture and movement in ways that were not part of his usual repertoire.

Note: *This ability to respond to facilitated movement indicated to the examiners that Ron had the potential to change his functional abilities and would be an appropriate candidate for NDT intervention. Indications of his ability to respond included: his ability to recruit muscles when conditions were optimal, even though he did not activate them under his "normal conditions," his willingness to try movements that he perceived as "unstable" when requested to do so by the therapist, his relatively good sensation, which allowed him to correctly perceive the therapist's manual input, and his ability to adapt in new situations.*

Coordination. Ron could not combine movements of the two sides of his body for bilateral or alternating movements even when the individual movements of these body parts were available. Movements that involved coordinating the entire body appeared awkward, uneven, and inaccurate. He could not perform complex tasks that required executing two movements at the same time, such as talking while moving from sitting to standing or washing his hands while controlling posture in a standing position. Sequential movements lacked fluidity and had the quality of separate steps rather than a continuous action.

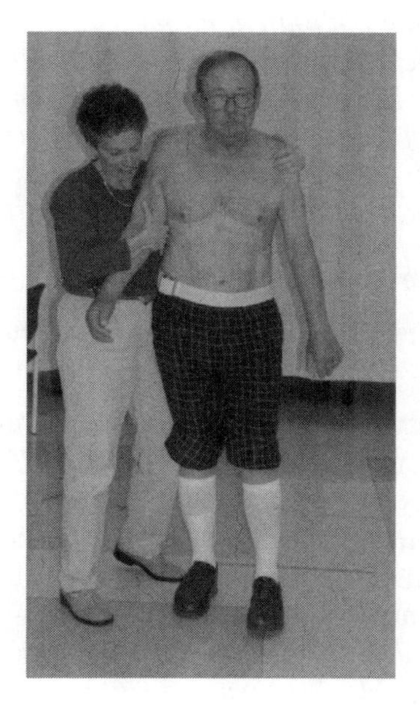

Figure 3.5. At 11 weeks post stroke, Ron shows instability of the right leg to support during stance and the inability to activate and time the muscle groups during swing phase.

Gait Analysis. Although Ron was not able to walk unassisted, gait characteristics are recorded here in order to have a baseline with which to compare changes as he recovers function. During ambulation, Ron was flexed at the neck, trunk, and hips, with his upper body mass shifted to the left and forward. The upper body shift increased when he was allowed to use the cane, and produced a forward rotation of the left side of his body. Step lengths were short, with a decrease in weight-bearing time on the right and a wide base of support. Stance on the right was characterized by overall instability and insufficient activation of all muscle groups, especially extensors. Variability was evident in the alignment of his body segments during right stance as he attempted to find a strategy to align his COM and recruit enough muscle activity to support himself during swing on the left. At late stance, the right hip remained in flexion with the upper body forward and the pelvis behind his BOS. There was little effective activation of the right LE against the floor to prepare the extremity effectively for swing. From this inactive position, he attempted to initiate swing of the right leg with various methods, often dragging or sliding his foot forward, and he had not yet developed consistent compensatory patterns. The most typical pattern was to lean more to the left with the upper body, dragging the rest of the body over to the left in an attempt to clear his right foot during swing phase.

Note: *The therapists used verbal and physical cues and feedback during this part of the examination and found that Ron had the capacity, when prompted, to change some of his motor patterns, such as alignment in anticipation of movement, weight shift, and adaptation of motor strategies to movement requirements. The variability of his movement strategies during gait indicated that he has potential to change, and he can be encouraged to try additional ways to solve some of his motor problems. His positive response to verbal encouragement and feedback regarding his successful attempts to change his movement patterns can be used as an additional strategy to assist with his motor relearning.*

Examination of Individual Systems

Neuromuscular system. Primary impairments directly related to the stroke were evident in the neuromuscular system.

Impairments in muscle activation. The problem of initiating and sustaining muscle activation was the greatest impairment Ron had at the time of this examination. He was unable to recruit the muscles of the trunk in patterns of co-activation, which placed a significant constraint on function. Postural activity in the trunk was insufficient to support symmetrical alignment or the active movements that he did attempt in sitting or standing. There was very little muscle activity in the trunk or right UE at rest. The right scapula and shoulder muscles were generally inactive, resulting in depression of the right shoulder and collapse of the trunk to the right and forward. His arm was heavy when the therapist moved it, and this heaviness contributed to trunk flexion because his postural control was not adequate to overcome the weight of the arm. This inactivity also contributed to the secondary impairments in the musculoskeletal system (see below), inappropriate compensations, and inefficient movement synergies.

Note: *In another client, the therapist might describe lack of movement as muscle weakness, but in the case of Ron, the therapists saw this as a primary impairment of recruitment and activation.*

Timing impairments. Ron could initiate, sustain, and terminate movements with the left extremities, however, he demonstrated difficulty with timing and sequencing postural control of the trunk with functional movements of the extremities to perform tasks efficiently. Although he had very little movement of the right UE, his attempts to move demonstrated a long latency before onset of the movement, followed by a short burst of activity that was not sustained. He often used momentum with repeated attempts when muscle recruitment was not available or attempted to coordinate movement components in a sequence that was ineffective. For example, in attempting to stand, he used excessive trunk flexion to bring his body forward, combined with inadequate hip flexion and insufficient activation of the muscles of the pelvic girdle and LEs to assist with support and movement of the COM. Ron also had difficulty timing and sequencing breathing with voicing, which resulted in inadequate support of long phrases or sentences, and low volume, especially at the end of a vocalization.

Inadequate force generation. As a result of impaired muscle activation, weakness was evident throughout the right extremities, more in the UE than the LE. Ron could not activate the muscles needed to complete the ROM at any joint of the right extremities. Weakness was noted in the face and oral-motor muscles contributing to the appearance of low affect. Inadequate activation was complicated by the secondary soft tissue stiffness that was developing in the right extremities. The inability to move against the resistance set up by this stiffness must be addressed in order to make a change in function.

Note: *In this examination, the therapists categorized the problem of force generation as a neuromuscular impairment rather than a musculoskeletal impairment because the client was only 5 weeks post stroke and showed little atrophy or joint contracture, which would indicate a secondary musculoskeletal weakness. They believed that the inability to generate forces for movement was directly related to the cerebral infarct, but they must also attend to the possibility of the development of weakness secondary to musculoskeletal impairments as well.*

Imbalance in muscle execution. In the trunk muscles, Ron did not use his extensors in effective patterns of co-activation with the flexors and did not sustain extensor activity when needed for sitting activities and maintaining standing postural alignment. There was more activity of the muscles on the left side of his body than the right, and he could not scale the amount of muscle response to adapt to postural instability or the force or temporal requirements of a task. This lack of sustained and dynamic extensor/flexor control also hindered selective control for speech volume and sustained voicing.

Musculoskeletal system

Range of motion. Passive ROM was limited by hypoextensibility and soft tissue tightness. Ron was developing stiffness and soft tissue tightness (as secondary impairments) in the right UE, especially distally, resulting in a position of flexion of the fingers due to lack of active movement. With lengthening and mobilization of soft tissues, passive ROM was within normal limits, with the exception of some limitation in the end ranges of the fingers. Active range was limited throughout the right side.

Sensory systems

Vision: Ron has little vision in his left eye, a condition he has experienced since infancy. He has worn glasses since his teen years. This vision defect may have contributed to his frequent lateral tilt in his head posture, because he needed to direct his right eye to see the entire visual field.

Auditory: Hearing appeared to be within functional limits.

Vestibular: Vestibular function did not appear to be impaired. Ron did not complain of dizziness, and when his posture or movements were corrected, he verbalized perception of an inability to control his position, rather than difficulty perceiving midline or verticality. His asymmetry in posture and movement appears to be a compensation for right-sided weakness and a realistic fear of falling, rather than a perceptual or vestibular deficit.

Somatosensory: Ron demonstrated appropriate body awareness. He was under-responsive to light or deep touch, particularly in the right UE, but he seldom "forgot" his hand and arm by the time of this examination for outpatient therapy. Initially decreased sensation did affect the safety of Ron's right UE. By report, while in the inpatient rehab unit, he occasionally caught his hand in the wheel of his wheelchair and was unaware of this.

Note: *The examiners were uncertain whether his inattention to his hand was related to allocating attention to multiple components of tasks that were complex, or to somatosensory deficits. Even though this problem was resolving, the need for integration between the two sides of the body and attention to sensation and movement of the right extremities will continue to be addressed during intervention.*

Regulatory system. Although he tired easily, Ron was alert and attentive throughout the examination. He was not distractible and his earlier lability, reported occasionally in the inpatient rehab program, seemed to be resolving.

Perceptual/Cognitive system. Ron demonstrated functional, although somewhat slowed, executive functions and motor planning that involved decision making, knowledge of the task, consequences of his actions, and logical planning for motor execution. The lack of success in tasks appeared to be related to his significant motor impairments, not to impairments in these cognitive functions.

Cardiovascular system. Ron has a history of cardiomegaly and Type II diabetes. At the time of this examination, there was edema in the right hand and foot with indications of poor distal supply in the right foot. Ron complained of cramping in both calves (L>R) with standing and walking and stated that he had had this problem prior to the stroke. On further questioning, he reported that he had been unable to walk more than 5 minutes on a treadmill at one time, but had consistently walked 20 minutes a day, with rests as needed, in the attempt to maintain overall cardiovascular endurance and distal circulation. In addition, he was noted to fatigue easily and have low endurance.

Note: *The examiners recognized that at least some of the fatigability might be related not only to his known cardiovascular conditions, but also to the demands of using a high level* *of attention and cognitive control to perform motor tasks that used to be automatic. The team will continue to monitor his fatigue over time.*

Respiratory system. Breathing rates were not measured during this examination, but activity did not seem to increase breath rate excessively. As mentioned, because of his decreased respiratory capacity, Ron did have difficulty timing and sequencing breathing and voicing and in sustaining vocalizations.

Multisystem impairments

Edema. As noted, Ron had edema in the right hand, which appeared to be related to both neuromuscular impairments (lack of muscle activation) and musculoskeletal impairments, (muscle stiffness, and soft tissue tightness). He was wearing a hand splint at night, which was partially effective in controlling the edema through the effect of improved alignment on venous return in the right UE. In addition, edema was occasionally evident in both feet and was thought to be related to cardiovascular impairments.

Pain. Ron complained of pain, particularly in the left LE, which occurred after exercise and appeared to be related to the cardiovascular system impairment. He had occasional pain in the right shoulder and hand, which appeared to be related to lack of active movement and the subsequent decrease in muscle length.

Evaluation

Client Strengths

1. Cognition, motivation, and interest. Ron indicates understanding of how motor impairments affect his function ("I can't turn the faucet on. My shoulder is weak. I can't reach my hand that far forward.") and an understanding of why intervention requires treatment of the motor components as well as practice of the function. He understands that regaining motor functions will improve his overall independence and ability to participate socially with family and friends.
2. Relatively good somatosensory abilities and perception of his body in space. Functional exteroceptive senses, appropriate for his age.
3. Memory of motor skills and ability to use verbal and manual cues and demonstration to adapt posture and movement to the task.
4. Evidence of potential for developing variability in muscle synergies to accomplish tasks by building on old synergies while adapting to the constraints of little muscle activation in the right extremities.

Contextual Facilitators

1. Supportive wife, able to balance helping with encouraging Ron's initiative and independence.

2. Availability of family and friends for support and assistance (e.g., transportation to therapy).
3. Wheelchair-accessible bathroom and house mostly on one level.

System and Motor Impairments that Limit Function.

Note: *The therapists have chosen to list those impairments that they hypothesize* ***currently most significantly*** *affect functional abilities, knowing that the relationships will change rapidly over the next few months, given that Ron is in the early stages of recovery from stroke.*

1. The inability to generate and sustain the muscle forces necessary to initiate, grade, and adapt appropriate muscle activity is seen as the major impairment in all motor functions that require combining posture with movement.
2. Inadequate postural control along with resulting poor alignment limits Ron's ability to use postures or perform functional tasks that require either proactive or reactive balance.
3. Imbalance of the patterns of motor activation governs his posture in sitting and standing, producing a dominance of flexion, poorly sustained extension, and lack of co-activation. This affects postural control in sitting and standing and all attempts at active movement.
4. Self-initiated compensatory movements offset limited movement on the right side and Ron's difficulty controlling his COM over the BOS. In the interest of regaining functional movement, Ron has learned to use his best solution to move and control his COM, leading with the head and left side, even though this is potentially limiting to development of a varied repertoire of movement patterns.
5. Secondary impairments of muscle hypoextensibility, joint stiffness, pain, and edema are already limiting movement in therapy and in home activities.

Expected Functional Outcomes (discipline-specific)

Physical Therapy

Short-term outcomes: 1 month

1. Ron will walk 30 feet in his home on uncarpeted level surfaces with a quad cane and minimal to moderate assistance by his wife.
2. Ron will stand up from and sit down in his wheelchair with only stand-by supervision, given adequate time and verbal cues for weight shift and weight distribution.
3. Ron will transfer from wheelchair to bed, chair, toilet, or car with stand-by supervision.

Long-term outcomes: 6 months

1. Ron will walk at home independently. He will not use a wheelchair in the house.
2. Ron will require stand-by assist to walk up and down one step to the living room using his quad cane.
3. Ron will walk with supervision in his community up to 500 feet in safe, predictable settings.

Occupational Therapy

Note: *Because Ron's right arm has limited movement, the short-term outcomes address functions that use the components of movement that are available but do not involve fine-motor use of the arm and hand. OT will (a) address functional ADL limitations in setting short-term goals, involving the right UE whenever possible, and (b) work at the level of impairment-related posture and movement goals in order to develop those components of posture and movement that will prepare for long-term outcomes that include functional use of the right arm and hand. Specific right UE function is not stated as part of a short-term ADL goal, but preparation of the right UE is included, anticipating functional use of the right UE as recovery continues.*

Short-term outcomes: 1 month

1. Ron will actively support his body weight on his right forearm while moving from a sitting position to/from supine getting in and out of bed, for improved safety and independence of this transition.
2. When seated at a table, Ron will rest his right UE on the surface to support symmetrical alignment in sitting and to aid changes in activation of the postural muscles of his trunk by inhibiting the downward pull of this extremity when he leaves it in his lap.
3. Ron will stand during dressing and pull up and adjust elastic-waist pants with supervision, due to improved dynamic postural control, allowing him to stand and perform an UE task involving significant weight shifts.

Long-term outcomes: 6 months

1. Ron will spontaneously use his right arm and hand for stabilization and gross manipulation of plates, glasses, and serving dishes from a position in which the right UE is resting on the table.
2. Ron will manage clothing while standing, using his right hand to stabilize clothing as he dresses.
3. Ron will stand at the sink and perform morning hygiene activities using his right hand to turn on the water. He will stabilize the toothpaste tube or deodorant with the right hand while he manages the caps with his left. He will wash and dry both hands and his upper body, managing the washcloth and towel independently.
4. Ron will resume dining out with friends and attending church with assistance from

his wife as needed, as an indicator that he has achieved a level of independence in mobility and personal management skills.

Speech-Language Pathology

Short-term outcomes: 1 month

1. Ron will speak sentences of 6 words with adequate volume for conversation from 10 feet away.

Long-term outcomes: 6 months

1. Speech therapy will be discontinued. Continued work for speech production and conversation will be incorporated into PT and OT.

Impairment-Related Posture and Movement Goals (all disciplines)

1. Demonstrate dynamic weight bearing in sitting and standing postures, re-establishing appropriate links between posture prior to and during functional movement sequences in sitting and standing.
2. Demonstrate balance between trunk flexors and extensors, resulting in a more active and upright posture during all functional activities.
3. Freely move the head independently from the trunk while using a variety of head and neck movements appropriate to support respiration and speech.
4. Demonstrate increased pelvic girdle activity and control, combined with increased hip flexion and trunk extension for improved control of the BOS in sitting and effective movement of the COM forward over the hips during tasks such as sit-to-stand or scooting sideways on the seat of the car.
5. Demonstrate co-activation of the trunk muscles to achieve a dynamic and upright sitting posture to allow depression and adduction of the scapulas, especially on the right, aligning the right shoulder girdle in order to facilitate activation of the right arm in weight-bearing and nonweight-bearing activities.
6. Use the right UE for weight-bearing activities, effectively pushing into the support surface (e.g., moving from supine to sitting or supporting weight on the right hand or forearm while using the left hand when standing).
7. Improve the timing and sequencing of muscle activation needed for variation in tasks, depending on the context.
8. Incorporate axial rotation when transferring from one surface to another and while walking to develop energy-efficient movements.
9. Increase the amount and variability of movements that incorporate both sides of the body in effective synergies.
10. Limit compensatory patterns and prevent learned nonuse by actively integrating both sides of the body for all daily living tasks.

Plan of Care

Ron and Lorraine have decided to pursue intensive therapeutic intervention on an outpatient basis, having seen improvements that have already occurred since his stroke and anticipating additional improvements. Lorraine will attend the therapy sessions as often as possible to learn what to practice at home and to encourage the appropriate level of independence. Each therapist will be responsible for functions related to their own discipline, but will be knowledgeable about the skills that the other professions are working on to support the best overall management. Co-treatment or overlapping treatment will be incorporated as appropriate to address common problem areas and to treat a number of movement problems at the same time for optimal use of time and resources. On an ongoing basis, the therapists will revise and upgrade those activities that Ron and Lorraine have been instructed to continue at home.

Ron's home program will include an ongoing educational component to focus on his responsibility for follow-through and to practice specific activities. He will be encouraged to find his own ways to be active at home; however, he will not be left on his own to figure out what he is able to do. Instructions for the home program will be very specific and whenever possible, the activity will be designed to be incorporated into Ron's daily routine. For example, Ron will be instructed to lie down by moving toward his right side, making sure to place his right forearm on the bed and support his weight on it before rolling back into a supine position. Because he takes an afternoon nap, he is to practice this maneuver twice a day, in the afternoon and again in the evening as he is getting into bed. Providing specific and time-event linked instructions assist with carryover, because even very motivated clients have difficulty figuring out what they can possibly do that is consistent with their level of recovery and practical for their lifestyle, given their limited movement and control. The intervention team takes the leadership in designing activities in treatment that will include what Ron is doing at home and provide feedback following his report on the ways that he incorporates the activities into his own setting.

For at least the next 2 months, Ron will receive PT and OT 3 times a week to take advantage of the rapid changes that are occurring. This frequency will be reevaluated in 2 months. The SLP will act in a consulting role. The PT and the OT will communicate so that, as appropriate, therapists can co-treat or overlap treatment. The therapists will include time in the rehab sessions for family teaching, evaluation of equipment needs, and practice with the therapists' supervision in a structured setting. The OT or the PT will make one visit to the home during this period to ensure transfer of skills in functional settings.

Note: *It would be ideal for intervention to take place in the client's home, however, Ron's insurance does not pay for this model of service. Recognizing this, the therapists will have to be diligent to make certain that the activities practiced in the rehab setting are as close to Ron's home setting as possible and design activities that address constraints posed by the physical environment of his home. For example, his home has a "sunken" living room and he could not negotiate the step at the time of this examination. The therapists need to address ambulation up and down one step as well as transfers that he would need in order to sit on the sofa once he gets into the room.*

On the positive side, his bathroom is wheelchair-accessible and does not currently pose constraints, so Ron can perform ADLs while he sits in his wheelchair, as he did in OT. However, the OT is faced with a different challenge; to prevent limitations in progress from the convenience of the wheelchair-accessible bathroom, the therapist may assign Ron the task of gradually performing more and more ADL tasks from a standing position.

The interdisciplinary team will informally reassess Ron to determine the need for this high frequency of intervention, the appropriateness of treatment strategies, and progress toward the stated outcomes and posture and movement goals. Formal examinations occur every 30 days, due to the requirement under Medicare and the documentation for billing. He will be re-examined with the FIM and other appropriate functional measures, such as timed walk and Get Up and Go Test.

Chapter Summary: A Guide for Organizing an Examination

This chapter describes and illustrates the NDT examination process. Because the NDT examination is a problem-solving process, there is no "one right way" to organize or interpret information about a client. NDT therapists use their best clinical judgment, experience, expertise, and the evidence that is available and meaningful to the client to make decisions during the examination process. NDT does believe that certain information must be included when examining a client and that information is classified in an NDT enablement model reflecting a systems approach to function and health. The examination information must be organized in a standard way that makes the information accessible and meaningful to other professionals. Although a common body of information is included in the examination of either an adult or a child, the organization of that information reflects the concerns of the client and family, the presenting problems, and reasons for referral. For example, an examination for the purpose of deciding on orthopedic surgery has a different focus than an examination to determine school placement or determining discharge from a rehab unit. Yet all examinations reflect the NDT principles of assessment described in this chapter. The following outline serves as a guide for organizing information, but is *not* an examination form. As demonstrated in the case studies, the examiner organizes the observations and analysis in the way that best communicates the data about a specific client.

Name:

Date of Assessment:

DOB:

Heath Condition:

Data Collection:

1. Reason for referral
2. Medical history and background
3. Overview of function

4. Family and environmental characteristics
    a. Daily routine
    b. Contextual factors/conditions and constraints on participation
        (1) assistive technology devices
        (2) splinting and orthotics
    c. Family concerns, expectations, and objectives

Examination

1. Morphology
    a. Body weight
    b. Height
    c. Limb circumference and length
    d. General skeletal structure
2. Examination of functional tasks/potential for change
    a. Gross motor/movements through space
    b. Fine motor/task-directed functions
    c. Communications
    d. ADL
    e. Oral-motor functions
    f. Social skills/Behavior
3. Tests and measures
    a. Norm-referenced
    b. Criterion-referenced
    c. Nonstandardized, self-referenced
4. Examination of posture and movement
    a. Alignment
    b. Relationship of BOS and COM
    c. Postural control and balance
        (1) anticipatory (proactive)/weight shift
        (2) steady-state balance
        (3) equilibrium (reactive)

d. Movement strategies and compensations

e. Muscle and postural tone/distribution of hyper- and hypotonia

f. Symmetry/Asymmetry

g. Kinesiological and biomechanical components of movement

h. Coordination

i. Descriptive analysis of specific motor functions (e.g., gait, handwriting, chewing)

5. Examination of system integrity and impairments

a. Neuromuscular

(1) muscle activation and execution

(a) timing, initiating, sustaining, terminating muscle activity

(b) generation of force/tension

(c) co-activation/reciprocal relationships

(d) intra- and interlimb dynamics

(e) modulation and scaling of forces

(2) coordination of postural stability with movement

(3) synergies

(4) spasticity

(5) extraneous movements

(6) fractionated or dissociated movements

(7) hypokinesia

b. Musculoskeletal

(1) range of motion; joint and soft tissue

(2) muscle extensibility, functional range

(3) muscle strength, endurance

(4) skeletal abnormalities

c. Sensory

(1) vision

(2) auditory

(3) gustatory

(4) vestibular

(5) somatosensory (tactile and proprioceptive)

(6) sensory processing and modulation

d. Regulatory

(1) arousal

(2) state regulation

(3) emotional regulation and control

e. Perceptual/cognitive

(1) intelligence

(2) attention

(3) memory

(4) adaptability

(5) motor planning (e.g., gestalt of task, perception of position in space and spatial relationships)

(6) executive functions (e.g., set goals, understand consequences of actions, inhibit impulsiveness)

f. Integumentary

(a) skin integrity

(b) skin color

(c) extensibility

g. Respiratory

(1) rate

(2) patterns

(3) breath control

(4) capacity

h. Cardiovascular

(1) heart rate

(2) blood pressure

(3) edema

(4) measures of fitness

(5) peripheral circulation (includes skin color and temperature)

i. Gastrointestinal

(1) control of bowel and bladder

(2) intake and tolerance (vomiting, choking)

(3) Signs of reflux (burps, odor, expression of pain)

j. Multisystem effects on motor dysfunction

(1) pain

(2) edema

(3) motor planning

6. Changes in performance and capacity, based on response to facilitation, modification of task, or environment

Evaluation

1. Strengths

   a. Client strengths

      (1) system integrities

      (2) motor functions

      (3) functional abilities

      (4) participation

   b. Contextual facilitators

      (1) family and community

      (2) environmental facilitators

2. Areas of concern linking impairments to function

   a. System impairments

   b. Ineffective postures and movements

   c. Functional limitations

   d. Barriers to participation

3. Summarize

   a. Hypothesize on relationships among impairments, posture and movement, and limitations in function.

   b. Consider which system impairments, posture, and movement components will have the greatest impact on development or recovery of function over time.

   c. Predict potential changes and secondary impairments based on intervention or lack of intervention and on available evidence.

4. Long-term outcomes
    a. Include time, measure, and specific context
5. Short-term outcomes
    a. Include time, measure, and specific context
6. Impairment-related goals

Plan of Care (based on clinical evidence, expertise, experience)

1. Frequency and duration
2. Client and family priorities and values
3. Equipment and assistive technology (orthoses and splints)
4. Model of care
5. Strategies of intervention
6. Role of family, medical, educational, and other professionals involved in care
7. Schedule for reexamination and evidence of achievement of goals and objectives

References

Adams, S. A. (1993). A study to test the scalability of the Rivermead Motor Assessment with acute stroke patients (abstract). *Physiotherapy, 79,* 506.

Adler, L. (2002). Batter up! Case study: Playing baseball to develop posture and reaching. *NDT Network, 9* (3), 1, 13, 14.

American Physical Therapy Association. (2001). APTA Guide to Physical Therapist Practice (2nd ed.). *Physical Therapy, 81* (1).

Barry, M. J. (2001, November). Evidence-based practice in pediatric physical therapy. *PT Magazine,* 38-52.

Bayley, N. (1993). *The Bayley scales of infant development* (2nd ed.). San Antonio, TX: The Psychological Corporation.

Berg, K., Wood-Dauphinee, S. L., Williams, J., & Gayton, D. (1992). Measuring balance in the elderly: Validation of an instrument. *Canadian Journal of Public Health, 83* (2), S7-11.

Berg, K., Wood-Dauphinee, S. L., & Williams, J. (1995). The balance scale: Reliability with elderly residents and patients with an acute stroke. *Scandinavian Journal of Rehabilitation Medicine, 27,* 27-34.

Bjornson, K. F., Grauber, C. S., Buford, V. L., & McLaughlin, J. (1998). Validity of the Gross Motor Function Measure. *Pediatric Physical Therapy, 10,* 43-47.

Bjornson, K. F., Grauber, C. S., McLaughlin, J. F., Kerfeld, C. I., & Clark, E. M. (1990). Test-retest reliability of the Gross Motor Function Measure in children with cerebral palsy. *Physical and Occupational Therapy in Pediatrics, 18* (2), 51-61.

Blaskey, J., & Jennings, M. C. (1999). Traumatic brain injury. In S. K. Campbell (Ed.), *Decision making in pediatric neurologic physical therapy* (pp. 84-140). Philadelphia: Churchill Livingstone.

Bly, L. L. (2001). A tribute to Mary Quinton. *NDT Network, 8* (2), 1-7.

Bobath, B. (1975). *Motor development in the different types of cerebral palsy.* London: Wm. Heineman.

Bobath, B. (1990). *Adult hemiplegia: Evaluation and treatment* (3rd ed.). London: Wm. Heinemann.

Bobath, K., & Bobath, B. (1979). Acceptance Speech (audiotape transcription), First Currative Foundation Awards Dinner, Milwaukee, WI.

Bruininks, R. H. (1978). *Bruininks-Oseretsky Test of Motor Proficiency: Examiners manual.* Circle Pines, MN: American Guidance Service.

Burden, R. L. (1980). Measuring the effects of stress on the mothers of handicapped infants. Must depression always follow? *Child Care Health and Development, 6,* 111-123.

Butler, N., Gill, R., & Pomeroy, D. (1978). Handicapped children: Their homes and life styles. Bristol, England: Department of Child Health, University of Bristol.

Campbell, S. K. (1997). Therapy programs for children that last a lifetime. *Physical and Occupational Therapy in Pediatrics, 17* (1), 1-15.

Campbell, S. K., Ostern, E. T., Kolobe, T. H. A., & Fisher, A. G. (1993). Development of the Test of Infant Motor Performance. In C. V. Granger & G. E. Gresham (Eds.), *New developments in functional assessment* (pp. 541-550). Philadelphia: W. B. Saunders.

Campbell, S. K., Ostern, E. T., Kolobe, T. H. A., Lenke, M., & Girolami, G. L. (1995). Construct validity of the Test of Infant Motor Performance. *Physical Therapy, 75,* 585-596.

Campbell, S. K., Wright, B. D., & Linacre, J. M. (2002). Functional movement scale in infants. *Journal of Applied Measures, 3* (2), 191-205.

Carlson, S. J., & Ramsey, C. (2000). Assistive technology. In S. K. Campbell (Ed.), *Physical therapy for children* (pp. 671-708). Philadelphia: W. B. Saunders.

Carr, J., & Shepherd, R. (2000). *Movement science: Foundations for physical therapy in rehabilitation* (2nd ed.). Gaithersburg, MD: Aspen Publications.

Carr, J. H., Shepherd, R. B., Nordholm, L., & Lynne, D. (1985). Investigation of new motor assessment scale for stroke patients. *Physical Therapy, 65,* 175-180.

Cook, A. M., & Hussey, S.M. (2002). *Assistive Technologies: Principles and Practice.* (2nd ed.). St. Louis, MO: Mosby, Inc.

Coster, W., Deeney, T., Haltiwanger, J., & Haley, S. (1998). *School function assessment (SFA).* San Antonio. TX: The Psychological Corporation.

DeRuyter, O. (2002). *Clinician's Guide to Assistive Technology.* St. Louis, MO: Mosby, Inc.

Diamond, M. & Cupps, B. (2002). NDT Framework for clinical decision making incorporating a disablement model. In M. Stamer (ED.), *Progress in Motion.* (pp. 13-29). Laguna Beach, CA: NDTA.

Diamond, M., & Schenkman, M. (1996). Use of the clinical decision-making process to achieve measurable improvement in function in a patient one year post CVA. *Neurology Report, 20* (2), 72-74.

Duger, T., Bumin, G., Uyanik, M., Aki, E., & Kayihan, H. (1999). The assessment of Bruininks-Oseretsky test of motor proficiency in children. *Pediatric Rehabilitation, 3* (3), 125-131.

Duncan, P. W., Propst, M., & Nelson, S. (1983). Reliability of the Fugl-Meyer assessment of sensorimotor recovery following stroke. *Physical Therapy, 63,* 1606-1610.

Duncan, P., Weiner, D. K., Chandler, J., & Studenski, S. (1990). Functional reach: A new clinical measure of balance. *Journal of Gerontology, 45,* M192-M197.

Dunlap, W. R., & Hollingsworth, J. S. (1977). How does a handicapped child affect the family? Implications for practitioners. *Family Coordinator, 26* (3), 286-292.

Erhardt, R. (1994). *Developmental hand dysfunction: Theory, assessment and treatment* (2nd ed.). Tucson, AZ: Therapy Skill Builders.

Floyd, F. J., & Zmich, D. E. (1991). Marriage and the parenting partnership: Perceptions and interactions of parents with mentally retarded and typically developing children. *Child Development, 62,* 1434-1446.

Fugl-Meyer, A. R., Jaasko, L., Leyman, I., Olsson, S., & Steglind, S. (1975). The post-stroke hemiplegic patient: 1. A method for evaluation of physical performance. *Scandinavian Journal of Rehabilitation Medicine, 7,* 13-31.

Girolami, G., Ryan, D. F., & Gardner, J. M. (2001). Treatment implementation, reassessment, and documentation. In A. Scherzer (Ed.), *Early diagnosis and interventional therapy in cerebral palsy. An interdisciplinary age-focused approach* (3rd ed., pp. 201-227). New York: Marcel Dekker.

Granger, C. V., Hamilton, B. B. & Kayton, R. (1989). *Guide for the use of the Functional Independence Measure (WeeFim) of the uniform data set for medical rehabilitation.* Research Foundation. Buffalo, NY: State University of New York.

Granger, C. V., Hamilton, B. B., Linacre, J. M., Heinemann, A. W., & Wright, B. D. (1993). Performance profiles of the Functional Independence Measure. *American Journal of Physical Medicine and Rehabilitation, 72,* 84-89.

Greiner, B. M., Czerniecki, J. M., & Deitz, J. C. (1993). Gait parameters of children with spastic diplegia: A comparison of effects of posterior and anterior walkers. *Archives of Physical Medicine and Rehabilitation, 74,* 381-385.

Grossman, F. K. (1972). *Brothers and sisters of retarded children: An exploratory study.* Syracuse, New York: Syracuse University Press.

Gudjonsdottir, B., & Mercer, V. S. (2002). Effects of a dynamic versus a static prone stander on bone mineral density and behavior in four children with severe cerebral palsy. *Pediatric Physical Therapy, 14,* 38-46.

Hadders-Algra, M. (2001). Early brain damage and the development of motor behavior in children: Clues for therapeutic intervention? *Neural Plasticity, 8* (1-2), 31-49.

Haley, S. M., Coster, W. J., Ludlow, L. H., Haltiwanger, J. T., & Andrellos, P. J. (1992). *Pediatric evaluation of disability inventory: Development standardization and administration manual.* Boston: New England Medical Center.

Howle, J. (1999). Cerebral palsy. In S. K. Campbell (Ed.), *Decision making in pediatric neurologic physical therapy* (pp. 23-83). Philadelphia: Churchill Livingstone.

Hsuch, I. P., Lee, M. M., & Hsish, C. L. (2001). Psychometric characteristics of the Barthel activities of daily living index in stroke. *Journal of the Formosan Medical Association, 100* (8), 526-532.

Jain, M., Turner, D., & Worrell, T. (1994). The Vulpe Assessment Battery and the Peabody Developmental Motor Scales: A preliminary study of concurrent validity between gross motor sections. *Physical and Occupational Therapy in Pediatrics, 14* (1), 23-33.

Jebsen, R. H., Taylor, N., Trieschmann, R. B., Trotter, M. J., & Howard, L. A. (1969). An objective and standardized test of hand function. *Archives of Physical Medicine and Rehabilitation, 50,* 311-319.

Johnson-Martin, N., Attermeier, S. M., & Hacker, B. (1990). *The Carolina curriculum for preschoolers with special needs.* Baltimore: Paul Brooks.

Johnson-Martin, N., Jens, K. G., & Attermeier, S. M. (1986). *The Carolina curriculum for handicapped infants and infants at risk.* Baltimore: Paul Brooks.

Jones, B. N., Molloy, I., Chamberlain, M. A., & Tennant, A. (2001). Factors determining participation in young adults with a physical disability: A pilot study. *Clinical Rehabilitation, 15* (5), 552-561.

Kolobe, T. H. A. (1992). Working with families of children with disabilities. *Pediatric Physical Therapy, 4,* 57-63.

Kolobe, T. H. A., Sparling, J., & Daniels, L. E. (2000). Family-centered intervention. In S. K. Campbell (Ed.), *Physical therapy for children* (pp. 881-909). Philadelphia: W. B. Saunders.

Law, M., Baptiste, S., McColl, M., Opzoomer, A., Polatajko, H., & Pollock, N. (1990). The Canadian Occupational Performance Measure: An outcome measure for occupational therapy. *Canadian Journal of Occupational Therapy, 57* (2), 82-87.

Law, M., Polatajko, H., Pollock, N., McColl, M. A., Carswell, A., & Baptiste, S. (1994). Pilot testing of the Canadian Occupational Performance Measure: Clinical and measurement issues. *Canadian Journal of Occupational Therapy, 61* (4), 191-197.

Levangie, P., Chimera, M., Johnston, M., Robinson, F., & Wobeskya, L. (1989). Effects of posture control walker versus standard rolling walker on gait characteristics of children with spastic cerebral palsy. *Physical and Occupational Therapy in Pediatrics, 9* (4),1-32, 1989.

Lincoln, N., & Leadbitter, D. (1979). Assessment of motor function in stroke patients. *Physiotherapy, 65,* 48-51.

Loewn, S. C., & Anderson, B. A. (1988). Reliability of the Modified Motor Assessment Scale and the Barthel Index. *Physical Therapy, 68,* 1077-1081.

Loewn, S. C., & Anderson, B. A. (1990). Predictors of stroke outcome using objective measurement scales. *Stroke, 21,* 78-81

Logan, L., Byers-Hinley, K., & Ciccone, C. (1990). Anterior vs. posterior walkers for children with cerebral palsy: A gait analysis study. *Developmental Medicine and Child Neurology, 32,* 1044-1048.

Lonsdale, G. (1978). Family life with a handicapped child: The parents speak. *Child Care Health and Development, 4,* 99-120.

Lunnen, K. Y. (1999). Children with multiple disabilities. In S. K. Campbell (Ed.), *Decision making in pediatric neurologic physical therapy* (pp. 141-197). Philadelphia: Churchill Livingstone.

Mahoney, R. I., & Barthel, D. W. (1965). Functional evaluation: The Barthel Index. *Maryland Medical Journal, 14,* 61-65.

Malouin, F., Pichard, L., Bonneau, C., Durand, A., & Corriveau, D. (1994). Evaluating motor recovery early after stroke: Comparison of the Fugl-Meyer Assessment and the Motor Assessment Scale. *Archives of Physical Medicine and Rehabilitation, 75* (11), 1206-1212.

Mann, W. C., Ottenbacher, K. J., Fraas, L., Tomita, M., & Granger, C. V. (1999). Effectiveness of assistive technology and environmental interventions in maintaining independence and reducing home care costs for the frail elderly. A randomized controlled trial. *Archives of Family Medicine, 8* (3), 210-217.

Mathias, S., Nayak, U., & Isaacs, B. (1986). Balance in elderly patients: The "Get-up and Go" test. *Archives of Physical Medicine and Rehabilitation, 67,* 387-389.

McMichaels, J. (1971). *Handicap: A study of physically developing children and their families.* London: Staples.

Miedaner, J. A. (1990). The effects of sitting positions on trunk extension for children with motor impairment. *Pediatric Physical Therapy, 2,* 11-14.

Montgomery, P. C. (2000). Achievement of gross motor skills in two children with cerebellar hypoplasia: Longitudinal case reports. *Pediatric Physical Therapy, 12,* 76-86.

Ottenbacher, K. J., Msall, M. E., Lyon, N., Duffy, L. C., Ziviani, J., Granger, C. V., Braun, S., & Feidler, R. C. (2000). The WeeFIM instrument: Its utility in detecting change in children with developmental disabilities. *Archives of Physical Medicine and Rehabilitation, 81* (10), 1317-1326.

Palisano, R. (2000). Decision making in pediatric physical therapy. In S. K. Campbell (Ed.), *Physical therapy for children* (pp. 198-224). Philadelphia: W. B. Saunders.

Pennington, L., & McConachie, H. (2001). Interaction between children with cerebral palsy and their mothers: The effects of speech intelligibility. *International Journal of Language and Communication Disorders, 36* (3), 371-393.

Persperin, J. (1990). Seating systems: The therapist and rehabilitation engineering team. *Physical and Occupational Therapy in Pediatrics, 10* (2), 11-45.

Peterson, P., & Wikoff, R. L. (1987). Home environment and adjustment in families with handicapped children: A canonical correlation study. *Occupational Therapy Journal of Research, 7,* 67-82.

Piper, M. C., & Darrah, J. (1994). *Motor assessment of the developing infant.* Philadelphia: W. B. Saunders.

Poole, J. L., & Whitney, S. L. (1988). Motor assessment scale for stroke patients: concurrent validity and interrater reliability. *Archives of Physical Medicine and Rehabilitation, 69,* 195-197.

Porch, B. (1981). *Porch Index of Communicative Ability (PICA).* Palo Alto, CA: Consulting Psychologists Press.

Public Law 100-407. (1998). *Technology-Related Assistance for Individuals with Disabilities Act of 1998.* Washington, DC: U.S. Department of Education, Office of Special Education and Rehabilitation Services.

Public Law 102-119. (1990). *Individuals with Disabilities Education Act (IDEA).* Washington, DC: U.S. Department of Education, Office of Special Education and Rehabilitation Services.

Public Law 105-17. (1997). *Individuals with Disabilities Education Act (IDEA) Amendments of 1997.* Washington, DC: U.S. Department of Education, Office of Special Education and Rehabilitation Services.

Rosetti, L. (1990). *Rosetti infant-toddler language scales.* Moline, IL: LinguiSystem, Inc.

Russell, D., Rosenbaum, P., Cadman, D., Gowland, C., Hardy, S., & Jarvis, S. (1989). The Gross Motor Function Measure: A means to evaluate the effects of physical therapy. *Developmental Medicine and Child Neurology, 31,* 341-352.

Russell, D. J., Rosenbaum, P. L., Gowland, C., Hardy, S., Lane, M., Plews, N., McGarvin, H., Cadman, D., & Jarvis, S. (1990). *Manual for the Gross Motor Function Measure: A measure of gross motor function in cerebral palsy.* Hamilton, Ontario, Canada: McMaster University.

Ryerson, S., & Levit, K.(1997). *Functional movement reeducation: A contemporary model for stroke rehabilitation.* New York: Churchill Livingstone.

Sackett, D. L., Rosenberg, W. M., & Gray, J. A. (1996). Evidence-based medicine: What it is and what it isn't. *British Medical Journal, 312,* 71-72.

Seelman, K. D. (1999). *What is assistive technology?* Washington, DC: U.S. Department of Education; National Institute on Disability and Rehabilitation Research.

Shankoff, J. P., & Hausen-Cram, P. (1987). Early intervention for disabled infants and their families: A quantitative analysis. *Pediatrics, 80,* 650-657.

Taylor, N., Sand, P. L., & Jebsen, R. H. (1973). Evaluation of hand function in children. *Archives of Physical Medicine and Rehabilitation, 54* (3), 129-135.

Thelen, E. (1994). *A dynamic systems approach to the development of cognition and action.* Cambridge, MA: Bradford Books/MIT Press.

VanDeusen, J., & Brunt, D. (1997). *Assessment in occupational therapy and physical therapy.* Philadelphia: W. B. Saunders.

Vulpe, S. G. (1979). *Vulpe assessment battery for the atypical child.* Toronto, Canada: National Institute on Mental Retardation.

Wade, D. T. (1992). *Measurement in neurological rehabilitation.* Oxford, England: Oxford University Press.

Wilson, B. N., Polatajko, H. J., Kaplan, B. J., & Faris, P. (1995). Use of the Bruininks-Oseretsky test of motor proficiency in occupational therapy. *American Journal of Occupational Therapy, 49* (1), 8-17.

Wilson, J. M. (1993). Selection and use of adaptive equipment. In B. H. Connolly & P. C. Montgomery (Eds.), *Therapeutic exercise in developmental disabilities* (2nd ed., pp. 167-182). Hixson, TN: Chattanooga Group.

World Health Organization. (2001). ICF: International classification of functioning, disability and health. Geneva, Switzerland: Author.

Zacharewicz, L. (2001). Predicting the patient's outcome: A review of measures for patients with stroke. *NDT Network, 8* (2), 10-11.

Zimmerman, I. L., Steiner, V. G., & Pond, E. R. (1991). *Preschool language scale* (3rd ed.). San Antonio, TX: The Psychological Corporation.

Chapter 4

Principles and Process of NDT Intervention

"Treatment has to be flexible and adapted to the many and varied needs of the individual. . . ." (K. Bobath & B. Bobath, 1984, p. 6)

Principles of Treatment

The strength of NDT has always been the clinical management of the sensorimotor problems resulting from ongoing analysis of system and motor impairments as the client develops or recovers from CNS pathology. Intervention consists of carefully planned treatment strategies directed toward improving function (Diamond & Schenkman, 1996). NDT therapists modify and adjust specific strategies throughout each treatment session as well as during a series of treatments, based on the client's response to the strategies selected and used. NDT utilizes an enablement model that considers all aspects of the person, the context and the task (see Figure 3.1) and structures intervention with principles derived from concepts of motor control, motor learning, and motor development applied to typical and atypical movement patterns. A number of specific principles, taught in all NDT courses, guide NDT intervention (Curriculum Committee, NDTA, 1996). The following paragraphs summarize these principles:

1. **Establish a treatment plan with anticipated outcomes that include specific, observable functions within a specific time frame under specific environmental conditions.** These goals will vary with age, family and client concerns, and the extent of signs at the onset of treatment. Establishing a reevaluation schedule is a critical part of the decision-making process. For example, a PT outcome for a independent, ambulating child with spastic cerebral palsy (CP) might be, "George will climb a full flight of stairs using one hand rail, at school, in a step-over-step fashion before the school year is over (8 months)." Movement goals and functional outcomes must be specific, consistent, and attainable, with standards high enough to foster improved performance, but not so high as to provoke discouragement by repeated failure (Larin, 2000).

2. **Design therapy to utilize the client's strengths, recognizing that each individual has competencies and disabilities.** Focusing on the individual's strengths builds self-esteem and centers everyone on the capabilities of the client at any point in the recovery or developmental process while providing the opportunity to acknowledge the individual characteristics of each client. For example, if a child has good imaginary play and language skills, storytelling can focus the child's attention, and imaginary play can provide a framework for moving. If an adult with stroke has a good sense of humor and can laugh at himself, he will tolerate mistakes in performance of tasks that he had performed easily before the stroke.

3. **Set anticipated outcomes and impairment goals in partnership with the family, the client, and the interdisciplinary team.** The intervention team, which includes the client and family, establishes desired functional outcomes and makes decisions concerning frequency, type, and context of treatment. Outcomes must be meaningful to the client and the family and are stated in terms of function. The individual team members may state these treatment objectives, which include impairment-related goal and functional outcomes, differently, but the goals always relate limitations in activities and participation in life to the underlying impairments. Even young, school-aged children are capable of participating in setting reasonable goals (Campbell, 1999b; Howle, 1999). For example, a 10-year-old child with hemiplegic CP wants to be able to kick a soccer ball. His family would like him to be able to play on the community YMCA team. His PT wants him to develop rhythm and coordination when walking. In order to reach these objectives, the PT identifies the underlying system and movement impairments, which might include (a) decreased strength on his left side, (b) inadequate postural control while standing on his left leg, (c) delayed initiation and inappropriate sequencing of patterns of muscle activation of either leg, and (d) inadequate interlimb coordination with overflow from the left leg to the left arm. The PT then develops treatment strategies directly related to soccer. Including the family and the child in the decision-making process will help the client and the family, as well as the clinician to focus on what is and what is not a reasonable expectation within a given time frame and to understand the process of relating goals to anticipated outcomes.

4. **NDT treatment constructs a purposeful relationship between sensory input and motor output.** The sensory systems contribute directly to the qualities of movement. Action depends on matching sensory and motor processes with perceived requirements of the task. Sensory input can be either facilitatory or inhibitory, depending on the internal state of the client and how the input is introduced (Girolami, Ryan, & Gardner, 2001). Therapeutic handling, which is an important NDT treatment strategy, provides very specific sensory input that grades the intensity, rhythm, and duration of somatosensory input while allowing the client to attend to other aspects of the task. Loud or vigorous auditory stimuli from the clinician's voice and visual stimuli from the environment can be useful in evoking attention or motivation or in producing forceful movement. A soothing voice helps an infant organize his behavior. Visual or auditory activities can stimulate an upright head position. Therapists must use multisensory stimuli carefully with highly distractible individuals or with infants and children who have regulatory system disorders. Low or high thresholds of tactile or vestibular input can have a profound effect on the effectiveness of the movement outcome. The therapist makes decisions to change the type, level, and location of sensory input according to the client's preferences and responses to specific input. Some clients enjoy touch and pressure, while others react with annoyance or irritation. Sensory stimulation must be paired with the client's ability to use the information and adapt motor responses.

NDT recognizes that sensory input is linked in two different ways to motor output, each affecting movement control. Sensory feedback uses sensory information before and after completing a movement to modulate, adjust, and fine-tune the movement relative to changes in the environment and task requirements. Feed-forward occurs as the client anticipates the postural and movement requirements for a task and instinctively prepares to fulfill requirements before the motor act begins. Feed-forward strategies are based on previous motor and sensory experience and require practice to become useful for the client (Bly, 1996; Whiteside, 1997). The NDT therapist uses the interplay between sensory feedback and feed-forward to help the client develop knowledge and instinct for efficient movement and respond to error detection and subsequent reorganization of functional movement that better matches the task goals and environmental demands.

> ***NDT Focus: The primary difference that separates NDT clinical practice from all other approaches is the inclusion of precise therapeutic handling, which includes both facilitation and inhibition as key interventions to achieve independent function.***

5. **Therapeutic handling is a primary intervention strategy that NDT therapists use to assist the client in achieving independent function.** It is the precision of therapeutic handling as a treatment strategy that differentiates NDT treatment from any other approach to the management of sensorimotor dysfunction in individuals with CNS pathophysiology. Therapeutic handling in NDT takes the form of *inhibition* or *facilitation of posture and movement* or, more often, a combination of these two features as needed to increase function. The therapist, through his or her hands on the client, can (a) direct, regulate, and organize tactile, proprioceptive, and vestibular input, (b) direct the client's initiation of movement more efficiently and with more effective muscle synergies, (c) support or change alignment of the body in relation to the base of support (BOS) and with respect to the force of gravity prior to and during movement sequences, (d) decrease the amount of force the client uses to stabilize body segments, (e) guide or redirect the direction, force, speed, and timing of muscle activation for successful task completion, (f) either constrain or increase the flexibility in the degrees of freedom needed to stabilize or move body segments in a functional activity, (g) sense the response of the client to the sensory input and the movement outcome and provide nonverbal feedback for reference of correction, (h) recognize when the client can become independent of the therapist's assistance and take over control of posture and movement, and (i) direct the client's attention to meaningful aspects of the motor task.

   Therapeutic handling has three essential interactive components:

   Hand placement–key points of control: The therapist places his or her hands purposefully and precisely on the client's body to specifically influence the area under the therapist's hands and indirectly influence other body parts. Mrs. Bobath called this *therapeutic handling through key points of control* (K. Bobath, 1959; K. Bobath & B. Bobath, 1964). The therapist monitors the client's responses to his or her handling and adapts the location, amount, direction, and type of input needed to obtain changes in alignment before and during a movement sequence to ensure effective response to this input. The therapist can place hands across a joint to gain alignment, initiate a weight shift, or stabilize that body part, or position hands directly on the muscles to enhance efficient, coordinated movement. Therapists choose proximal or distal key points of control depending on the intent of handling, with the understanding that the role of each hand may shift several times during a movement sequence.

Proximal key points, located on the trunk, including the shoulder and pelvic girdles, are used to influence patterns of posture and movement in all three planes (sagittal, frontal, and transverse). Distal key points are the head and the upper and lower extremities. A therapist can use proximal or distal key points to inhibit or facilitate posture and movement in sequence or simultaneously. Key points are used interchangeably and in combinations (such as right shoulder and left side of pelvis) because each client responds differently and the therapist must adapt his or her handling to the client's reaction at that moment in time. It is essential for the therapist to withdraw control gradually as the movement proceeds or when it is evident that the client is able to perform a task unaided. This allows the client to detect errors and solve problems when executing movement.

Facilitation: Facilitation is the strategy of therapeutic handling that makes a posture or movement easier or more likely to occur. Clinicians utilize facilitation to gain functional, meaningful activities. During the examination, the therapist identifies those components of posture and movement that are needed to reach the functional goal, then incorporates facilitation as a treatment strategy to increase the client's access to repertoires, combining postures and movements in anticipation of and during functional activities. Facilitation modifies postural control by increasing degrees of freedom, supporting a body segment during an activity, and activating the postural system to produce change in alignment of the body relative to gravity or the BOS. Facilitation is frequently used to activate, change, or grade the speed, direction, magnitude, or timing of active movement. During treatment, the therapist sets up the environment, varies the task, and decides which components of the posture or movement can be made easier through facilitation to complement the motor learning process.

Facilitation requires planning and practice by the therapist so that he or she can instantaneously follow or lead the client. Done well, it looks simple. For example, a child with CP attempting to play with a toy, must roll over, sit up, and use both hands to manipulate the toy. If the child is unable to do this, the therapist places hands on the child *at the same time* that the child initiates the movement. The therapist changes handling from one key point (or more) on the child's body to another, to maintain alignment and facilitate smooth transitions and coordinated patterns of activation while altering speed, direction, or timing as necessary for the child to move efficiently. Simultaneously, the therapist inhibits abnormal stiffness and ineffective motor synergies that interfere with completion of the task. The therapist is always feeling the client's muscles and movement response to facilitation and modifying input, unobtrusively gauging when to assist the child and when to give full control so that the child experiences the consequence of his or her movement (and errors). This promotes the child's ability to problem solve his or her own solution for the task. The therapist does all this while engaging the child in activities appropriate for the developmental age, including language, play, and socialization. In addition, the therapist must also provide as wide a variety of sensorimotor patterns as possible during treatment so that the child can build movement repertories and adapt posture and movement for similar functions in other contexts.

Inhibition: Therapists use inhibition to restrict the client's atypical postures and movements that prevent the development of more selective motor patterns and efficient performance. Originally in the Bobath Approach, the term *inhibition* referred to reducing tone and abnormal reflex activity resulting from CNS dysfunction (see Chapter 5). Currently, this term in NDT refers to the reduction of specific underlying impairments that interfere with function. For example, elongating a shortened muscle reduces the effect that tightness will have on posture and range of motion (ROM). Inhibiting excessive co-activation patterns allows dynamic stability for more effective postural control. A clinician will utilize inhibition in treatment to (a) prevent or redirect those components of a movement that are unnecessary and interfere with intentional, coordinated movement, (b) constrain the degrees of freedom, to decrease the amount of force the client uses to stabilize posture, (c) balance antagonistic muscle groups, or (d) reduce spasticity or excessive muscle stiffness that interferes with moving specific segments of the body. Most often in NDT treatment, inhibition is used in combination with facilitation through therapeutic handling from key points of control.

6. **Treatment strategies often include preparation and simulation of critical foundational elements (task components) as well as practice of the whole task.** In an NDT approach, clients with CNS pathology are not expected to improve function simply by practicing the skilled activity because they cannot select or activate the appropriate patterns of motor coordination to link the posture and movements needed for complex skills (B. Bobath & Finnie, 1958). Although practice and repetition alone might work for persons with normal CNS, even athletes prepare for specific activity by stretching and warming up. In order to complete a task, a client might need to learn and practice posture and movement components outside the functional task, in a less challenging position, with less demand for timing or speed, or with physical assistance to support the posture or activate muscles. For example, infants and young children might lack experience in the movements necessary to complete a particular functional task, or adults in the early stages of recovery from stroke might have lost motor memory and need to be prepared with activities that increase

sensation of posture and mobility in settings that approximate these everyday, real-life tasks. (Davis 2002). A client of any age can lack joint or muscle mobility, patterns of postural activation, alignment, or strength, any of which can affect performance. Often the components of a movement sequence must be prepared before the client can put them together in a functional sequence. The anticipated outcome might be to move from supine to sitting up at the side of the bed, but the preparatory therapeutic activities might include passive elongation of the muscles of the trunk for lateral and rotational trunk movements, facilitated reaching across the body, supporting weight on elbow and forearm in the sidelying position, and learning to push away from the support surface to raise up to support on the hand. All of these components will eventually come together to produce a function–in this case, getting out of bed. Whenever possible, treatment strategies include preparation of critical elements of a task within the functional context. For example, the therapist might have more success elongating the muscles of the trunk and mobilizing the scapula on the thoracic wall, if the client is actively reaching overhead to retrieve a book from a high shelf or to clean the mirror above the bathroom sink.

NDT Focus: The NDT approach analyzes the entire task, the various system impairments, and the specific postures and movements needed, then provides practice of the critical foundational elements, and finally puts these components together and gives the client opportunities to practice the total skill. However, in any one treatment session a client might practice separate motor components as well as functional tasks.

Simulation–learning and practicing components of a task through motivating activities that ensure success–is a useful tool in preparing a client for function. These activities are at a lower level of difficulty, often incorporating therapeutic handling needed to obtain sensation of the desired posture and movement components while inhibiting habitual and compensatory patterns (Adler, 2002). For example, prior to attempting the task of actually putting on real socks or pants, a client might "pretend" to put on the garments by holding a small hoop with both hands, placing a foot through the hoop, then pulling the hoop up the leg to practice dressing. The important part of simulation during NDT intervention is remaining focused on the functional skill: the client is pretending to pull on pantyhose or pants and is not simply putting a foot into a hoop while holding it with two hands. Simulation places the posture and movement into the function and focuses the client (and the clinician) on the intent of the task.

7. **NDT intervention is designed to obtain active responses from the client in goal-directed activities.** NDT uses active movement to produce change in movement patterns and motor performance. Active participation by the client is critical for motor learning (Schmidt, 1991) and includes both self-initiated voluntary movement and

therapist-facilitated postural reactions performed within the context of goal-directed activities. Postural control, which requires moving in all three planes and is performed automatically during balance activities, requires a great deal of mobility, strength, endurance, and strategy for control. In addition, postural control is a necessary element for all functional activities. NDT therapists have the option to work with a client in either a feedback or feed-forward mode, whichever is most effective in obtaining the desired responses by the client. Active feed-forward movements are effective for young children or individuals who cannot understand or are unable to cooperate with methods that utilize cognitively directed movements. The NDT therapist provides an optimal balance between conscious attention and automatic execution according to the demands of the functional task.

8. **Whenever possible during treatment, movement is initiated and actively performed by the client.** The therapist makes decisions or adjusts the strategies to best achieve the outcome even when the client leads the treatment by initiating the execution of the movement sequence. For example, if the goal is to improve reaching in a sitting position, the therapist sets up the environment, placing the child in a secure seated position and providing motivating toys in various positions. (see fig. 1.2, Chapter 1) This structuring of the environment and thoughtful placement of the toys requires the child to change, adjust, and correct muscle length and alignment of the joints and stabilize the trunk, shoulder, arm, and hand as he or she moves through space and provides active opportunities to develop accuracy in reaching while engaging in play with these various items. The therapist offers this guidance subtly, so that the child is often unaware that the therapist has provided the structure. In addition, the therapist's hands might rest lightly but purposefully on the child's trunk, shoulder, or hand, available to facilitate or inhibit during the activity to improve or ensure success in the motor performance.

9. **NDT intervention includes planning and solving motor problems.** NDT therapists, because of their strength in analysis of motor problems, can help the client in motor planning. Motor planning begins with one-step, goal-directed problems and progresses to multistep, open-ended functions, as demonstrated by the progression revealed in first asking, "How are you going to get your arm in your sleeve?" then later asking, "How are you going to get dressed in time for breakfast?" Self-initiated problem solving transfers the responsibility and ownership of movement sequences from the therapist to the client. Each client must eventually work out ways to perform various tasks based on his or her own system integrity and limitations as well as motivation, priority, and necessity for the task. No two people plan and carry out motor sequencing tasks in exactly the same way, and every individual alters the plan and solution for a motor problem according to the specific task conditions and environmental constraints at the moment. For example, while generally the same, the requirements for placing the arm and hand through a stiff jacket sleeve are different from those for placing the arm and hand through a tight, flexible sweater sleeve; and placing the hand in a glove is different from placing the hand in a mitten.

10. **NDT intervention allows the client to learn from errors that occur during movement.** Error awareness is part of the motor learning process. Learning takes place when errors occur and individuals evaluate the knowledge of results, then correct their own errors (Gentile, 2000). In NDT treatment, this means that the therapist must allow time for the client to assess the situation and attempt a variety of movement plans to achieve the goal. However, the therapist may limit the possibilities so that the client reaches a successful conclusion without unnecessary frustration and disappointments. When learning new skills or attempting skills in a novel situation, the client might take a longer time to solve the problem, and the clinician must build this time into the treatment session. The therapist continually introduces new activities in therapy that require the client to attempt new movements, even when errors are likely. It is an ongoing challenge to the NDT therapist to decide when to allow the client to select and use available motor patterns even when execution is ineffective, and when to guide the client to a more adaptive outcome. Clinicians constantly make decisions regarding error in performance and allow "successful failures," understanding that making and correcting errors is important in skill learning (Magill, 1998).

11. **Repetition is an important component in motor learning.** Motor activities that are task-specific, repeated throughout a session with variability, and included in functional ways at home have a better chance of becoming part of the client's habitual repertoire than infrequently practiced skills. This is an important concept in neuronal group selection theory and has always been part of the Bobaths' teachings (see Chapter 5). Therapists need to wait, observe, and analyze while a client "practices" an activity during therapy. Clients can be encouraged to find "another way" or "more ways" to do a task. Repetition is important but does not need to be boring. Repetition does not necessarily mean doing the same thing the same way, but rather finding a variety of strategies to accomplish functional objectives. For example, the therapist might ask a client to find a way to get up from sitting on a chair while holding a large object or a cup of water in both hands, with bare feet or with shoes, or without using the chair for support. Practicing with variety can include silly, awkward, and inefficient motor plans ("Stand up with your feet crossed" or "Put your shirt on backward") to help the client develop originality when solving problems. Larin (2000) calls this "creative behavior," which includes the components of movement variability, flexibility, and elaboration.

12. **Create an environment that is conducive to cooperative participation and support of the client's efforts.** The enablement model of NDT considers the environment to be a strong stimulus for eliciting and changing motor behavior. The concept of environmental affordances, first suggested by Gibson (1966, 1979), describes the specific actions that result from the relationship between a person and the specific environment in the physical world. A supportive environment can motivate clients to move in ways that achieve the therapeutic objectives even when these goals are difficult and energy-consuming (Fetters, 1991). The environment can

motivate the client to engage in exploratory, self-initiated activities and provide reasonable opportunities to practice preferred movement patterns even when the therapist is not available to supply feedback.

The concept of environmental affordances includes not only the physical conditions but also the attitudes, beliefs, and approach of individuals toward their environment. The NDT approach views therapy as an ongoing part of the life of a client with CNS dysfunction, and as such, therapy should be a positive experience. NDT therapists believe that their clients will improve and convey this attitude to their clients in their positive approach to health-related issues. If clients enjoy movement, they will be more inclined to make movement a part of their lifestyle through exercise and recreation, to prevent disability in daily life roles. Health-related fitness is important for health promotion and prevention of secondary impairments. Teaching clients to understand and be responsible for their physical fitness helps to prepare individuals for the maximum degree of self-determination attainable.

13. **Knowledge of the development of posture and movement components is used in designing treatment strategies.** NDT therapists have a strong foundation in how posture and movement are linked in motor development, especially relating to the contributions and interactions of the neuromuscular, musculoskeletal, and sensory systems in producing efficient motor skills. The knowledge of the development of the different components of posture and movement (and the systems that produce these components) leads to intervention strategies that effectively match movement ability to the various stages of development or recovery for adults and children. This understanding of typical development of posture and movement also allows therapists to recognize components that might be missing or atypically performed in a variety of movement patterns. For example, an adult who has low voice volume might speak in short phrases because he or she has not developed adequate co-activation of the trunk flexors, extensors, and rotators to support the rib cage when speaking while sitting unsupported. Knowing what components of movement are needed to support the rib cage during speech production leads the therapist to develop intervention strategies that will link co-activation of the trunk muscles with stable posture and transitional movements (Massery & Moerchen, 1996).

14. **A single treatment session progresses from activities in which the client is most capable to activities that are more challenging.** Within each treatment session, clients should have opportunities to work with activities at which they are successful and that are appropriate to the stage of recovery, development, and age. The therapist must control the progression from one activity to another so that the force of gravity, speed, or effort required provides the "just-right" challenge for the client. In this way, the client continues to produce movement directed toward broadening the options for functional change. Through experience with an individual client, a therapist discovers the activities that have a positive effect on the client's movement. The clinician presents these activities early in a treatment session to give the

client control in positions in which movement is easier for the individual, before attempting movement in positions that are difficult or new or before practicing within a functional task. Motor learning shows that individuals will persist in attempting difficult movements if they first experience success with less difficult movements. *The NDT therapist must wait for the client's response* before deciding to limit or change the possibilities in a movement sequence so that the client can perform without gross errors of execution that might lead to further abnormal strategies. This interchange between client and therapist takes time and experience. Treatment should end with activities that are functional for the client.

One of the ongoing challenges for the NDT clinician is knowing when to push for difficult aspects of movement control and when to back off. Often the state of the client affects motivation and motor control, and the therapist will need to make changes within a treatment session and from one treatment session to another even when the therapist (and often the client as well) lacks knowledge of other life factors that hold the reason for a change, either better or worse, in performance. An experienced clinician picks up on these daily changes and alters the treatment progression accordingly.

15. **NDT therapy sessions provide motivation and purpose to engage the client fully in developing and reinforcing movement responses.** Clients need to engage in pleasurable activities in order to be motivated for very difficult tasks. Play is integrated into treatment with children who have CP, to motivate but not to overstimulate to the point of distraction from therapeutic goals. Finding the balance between spontaneous play by the child (which involves problem solving and initiation of new motor behavior) and structured play guided by the therapist is an ongoing challenge. Simulated sports or dance is appropriate play for school-aged children and teens. Older teens and adults might enjoy developing their tennis or golf swing, or card playing, cooking, or gardening skills. Music develops rhythm, timing, and endurance and can be motivating for children and adults. These activities are highly motivating and are functionally oriented. One factor in producing successful outcomes is the clinician's ability to know the interests, both work and leisure, of the client, improvise in the choice of activities, and change them appropriately during a treatment session while keeping the therapeutic goals in mind (Embry & Adams, 1996). For example, a teenage boy brings his car magazines to PT. He wants to sit in his wheelchair and show his favorite cars to his therapist. The therapist wants movement and motor planning. Knowing that the magazines provide motivation, the therapist takes his magazines as the boy comes into the room to take off his coat, and places them on a table near the door. The PT then requires the boy to transfer out of his chair, walk to the table, retrieve a magazine, return to sit on a bench, cut out a photo, stand, tape the photo on the wall lining up his favorite cars as he describe the make, model and special features. The therapist assists these postures and movements as needed, to ensure successful outcomes for the therapist and the client.

16. **NDT intervention methods include modifying the task, or the environment, to take into account the current level of the client's performance and capacity for function.** The goal of NDT intervention is to permit the client to function independently in his or her real-life settings. However, in the various stages of recovery or when learning new tasks, the client can have weakness, lack of control of posture or movement, or other system impairments that prevent this possibility. The therapist might simplify the task of climbing stairs step-over-step by modifying the stairs, using only a 4-inch rise with a four-step limit, or might allow the client to hold onto two railings if balance problems limit safety and the security the client needs to focus on the reciprocal pattern of lower extremity (LE) movements. If a client cannot swallow thin liquids, the therapist might thicken the liquid, which would make the task easier as the person works to gain control of oral-motor mechanisms. Modification of the task and the environment to increase function might also include adaptive equipment such as standers, walkers, powered mobility, special adapted seating, adapted self-care products, assistive technology (including switch-operated devices, computers, and communication aids), orthotics, and splints for positioning and mobility. This is a natural part of NDT intervention and is used separately or in combination with facilitation, depending on the task objective and capabilities of the client.

17. **As a client is able to perform movements independently, the therapist provides time during a treatment session for the client to move freely.** Information from motor learning theory indicates that it is important for clients to feel movement produced through their own efforts without input from the therapist. Only in this way will clients incorporate these movements into daily living. It is equally important not to interrupt the client's spontaneous activity in order to adhere to a planned sequence of therapeutic activities. The NDT therapist is always prepared to abandon the agenda in order to accommodate and utilize the client's changing interests and motivations. Clients need to work out their own strategies for accomplishing activities, and therapists must accept their clients' ability to find "the best way" for themselves at that time, even when skill execution deteriorates. Allowing self-initiated and self-controlled movement gives the message that clients are in control of their world and can learn from their own activity.

18. **Individual treatment sessions are designed to evaluate the effectiveness of treatment with the session.** NDT therapists change intervention strategies based on the client's response to treatment; therefore clinicians integrate assessment and treatment throughout the sessions and over time. Each session is designed to evaluate the effectiveness of treatment informally by motivating the client to demonstrate an activity, movement, or posture at the beginning of treatment, throughout the treatment, and again at the end in order to determine whether changes have occurred. For example, if the goal is to develop postural control to support movements of the upper extremities (UEs) for dressing and grooming, at the beginning of a session the therapist might ask the client to stretch the arms overhead, out in

front, and to the sides, then compare these movement patterns at the end of the session. If dressing is the desired outcome, the skill of dressing must be the pre- and post-test. The pre- and post-tests might include how long it takes for the client to dress, for example. If the client cannot do the movement unaided, the pre- and post-tests might examine the amount of manual assistance or verbal guidance needed at the beginning and end of the session. Knowing what changes have occurred is motivating to the client and reinforcing for the therapist and the family.

19. **Recognize and respect the communicative intent of the client's motor behavior.** The ability of a therapist to interpret nonverbal communication is critical when treating infants, children who are too young to speak, or cognitively impaired clients or adults with aphasia or apraxia. Movement or the refusal to move might be communicating fear, insecurity, lack of understanding, or physical discomfort. For example, an adult who refuses to feed herself might have oral hypersensitivity. An increase in muscle stiffness might be an adaptive compensation due to fear of falling, not a deterioration in a system impairment. An adult who refuses to try to descend stairs could be expressing an impairment in visual perception. A crying child might be experiencing physical pain if those muscles that cross the hip have not been prepared prior to attempting functional activities in long sitting. Boehme (1998) described many of the reasons that children cry in therapy and suggested that by creating a partnership with the child and using therapeutic tools sensitively, NDT therapists have the opportunity to shift fear into excitement as new movements become familiar and meaningful to the child. When using therapeutic handling, therapists communicate acceptance, caring, and respect for the client's effort, which helps build self-esteem in the client and cooperative participation in the NDT program.

20. **Families receive information regarding the client's problems and management of those problems as they are able to understand and assimilate the information.** In an NDT approach, the role of the family, both with children with CP and adults with hemiplegia, is critical. Families adjust to the knowledge of disability and its impact in different ways at different times. For example, if the birth of a child with CP is uneventful with no recognizable problems, as is often the case with hemiplegic CP, a family might view the birth as no more disruptive or stressful than the birth of any additional child. If, however, the child was born prematurely, is medically fragile, and requires extensive hospitalization, the parents might need greater levels of support to understand the special needs of their infant. Families need to receive the information that allows them to understand the strengths and the problems their child currently has and to adjust their patterns of parenting to manage their responsibility toward this child, as well as toward other family members. When the child reaches school age, attends public school, and is visible in the community environment, the family will have a new set of limitations to confront concerning the child's rate of progress, ongoing disability, and plans for the future. In another example, the wife of a man who has had a stroke might find it extremely difficult to adjust initially to the loss of his role as financial provider and decision maker and to the changes that

she must now make from her previous role of homemaker or professional. She needs information not only about his physical disability, but also about the impact of his condition on their life roles and the modifications that will be needed in their home environment. Not all persons with stroke are elderly, and many couples find themselves reassessing professional ambitions and investment and retirement plans. The adjustment process in chronic health conditions is ongoing and constantly changing with recovery, development, and aging. The ability to adjust reflects the individual capabilities of the family and their particular pattern of response to life stresses.

21. **In an NDT approach, suggestions to the family are as practical as possible.** Therapists must remember that families have responsibilities toward other family members, to jobs, and to their community, as well as to the family member with a disability. NDT includes therapeutic activities that the family can easily incorporate into the daily care routines of the individual with a disability. These interactions are particularly "therapeutic" because they occur within the family and home structure and are directly related to goals for function in a meaningful environment (Davis, 2002). This home intervention is *not* an "adjunct to therapy," but is equal in importance to the therapist-generated activities in the total program. For example, ROM of the UEs can become part of the routine when the client stretches out an arm to put on a coat or pull off a T-shirt. Massage to express edema of the hand can be done each time a woman applies her moisturizer. A parent can incorporate facial muscle stimulation and movements for oral-motor control while washing the child's face or brushing the child's teeth. Activities that are done in the home or with the family in various environments take advantage of principles of motor learning by providing additional practice time with repetition and variability in functional settings. Nancie Finnie (1997) was instrumental in adapting the therapeutic ideas of the Bobath Approach for use in home and school environments, stressing the practical application of these ideas in meaningful contexts.

22. **NDT recommends an interdisciplinary model of service.** Mrs. Bobath taught that although multiple disciplines, with their own specialties, were involved with each client, it was important for all members of the treatment team to understand and approach each client's problems from a similar point of view. However, each profession's degree of involvement varies depending on the client's age, level of development or recovery, the physical setting, and the system of service delivery. For example, Indredavik, Bakke, Slordahl, Rokseth, and Haheim (1999) showed that the level of integration of PT with the approach used by nursing positively influenced outcomes of clients in a stroke unit. Research on infant development and the stress of neonatal intensive care noted that the infant's primary nurse typically takes the lead role, and along with the infant's developmental therapist (physical or occupational therapist) must support and educate the parents as long-term caregivers, in order to enhance infant and family outcomes (Campbell, 1999a; Lawhon, 1997; Sweeney, 1994).

23. **Coordinate with the goals and activities of all other medical, therapeutic, social, and educational disciplines to ensure a life-span approach to solving the client's problems.** At different times in the client's life, the focus and importance of the various disciplines will change, with one discipline assuming a greater importance than another. For example, as a client following stroke is preparing for discharge, the OT and the social worker will have important roles in examining the client's independence and the support of the home environment. If a family is considering selective dorsal rhizotomy as an intervention for their child with spastic diplegia, the neurosurgeon and the PT will take on more significant roles. If a school-aged child is being considered for an augmented communication system, the SLP and the OT will have more important roles. If a family moves or another child is born, the family might decide to withdraw from an ongoing therapeutic program until the stressors are reduced. A teenager might decide that swimming with friends is more important than weekly PT. Collaboration between professionals and the family with a child having a disability has been mandated by law in the United States (Public Law 102-119, 1990). This law empowers the family to act as advocates for their child through active participation in decision-making regarding the prioritization of treatment goals (Effgen, 2000). Each NDT clinician must recognize that the services he or she provides may not always be a high priority for any individual family or client and must respect and support that decision.

The Problem-Solving Process in NDT Intervention

Two photo case studies summarize the principles of intervention by illustrating the treatment planning and implementation processes. The two case studies were selected to highlight different aspects of the NDT process. The first case is a child with diplegic CP and demonstrates the issues involved in planning, sequencing, and implementing a single PT treatment session.

The second case is a man with hemiplegia following stroke and illustrates the NDT decision-making process as strategies and methods change with recovery over 9 months of PT and OT intervention.

Case 1: Child With Cerebral Palsy

Summary of Data Collection

Chiara is a 4-year-old girl with a diagnosis of spastic diplegic CP secondary to prematurity. She was born at 29 weeks gestation with a birth weight of 2 lb. 6 oz. She was in the NICU for 3 months and on a ventilator. She now lives at home with her mother, who is a single parent. She has an active, extended family, including grandparents, aunts, and uncles. When her mother is at work, Chiara attends a community-based preschool with children who are developing typically. She has age-appropriate language and is very verbal and social. She loves pretend play.

Examination of Functional Skills

Gross motor/movement through space: Chiara's motor disability is classified as level III according to the Gross Motor Function Classification System. She can sit independently, crawl on hands and knees, pull to stand, and walk with a walker or with the support of furniture. She cannot walk independently, even at a household level. She cannot assume standing without external support. She uses a posture walker outdoors and for distances but prefers to crawl in the house and at school. She wears AFOs.

Fine motor/manipulation: She can remove simple clothing independently and assists with dressing. She can feed herself independently with silverware. She has a wide variety of patterns of grasp, preferring the right hand for manipulation. She can draw age-appropriate figures and color, and is beginning to cut with scissors, although this is difficult because of limited assistance from the left hand. She has difficulty with bimanual tasks.

Communications: She speaks well in full sentences but tends to hold her breath and retract her upper lip and tongue and forcefully extend her jaw to increase proximal stability. For this reason, she does not speak and move simultaneously and at times has difficulty with volume control and intelligibility when speaking to unfamiliar people.

Observations of Posture and Movement

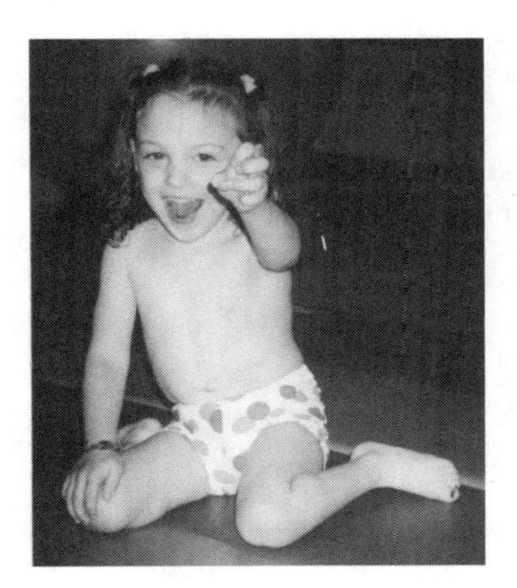

Figure 4.1. Chiara's sitting posture of choice is W-sitting with more weight on the right than the left. In general, she has more stiffness and less variety of movements in the LEs than the UEs, with more obvious motor impairments on the left side. This functional position allows her to have a stable base and use the left hand for play. However, this position prevents weight shift, trunk symmetry, and easy transitions to other postures, and limits bilateral use of her hands. These limitations reinforce the secondary impairments of hip internal rotation and tibial torsion.

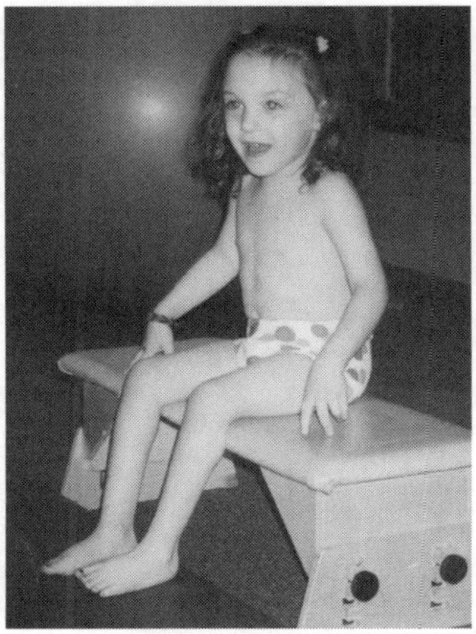

Figure 4.2. Chiara can sit independently on a small bench, but she is insecure, which further limits hand use. To assist her proximal stability, she keeps her tongue against her bottom teeth, holds her breath, and maintains her jaw in an open posture.

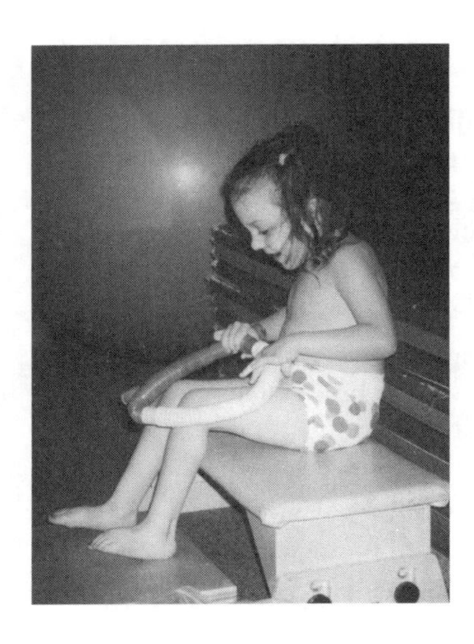

Figure 4.3. Chiara can play with items while sitting, but uses excessive muscle activity to maintain postural stability. Her attempts to maintain a stable posture produce secondary musculoskeletal impairments, including posterior pelvic tilt, increased thoracic flexion, and decreased mobility of the rib cage and scapula. She cannot reach into space due to the decrease in the freedom of the scapular muscles for mobility. She does not use the floor to assist stability, and her feet often do not even contact the floor but are part of a tightly-linked flexion synergy. As seen here, the effort to push the flexible tubes together increases overall flexor stiffness in sitting.

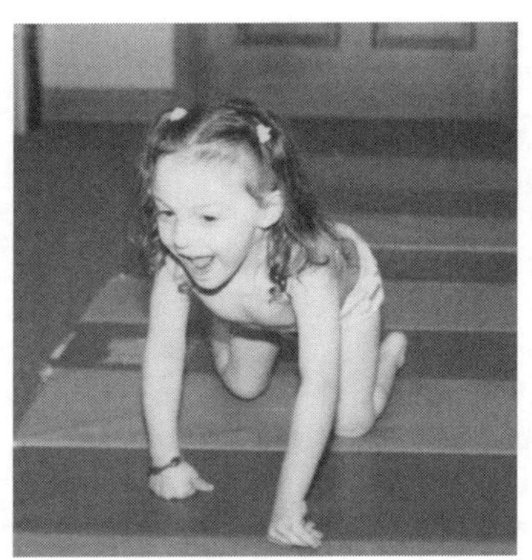

Figure 4.4. Chiara can creep reciprocally, but prefers to "bunny hop," a strategy she uses to increase her speed and efficiency. The active movement excursions of the LEs are very limited so that the hip flexors are activated in their shortened range. Again, the total flexor synergy of the LEs is evident. Her hands are frequently fisted, and she takes weight on her metacarpal heads. There is no smooth rotation along the spine or between the scapular and pelvic girdles.

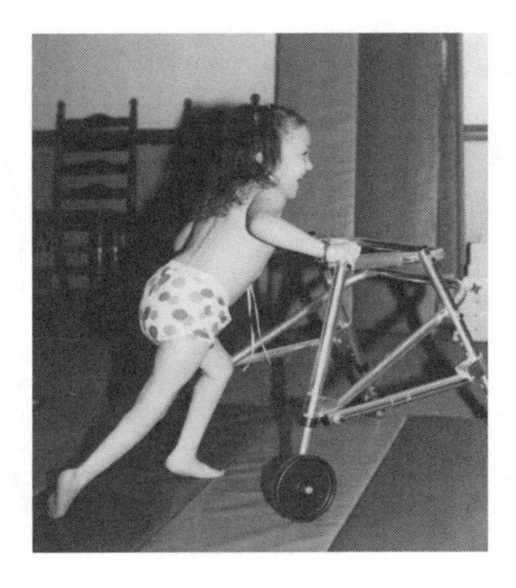

Figure 4.5. Chiara can pull to stand at her walker through a modified half-kneel. Her feet plantar-flex as the hips and knees extend. The back extensors are active, but not in patterns of co-activation with the abdominals. There is excessive use of the arms to pull to standing.

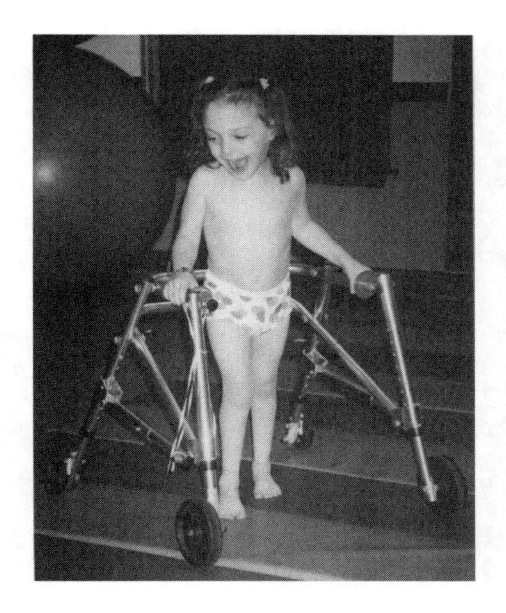

Figure 4.6. Chiara turns and positions herself in the walker. She walks well on level surfaces, but her base of support is narrow, cadence is slow, and she relies heavily on her arms for weight bearing. As she steps, her stride is short and she shifts her entire upper body laterally over her weight-bearing leg to step with the contralateral leg. In order to maintain extension for standing, she uses minimal hip and knee flexion during swing phase. She has increased shoulder girdle and rib cage elevation with increased UE flexion, internal rotation, and pronation. Without her AFOs, it is obvious that the muscle belly of each gastroc is higher than average and atrophied secondary to constant wearing of orthotics. Earlier photos showed the limitation in ROM at the ankle, which is also secondary to the AFOs.

The treatment illustrated here will consider both the person and contextual issues involved in planning an individual PT treatment session. This case study utilizes the NDT problem-solving model diagrammed in Chapter 3 (see Figure 3.1) and incorporates the NDT treatment principles discussed in this chapter. The focus is not the specific strategies utilized, but rather the decision-making process, which is the key to the NDT approach. The same process can be used in an OT or SLT session.

The proposed functional activity outcome for this PT session: Chiara will carry an item in both hands while walking independently, 12 feet across the treatment room, after 1 hour of PT intervention.

The thought process underlying this decision follows. This outcome was selected because it is a parental objective that Chiara will ambulate at home and in her preschool, transporting her play or learning materials with her. It is important to Chiara because she likes being independent, and she is moving toward a total-inclusion educational program. The therapist also anticipates that the secondary musculoskeletal impairments (i.e., decreased ROM and skeletal deformities) will be made worse by prolonged time crawling on the floor with continual action of the hip and knee flexors in their shortened range. In addition, W-sitting is the easiest transition from crawling, and this too increases the time spent with hips and knees flexed and internally rotated. Chiara and those around her (family, teachers, and classmates) need to perceive her as an "ambulator" rather than a "crawler," which would match other activities expected of a 4-year-old girl. Although she will most likely be able to walk and carry an item requiring two hands in PT, she probably would not be able to carry this over into her classroom setting at this time, due to the distractions of other children and obstacles in her path. Once the function is established in a controlled treatment setting, it will be integrated into other environments.

Impairment Goals Related to Functional Outcome:

1. Recruit trunk muscles in patterns of co-activation to free the shoulder girdle to control movement of arms in space.
2. Improve timing and adaptability of inter- and intralimb movements to coordinate synergies needed for gait.
3. Improve selection and execution of appropriate synergistic and reciprocal muscle action of both upper and lower extremities.
4. Increase ROM of hips and ankles for active functional range.

Posture and Movement Goals Related to Functional Outcome:

1. Develop appropriate trunk alignment during movement sequences.
2. Develop weight shift prior to movement so that either side can initiate movement.
3. Develop weight bearing of appropriate body part, using the support surface to organize anticipatory weight shift.
4. Decrease reliance on upper body for support while sitting and standing.
5. Develop transitional movements with weight shift and axial rotation.
6. Improve steady-state balance and postural control in sitting and standing.
7. Grade stiffness in the LEs to switch quickly and smoothly between swing and stance phase of gait.

Contextual Considerations

Chiara enjoys dressup, makeup, and social interactions. She is nervous and a little self-conscious about having her picture taken, so is being "paid" for her participation with a makeup kit for young girls. The session will include applying the makeup and modeling, then she will take the kit home. The makeup kit will be the item she carries when walking independently at the end of the session. She is very vested in the activity and is motivated to do well throughout the session by the knowledge that she will take home the makeup kit as a result of her work. She is pleased that her uncle, who does not typically observe PT sessions, will be present today. These factors outweigh her shyness and facilitate optimal cooperation and performance. This PT session immediately followed her regularly scheduled OT session, which was 1 hour in length and addressed independent dressing activities while in bench sitting, as well as the components of movement needed for dressing skills.

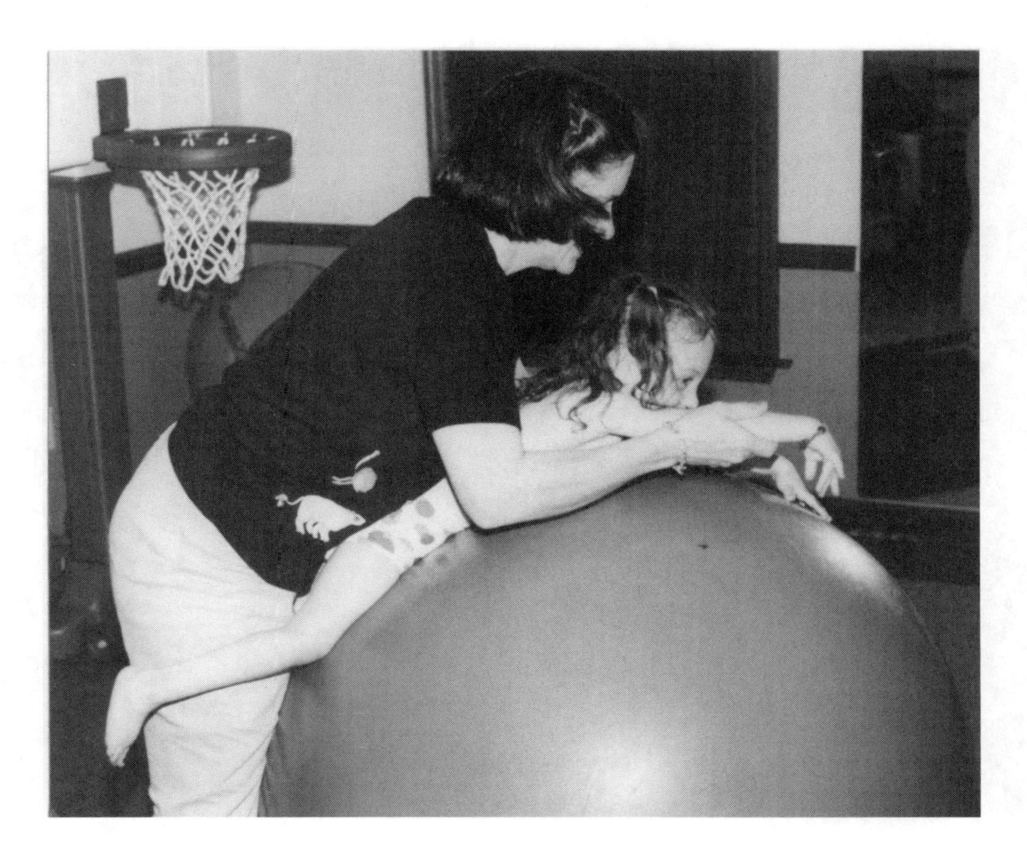

Figure 4.7. The PT session begins on a large ball at Chiara's request. She enjoys responding to the movement of the ball, particularly if the ball is moved rapidly. It is an activity with which she is familiar and that she can follow easily. The therapist uses this equipment to address system impairments and posture and movement goals. The position in prone allows isometric, sustained holding of the trunk extensors to improve postural control while allowing rapid movement through the UEs to decrease dynamic stiffness, which is largely compensatory for lack of co-activation of the trunk. The UEs are taken to the ends of ranges of shoulder flexion with elbow extension, which prepares the muscle length needed for later functions while the trunk is used for postural control. Beginning by combining postural control with distal movement provides carryover from the functions practiced in OT but in a new position. The movement helps to modulate arousal and attention through vestibular stimulation. Working on the large ball positions Chiara in relation to the therapist, permitting better body mechanics for the therapist as she works with Chiara in a prone position. However, this position keeps Chiara working in the sagittal plane. Therefore, as soon as the therapist feels that Chiara has gained the range and activated the trunk extensors, the therapist facilitates transition to sidelying in order to work on abdominal obliques in their shortened range and the transitions to a sitting position. The therapist also uses this time to distract Chiara from the photography and focus her attention on the play goal.

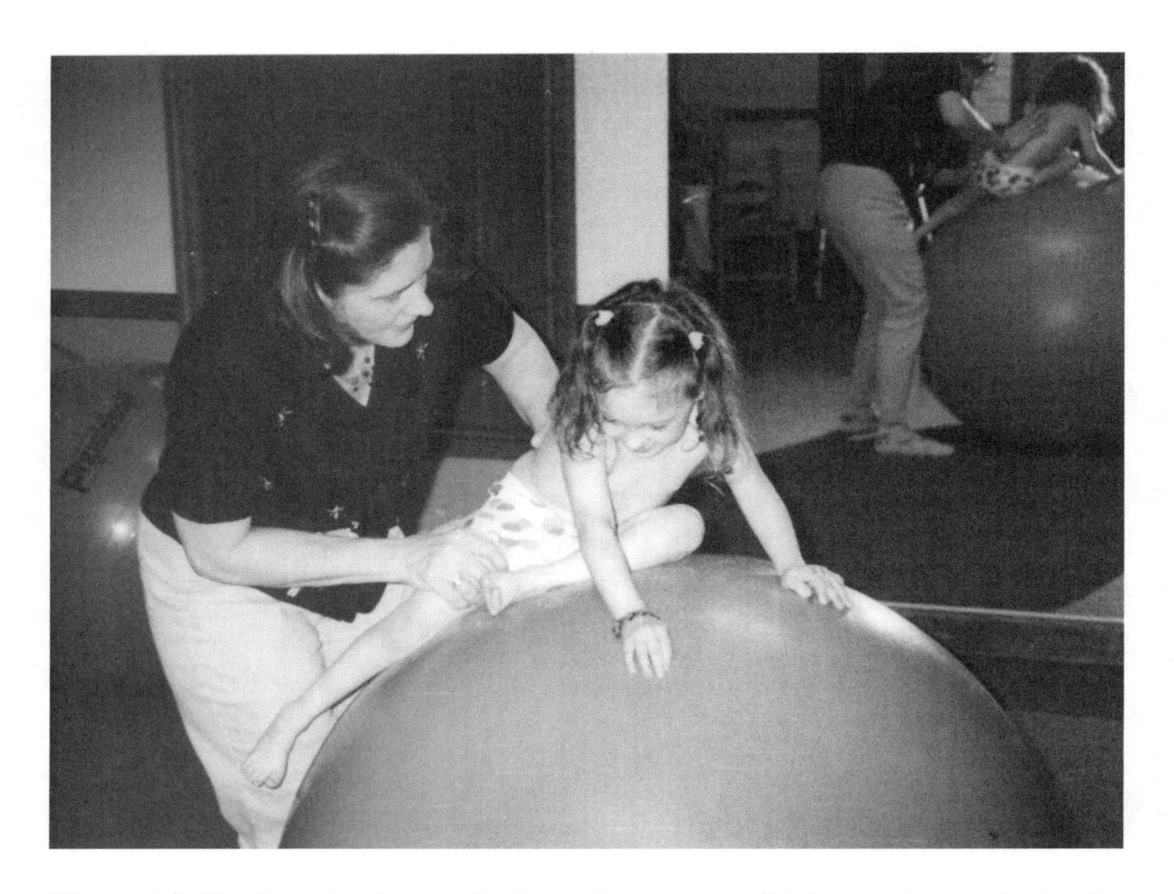

Figure 4.8. The therapist changes the key points to more distal control to emphasize the weight shifting caudally and diagonally, increasing the potential for axial rotation with exaggerated interlimb control of the LEs. The left LE is in flexion with abduction and external rotation, and the right is in greater extension, adduction, and internal rotation. This interlimb organization will be necessary during ambulation and is difficult for Chiara to recruit. The therapist's hand on Chiara's back facilitates trunk extension with scapular stability on the thoracic wall while Chiara actively pushes up through side sitting to a sitting position. The therapist can either increase or minimize the impact of gravity on Chiara's relationship to the weight-bearing surface by moving the ball. Gently shifting weight decreases the amount of shoulder elevation that occurs during the transition. The vestibular, visual, and somatosensory systems are simultaneously stimulated in ways that are typical for her age. The therapist can alter speed, direction, and rhythm of movement to allow Chiara to anticipate and respond to unexpected perturbations in her balance. This is hard work for Chiara, and she occasionally retracts her upper lip and loses saliva control during the transitions.

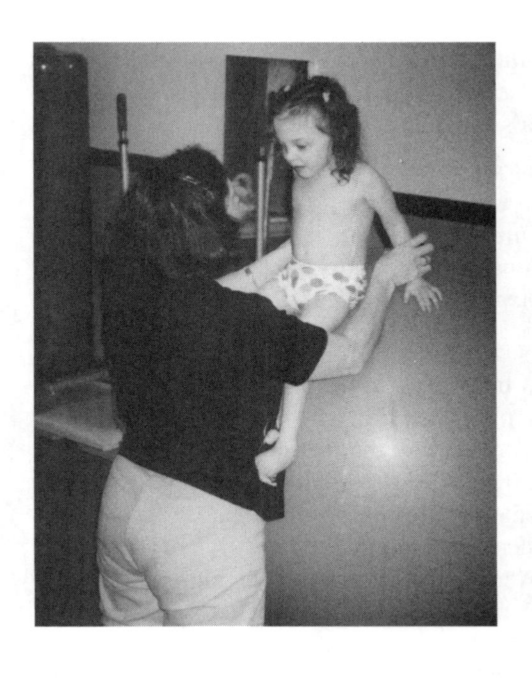

Figure 4.9. Now in sitting, Chiara's trunk is symmetrical, head aligned, chin tucked, and mouth lightly closed. The therapist moves the ball so that Chiara's weight is shifted forward to increase the demand for trunk extension with simultaneous hip flexion. This also brings Chiara into more erect alignment than was seen initially in bench sitting. The key points are distal on Chiara's forearms to encourage weight-bearing on her open hands. Chiara's hands must accommodate to the constantly changing surface of the ball. This posture activates the scapular adductors and influences the contour of the rib-cage by increasing thoracic extension. The therapist is positioned below Chiara's eye level to help with the head, neck, and eye position. The therapist and Chiara discuss how a model applies her makeup. At this time, there are less stringent requirements of the extremities, but strong requirements of the postural muscles. This allows Chiara to use the respiratory muscles in isolation from postural control, and she speaks in long sentences that require respiratory control. Conversation allows the therapist to listen to changes in Chiara's voicing and breathing.

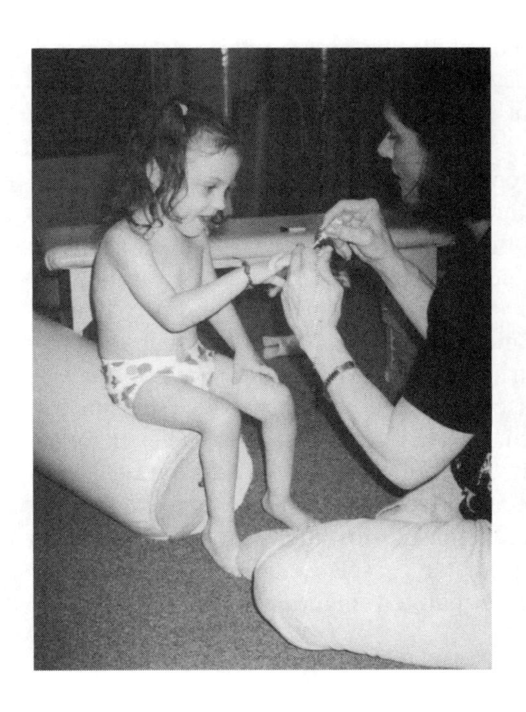

Figure 4.10. Chiara transitions from the ball onto a slanted bolster (reversing the pattern shown in figures 4.7 and 4.8) to have her nails polished. The position was selected to build on the components linking postural control with movement of the extremities developed on the ball. The position of the bolster assists in a vertical alignment of her pelvis and symmetry of her trunk. Her weight shift forward now places weight on her feet so that her feet are part of her base of support (BOS). The slanted position of the bolster promotes the trunk extension that was developed on the ball, but decreases the input from the vestibular system. With only verbal cues to "sit tall like a model" and her focus on admiring the lovely purple color she has selected rather than on her posture, she loses some of her trunk extension and vertical pelvis as she lifts her right hand for nail polish. Notice

also her oral posture, which is indicative of postural insecurity and the stress of the task. In this position the therapist can use strategies to increase soft tissue mobility and increase somatosensory awareness in the LEs while Chiara's toenails are painted.

Note: *The therapist notices that the interactions of the neuromuscular, musculoskeletal, and sensory systems linking posture with UE movements are particularly difficult for Chiara when she is engaged in a highly motivating function. Throughout treatment, the PT will alter the demands of each of these elements to determine how best to combine function, posture, and movement components and underlying body systems to ensure the best possible performance.*

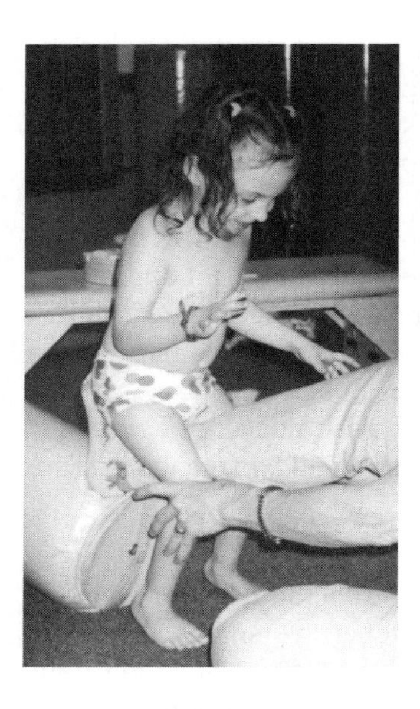

Figure 4.11. Chiara transitions to standing to allow the therapist to blow on her nails to aid drying and to show off their beauty. This demonstrates how the therapist uses play to gain motor components. The therapist controls hip adduction and internal rotation of the LEs by positioning her leg in between Chiara's legs. The therapist's foot facilitates forward translation of Chiara's trunk over her feet and activates hip extension as Chiara initiates the appropriate strategy, taking weight on her feet and pushing to stand with her legs without using her hands on the support, a strategy she does not usually initiate. Because Chiara's nail polish is not dry, she is highly motivated not to put her hands on any support. The therapist's hands above Chiara's knees allow the PT to increase the downward pressure to heighten Chiara's awareness of weight bearing through the feet, assist in the forward translation of the tibia over the talus for dorsiflexion, and inhibit the tendency for hip internal rotation and adduction, all movement components that Chiara will need for walking.

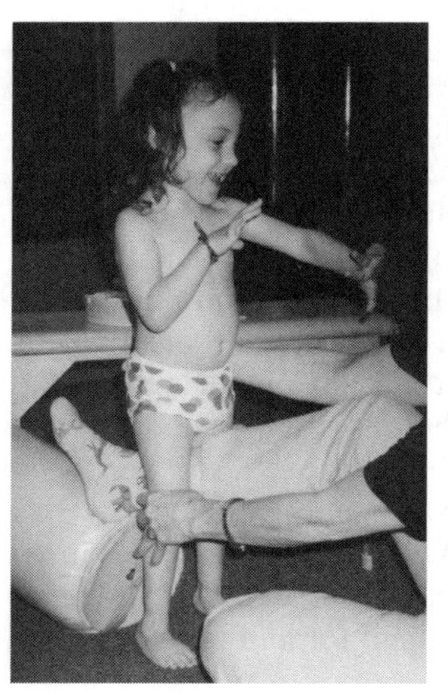

Figure 4.12. Work continues to focus on graded control into terminal extension at the hips and knees with symmetrical weight bearing on the feet by repetitions of the transition between sit and stand. The therapist changes key points to facilitate trunk extension, placing her right hand on Chiara's mid-thoracic spine and her left hand on Chiara's right quadriceps. With symmetrical alignment and improved co-activation of the trunk muscles, the therapist can reduce the amount of assistance as Chiara takes over the work. The therapist stresses graded control through the LEs in and out of terminal extension. Concentric work through the range, including the end of the range, increases movement control of the LEs. The action of the scapular muscles can support the distal activity of admiring her painted fingernails.

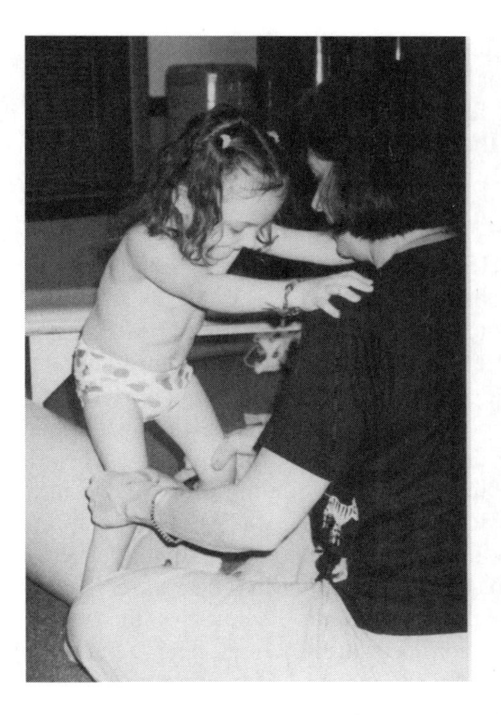

Figure 4.13. Moving back to sitting requires eccentric grading of the quadriceps, a particularly difficult task for Chiara. The therapist modifies the task to give Chiara a stronger sense of the forward flexion from the hips necessary to maintain trunk alignment with weight firmly over her feet throughout the descent. With Chiara's hands lightly resting on the therapist's shoulders, the PT can determine which part of the range Chiara can control and when she might collapse into sitting. The therapist's hands on Chiara's quadriceps and hamstrings control the speed of descent and allow the therapist to stop the motion so that Chiara remains active throughout the range. Although rising and sitting are not major functional outcomes for this session, they are important actions if Chiara is to ambulate independently, and control of the quadriceps and hamstrings in reciprocal relationships is important during walking.

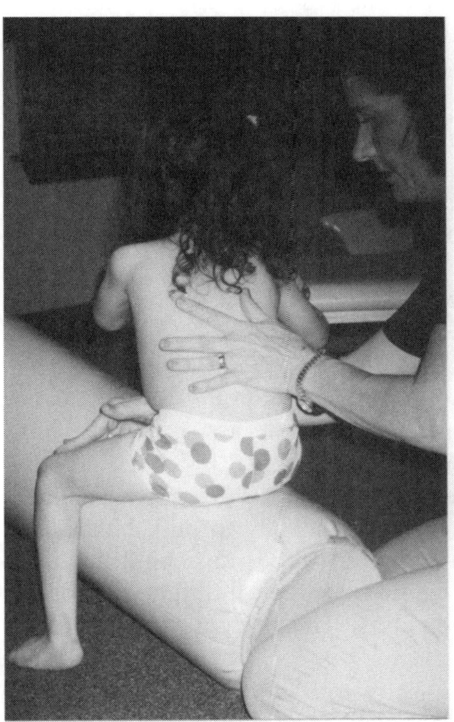

Figure 4.14. Chiara turns around on the bolster as the makeup kit is repositioned to allow selection of eye shadow, blush, and lip gloss. Even though this position encourages backward tilting of the pelvis and compensatory thoracic rounding, the therapist and Chiara together work to counter these biomechanical factors. The bolster facilitates symmetrical weight bearing across the hips, giving Chiara an appropriate BOS. The therapist's left index finger, thumb, and palm assist thoracic extension, which is used with abdominal obliques to align the rib cage over the pelvis. The third and fourth digits aid rotation of the ribs in an isolated, graded fashion. The PT's right hand works to preserve foot-ankle alignment with LE abduction and external rotation and to maintain the weight bearing on Chiara's left foot. Chiara gradually shifts her weight to the left and rotates to the right to select the blush she plans to apply. This position allows the therapist to observe the scapula stabilizing against the thoracic wall and moving appropriately to support

the UE as Chiara directs her attention to the right. The mirror in front of Chiara allows the therapist to view Chiara from the front simultaneously. By leaving her hands in place even when she is not facilitating movement, the PT can feel when Chiara increases the amount of lower body weight bearing to free her UEs for the fine motor work as the session progresses.

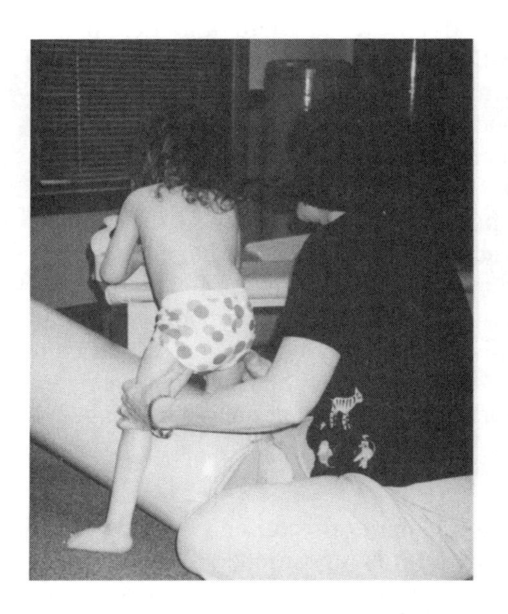

Figure 4.15. Chiara spontaneously stands as the therapist shifts her hands to facilitate extension at the hips and feels Chiara move her pelvis forward over her feet, a movement that she will need to perform rapidly during walking. Again the UEs are free from postural work as she applies blush to her face. The therapist can palpate the femoral heads with her thumbs to see if the hip joints move into full extension as Chiara stands. The effort to apply blush produces lateral flexion to the weight-bearing (right) side. At this point in the session, Chiara and the therapist are jointly deciding on the transitions and specifics of the activities. The therapist is focused on the impairment of posture and movements that appear to limit function, while Chiara is focused on moving in order to play. These are compatible goals.

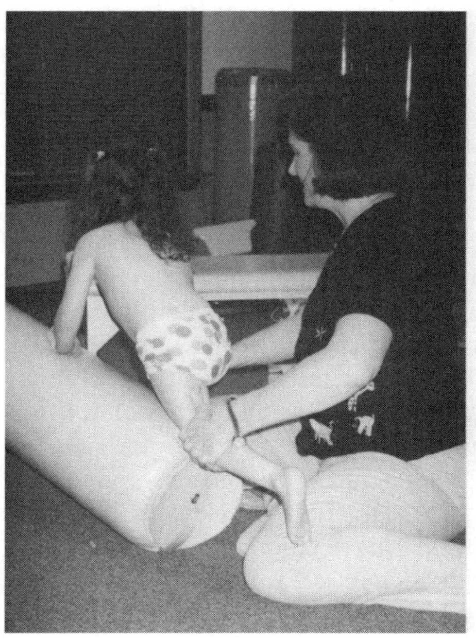

Figure 4.16. As trunk stability increases, the therapist challenges Chiara's trunk movement more by changing the BOS to the right LE and left UE. The therapist can slowly roll the bolster, which requires accommodation to changes of the points of weight bearing. The scapular muscles on the left must accommodate to the shape and movement of the bolster while maintaining stability for weight bearing through the left hand. The therapist's two hands assist LE interlimb coordination. Chiara's right LE is flexed at the hip and knee while the left is extended. The therapist can feel any tendency to pull the left hip into flexion. Chiara still has difficulty maintaining the elongation between the right side of the rib cage and pelvis as her weight is shifted to the right LE.

Note: *The therapist at this time must balance Chiara's desire for function and play with concerns about the impact of atypical posture and movement and reinforcement of current impairments on future function along with possible emergence of secondary impairments. For example, is this lateral flexion an acceptable deviation during the performance of a difficult activity, or is it the foreshadowing of the development of a scoliosis, when Chiara becomes a teenager, secondary to the consistent use of asymmetrical postures when she is challenged? It is only by repeated, careful observation, analysis, and documentation based on interpretation of clinical evidence that a therapist can make the best decision, matching function with movement components.*

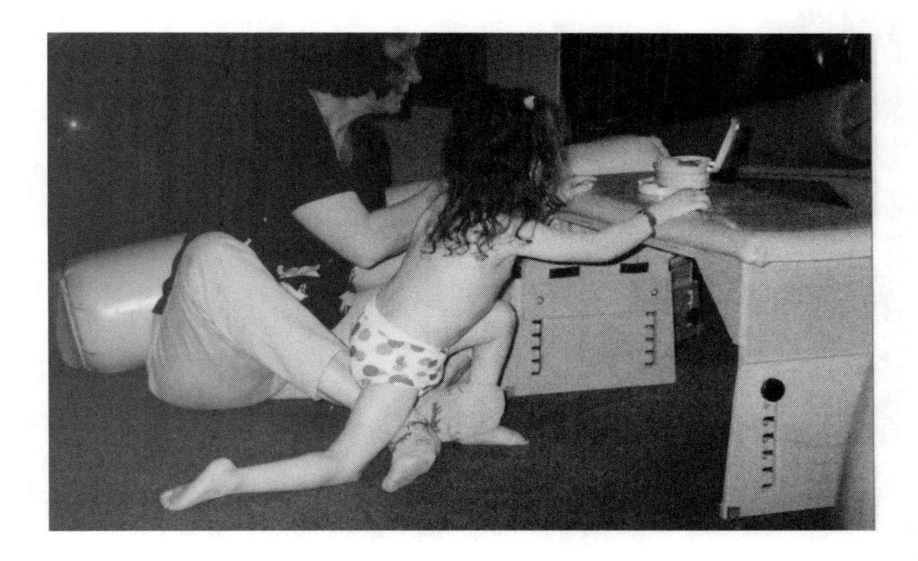

Figure 4.17. The therapist modifies the environment by removing the bolster, leaving the makeup kit on a high bench. The therapist makes this decision in the belief that Chiara has sufficient proximal stability to permit isolated control between the LEs with weight shifts needed for her to rise to standing. The therapist uses her left foot to align Chiara's left leg with the tibia over the talus and the hip and knee flexed and slightly externally rotated. The therapist uses her right foot to slow the movement of Chiara's right LE as it pulls into increasing hip flexion. Chiara maintains trunk alignment and is able to bring her arms forward and upward onto the support surface. She is supporting herself on the table, but does not increase the use of the latissimus or pectorals for the stability. Chiara experiences appropriate trunk alignment and UE movements without the input from the therapist to those body parts. Although this is a difficult transition for Chiara, her attention continues to be focused on the selection of lip gloss, and she carries on lengthy negotiation with her therapist regarding an appropriate color to wear for her return to the daycare center. Chiara wants bright red; the therapist negotiates for light pink. Once again, Chiara demonstrates the proximal control for the difficult posture and movement requirements and the use of the respiratory muscles necessary for controlling voicing with meaningful inflection.

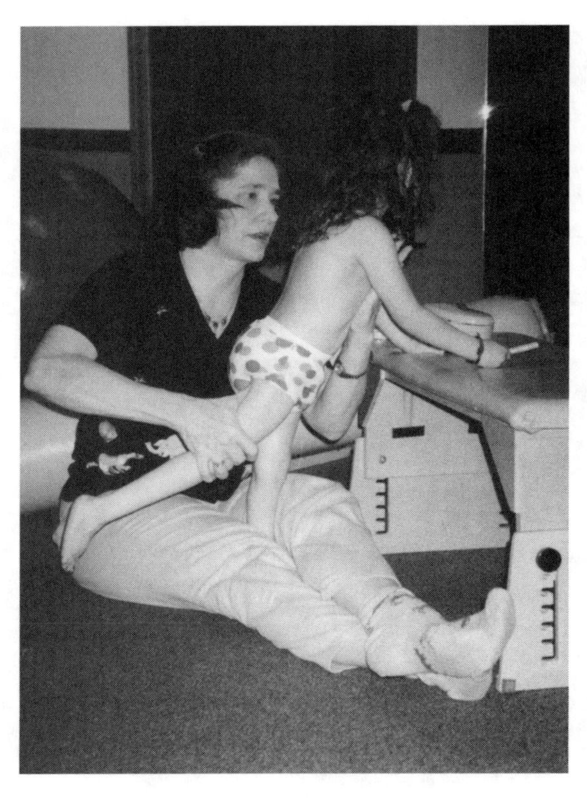

Figure 4.18. To apply her lip gloss, Chiara shifts her weight forward and pushes up with her left leg, gradually increasing the load on the UEs. The therapist modifies the transitions by these key points.

* The therapist's right hand increases the isolated movements between the LEs by slowing the movement of the trailing leg, adding slight traction and vibration during the transition and accentuating the terminal ranges of the hip and knee extension on the left.
* The therapist's left leg helps to keep Chiara's left leg and ankle positioned and to allow the pelvis to move forward over her left weight-bearing leg. These are critical posture and movement components necessary in gait. In addition, the UEs are in the appropriate position for carrying items in two hands. Note that slight external rotation with forearm supination is apparent in the UEs.
* The therapist's left UE provides a variety of inputs. The forearm and heel of the hand help with rib cage orientation and alignment as Chiara moves. The hand is reaching upward and can, as needed, decrease lip retraction and assist in lip closure.

In this sequence, the therapist returns to a great deal of physical handling because it is a time of emotional stress (negotiating color of gloss) and excessive muscle exertion for Chiara. The therapist does not want Chiara to lose the control of posture and movement that she has gained in this session. A precise fine motor task (selecting and removing one lip gloss from a long tube) is combined with a challenging gross motor transition (moving from half-kneel to stride position) while coping with emotions that accompany her conceding to wearing the subtle pink shade. This activity is indicative of the complex linking among various systems (cognitive, sensory, motor, and limbic) that is a hallmark of independent life and of the "just-right" challenge that is presented in therapy.

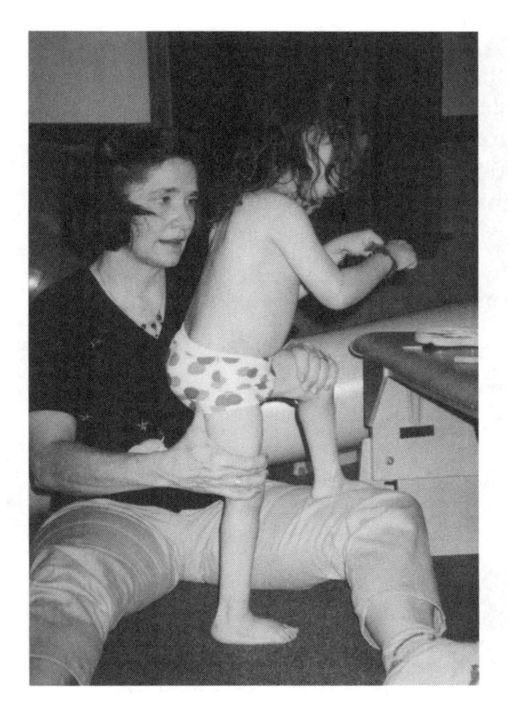

Figure 4.19. Chiara selects the tube of gloss she will apply. The activity requires that she stabilize with the left hand as she twists and pulls off the cap. This activity reinforces the work that had occurred in her OT session during which she had to use her hands together, but for different actions while dressing. Although this activity is highly motivating to Chiara, it is very challenging. The therapist utilizes an alternate LE position that continues to require interlimb dissociated postures. The therapist facilitates hip extension and inhibits left LE adduction and internal rotation. Chiara's weight is shifted slightly forward over her feet. The effort is obvious in the UEs, with shoulder elevation and a slight pull into flexion with increased dynamic stiffness, and in the open mouth posture. Chiara does not revert to the breath-holding strategy noted earlier in the session and is able to continue active co-activation of the muscles of the trunk. She talks freely about her choices throughout the activity.

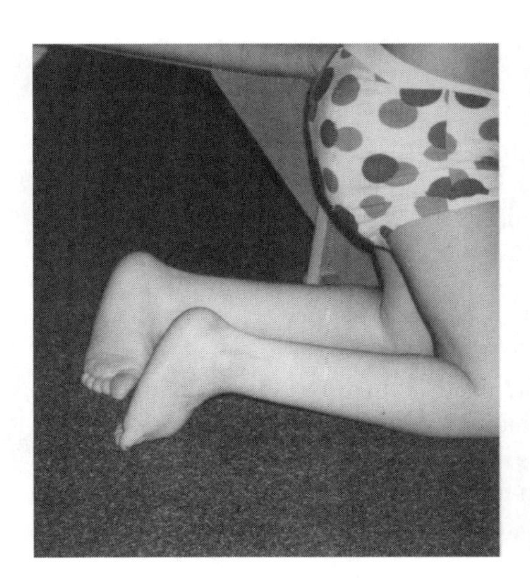

Figure 4.20. Up to this point, the therapist has chosen to have Chiara to work without shoes, socks, and orthotics even though much of the session has involved weight bearing on the LEs. With all the changes in posture and movement, Chiara's LEs evidence stiffness, especially at the ankles and feet, that increases with effort and emotion. In addition, it is extremely difficult for Chiara to isolate ankle movements from toe movements so that ankle dorsiflexion is consistently coupled with toe flexion or curling. This tendency significantly limits the forward weight shift across the foot and will interfere with independent walking. There is also indication of a slight subluxation at the talocrual joint with associated malalignment throughout the entire foot. As is evident in this photo, when Chiara flexes her knees to kneel next to a bench, dorsiflexion and toe flexion occur and the dorsum of her feet have decreased contact with the support surface. Because the PT intends to place additional demands on Chiara in the upright position, she decides to put Chiara's AFOs on·

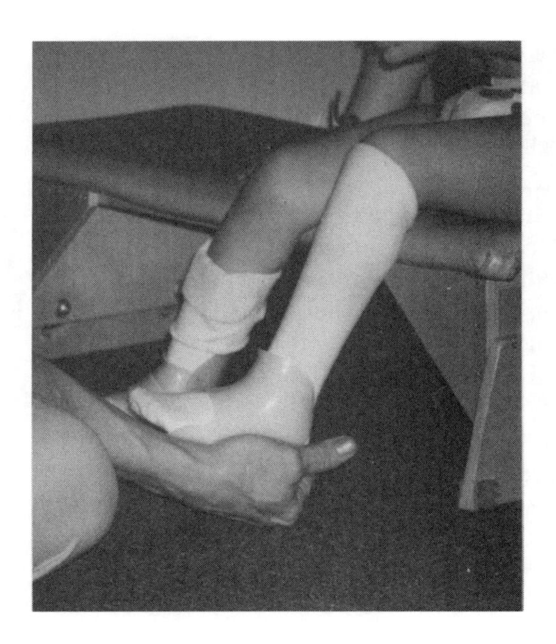

Figure 4.21. At this point in the session, the therapist puts on Chiara's AFOs as Chiara sits independently on a small bench. Although somatosensory input decreases when the orthotics are worn, the improvement in foot/ankle alignment is significant. In addition, Chiara typically ambulates in her orthotics on a daily basis and is more familiar and comfortable wearing this support.

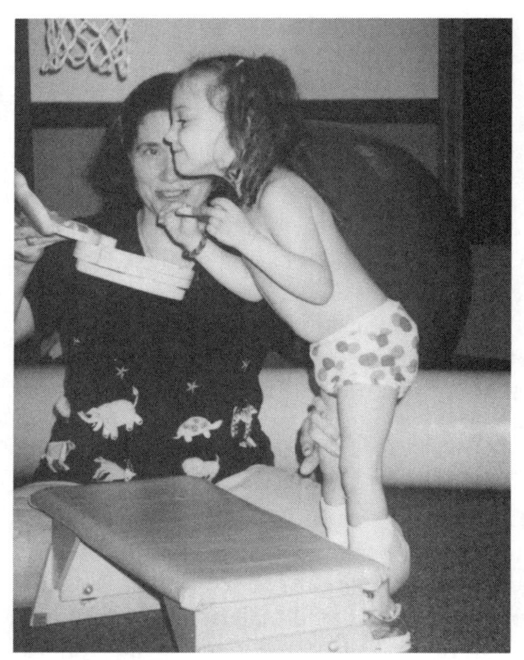

Figure 4.22. Once her orthotics are on, Chiara returns to some simple standing activities with the modification of alignment. Here she checks her lip gloss in the mirror. This helps to get some lip closure, but she demonstrates increased hip flexion and lacks sufficient hip extensor activation to align her body appropriately over her feet in the sagittal plane. However, she is able to stand independent of any support while using her hands for a fine motor function (putting on lip gloss) with her weight distributed evenly between her LEs when viewed in the frontal plane. It is likely that the therapist has created a situation by placing the mirror of the makeup kit in a way that encourages forward leaning because, given time, Chiara momentarily improves her alignment and does not return to the pretreatment strategies.

Note: *This is another decision point for the therapist. Although Chiara is not standing perfectly aligned, the therapist believes that, rather than trying to perfect Chiara's posture in this position, they can move on to gait activities.*

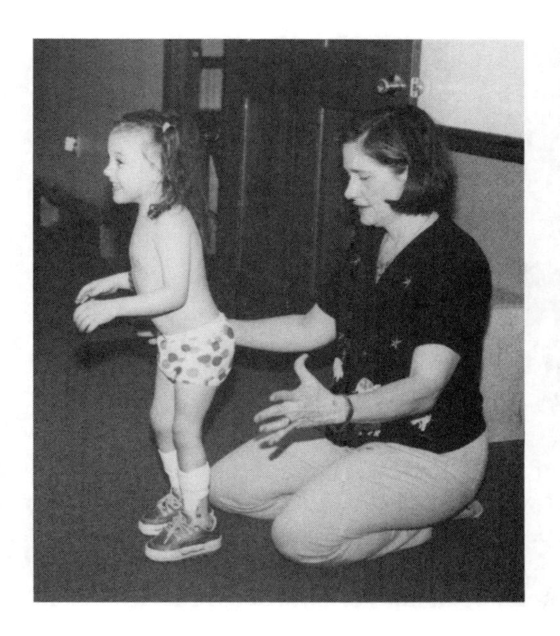

Figure 4.23. Now fully "made up," Chiara stands independently, showing her uncle her new face and body makeup. As Chiara gets the feeling for "standing straight like a model," the therapist can evaluate Chiara's ability to correct her own alignment and weight bearing and use her postural reactions without manual guidance. Although Chiara still has some shoulder elevation, increased stiffness in the UEs, and increased hip flexion, she does have her arms in front of her body and her weight forward as necessary for walking. She can talk as she stands.

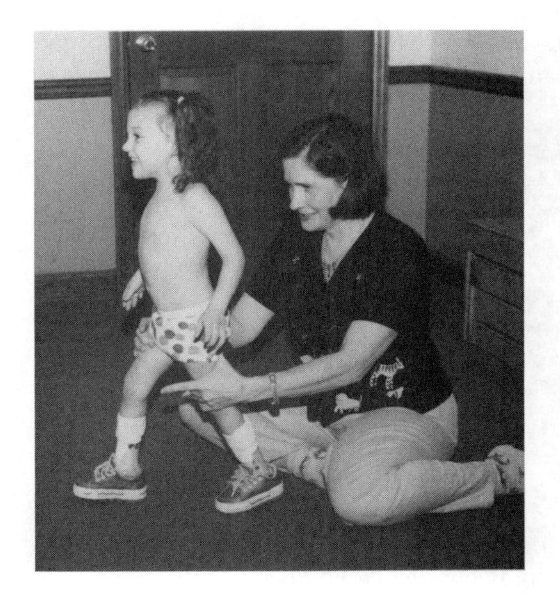

Figure 4.24. Gait training begins as Chiara walks "down the runway." Compare her posture and stride to her pretreatment photos (see Figure 4.6). Her posture and stride reflect her ability to isolate the movements of one leg from the other, shift her weight from her BOS while maintaining trunk symmetry, take all her weight on her feet, and begin to push against the floor to get the rocker action of gait from heel strike to forward transition of weight across the foot toward the toes. Proximal instability is still evident in the posture of her scapula and overuse of trunk extensors with the relatively reduced use of the abdominal obliques. She used a similar strategy in Figure 4.18 as she moved from half-kneel to stand. Also evident is an emphasis on increasing the control of knee extension coupled with dorsiflexion during the late stages of stance. At this time, though, the PT uses her left hand to help correctly position the patella over the joint space to increase the efficiency of the quadriceps during gait. There are many aspects of gait training that might be included in other sessions, such as treadmill work, taping to position the patella, and use of different assistive devices. (These activities reflect only a small sampling.)

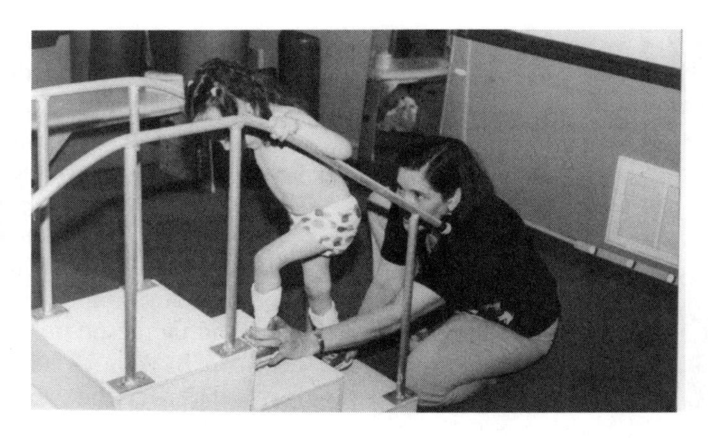

Figure 4.25. Chiara chooses to climb onto a platform to receive an award for being the "best model ever." This activity requires rapid shifts of weight from one foot to the other, activation of different muscle groups in each leg simultaneously (hip flexors on one side with hip extensors on the other), and a rapid change of activity in one muscle group to another within the same LE. Although this skill is beyond her comfortable motor performance, Chiara wants to repeat this activity over and over. The therapist must then find how to make the activity match the posture and movement goals and address the impairments that limit this function. Stair climbing was not in the therapist's plan, but is clearly in Chiara's. The therapist decides that stair climbing does allow a forward weight shift, work on placement and strengthening of the LEs, and eccentric LE work necessary for gait, and does not interfere with Chiara's plan.

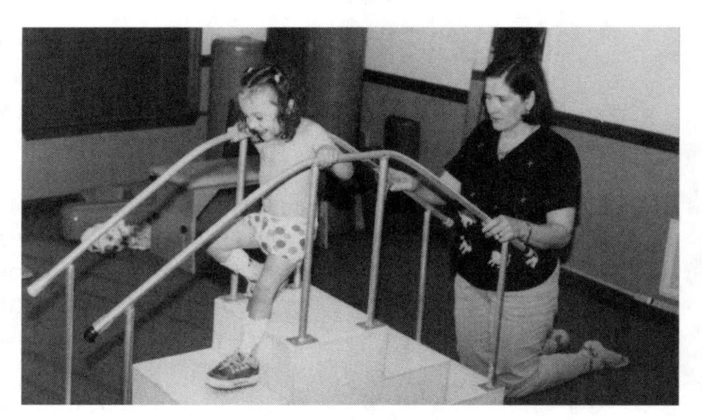

Figure 4.26. Descending is much more difficult for Chiara, evidenced as a deterioration of her overall performance with poorer trunk and UE alignment, increased dependence on the UEs for support, increased upper lip retraction, and the inability to align her pelvis and trunk over her femurs. However, she is able to grade LE stiffness and coordinate placement of her hands on the handrails while isolating intra- and interlimb synergies to complete the task safely. The joy of descending stairs on her own is apparent, and the therapist decides not to interrupt, recognizing that we all learn while performing tasks that are outside our ability limits.

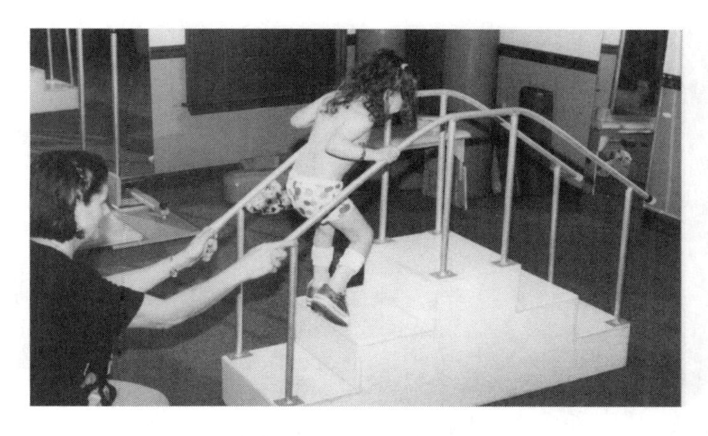

Figure 4.27. Chiara tries several different strategies using trial and error, independently experimenting and practicing her own solutions to the problem of stair climbing. This aspect of the session is very challenging and energy consuming for Chiara, but she is totally self-driven. The therapist alters only those aspects that she perceives to be dangerous for Chiara. Soon Chiara is ready to move on to a less-demanding activity, and the therapist is relieved that she did not have to intervene and redirect Chiara's efforts.

Note: *Upon returning to ambulating on the floor, Chiara demonstrates the patterns of movement seen earlier in this hour, indicating her ability to select effective synergies for walking when the setting is less tressful.*

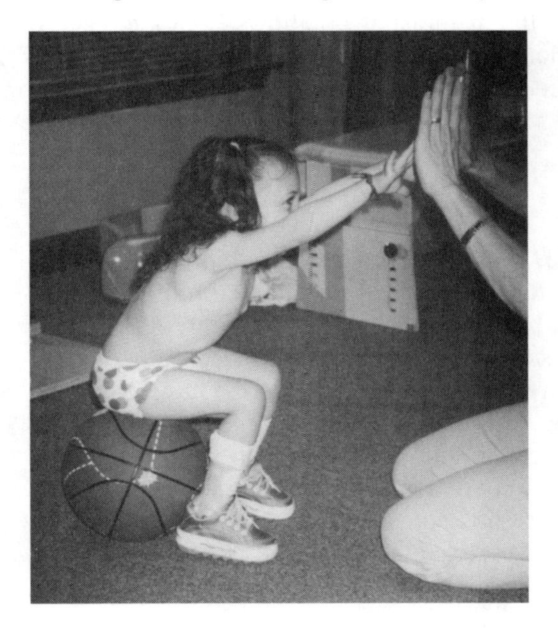

Figure 4.28. Tired from her "award ceremony," Chiara decides to sit. The therapist provides a "silly seat," a small basketball instead of the bench, as a way to repeat many of the previous seated activities but with variation. Sitting on a small ball retains co-activation of the LE musculature and muscles around the pelvis for postural stability and reaffirms Chiara's perception of her lower body and LEs as her dynamic BOS. Seated on a ball rather than a stable seat, Chiara must adapt weight shifts to a moving surface and shift her pelvis forward over her femurs–a pattern she had lost during stair climbing. Now, the therapist wants to regain the UE freedom of movement Chiara had shown prior to stair climbing. Chiara gives a "high five" for her excellence in modeling and demonstrates her ability to quickly activate and time her arm movements through space to precisely place her hand in the therapist's, indicating the stability of these UE patterns, once stress is reduced.

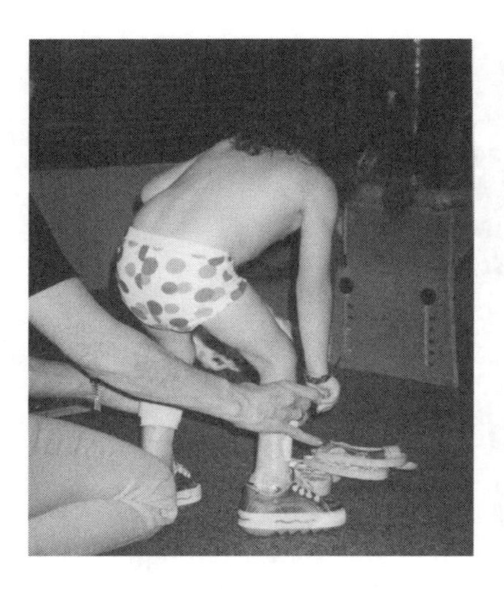

Figure 4.29. To reestablish the synergies of movement needed to get up and down from standing, the PT uses a more demanding setting (compare to figures 4.10-4.13). The therapist controls only the alignment of Chiara's tibias over the talus, and Chiara is responsible for graded control of her hips and knees. During these transitions, Chiara selects and applies eye shadow as tummy makeup (which won't be visible at school). The LEs provide the stability for her BOS so that her arms and hands are free to reach and grasp. Multiple transitions to and from the floor as she paints her tummy increase Chiara's comfort in standing, decrease the fear of falling during ambulation, and increase her overall ability to move in a standing position.

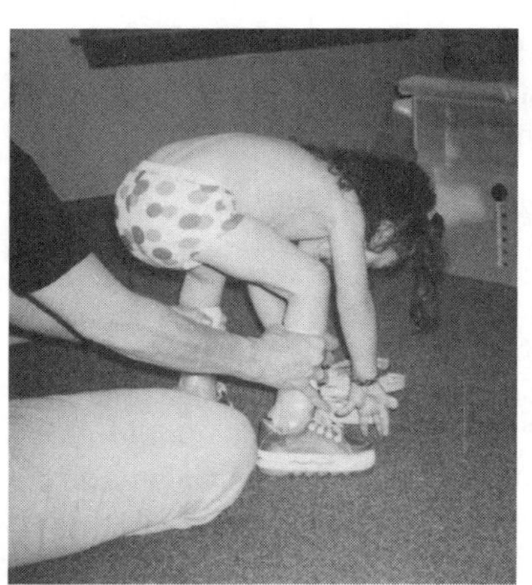

Figure 4.30. Chiara maintains a partial squat position while she puts together all the trays of her makeup kit. She is able to demonstrate control of eccentric and isometric contraction and co-activation of the quadriceps and hamstrings, as well as hip flexors and extensors. Assistance from the therapist's hands helps to keep her center of mass (COM) forward over her BOS. In these transitions, the therapist again allows Chiara to lead in the transition while assisting only with issues of alignment as needed.

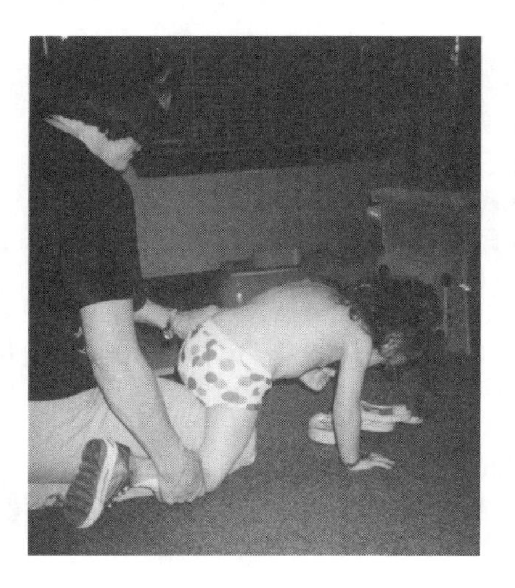

Figure 4.31. As Chiara goes to the floor, the therapist facilitates the extremes of dissociated movements of the LEs. Chiara stabilizes with the right UE, demonstrating a stable shoulder girdle, graded elbow extension, and weight on an open hand. She has refined the use of the left UE to hold an eye shadow wand between the index finger and thumb in this complex posture. She continues to talk through all transitions, developing creative ideas of how to use her new makeup–including some that may not be appreciated at home!

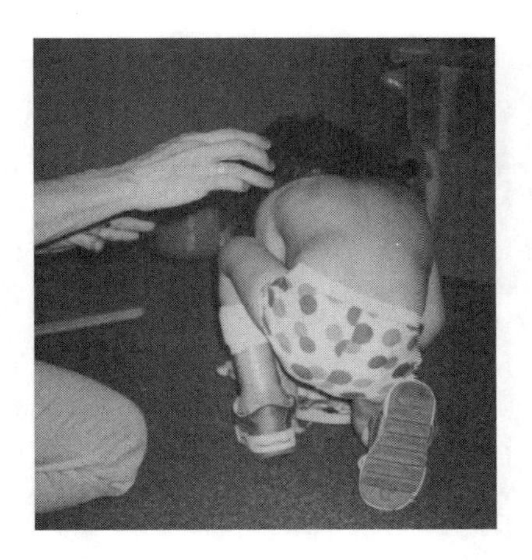

Figure 4.32. Chiara is able to hold this rather precarious posture independently as she completes a precise task with the UEs. She successfully uses co-activation of her trunk muscles for stability with dissociated movements of the LEs. In this position, she packs up her kit with one hand while using the opposite hand to help with balance. With only fingertip assistance from the therapist, Chiara rises to standing while holding her kit.

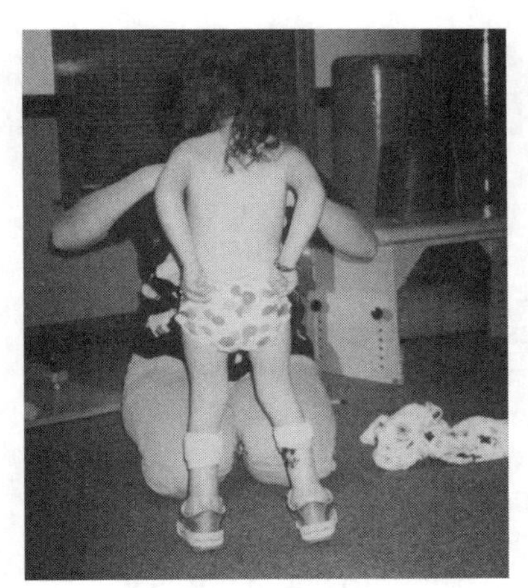

Figure 4.33. After Chiara hands the kit to the therapist, she dresses to return to preschool. She is able to stand, and spontaneously reaches back with both hands to adjust her clothing. She demonstrates the ability to use the UEs in backward space while keeping her balance and alignment in standing and completing a part of the task of dressing (OT functional outcome).

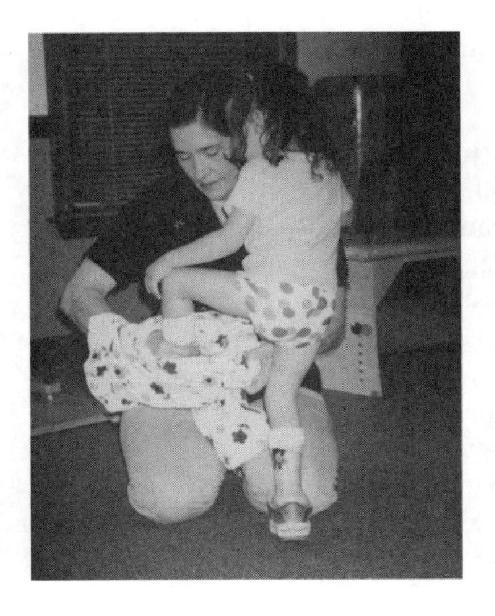

Figure 4.34. At this point, the PT incorporates dressing into Chiara's treatment sequence. The therapist assists lower-body dressing, conducting the activity while standing (as is age-appropriate) and reinforcing the same components of proximal control: weight shift from one LE to the other, axial rotation, and interlimb dissociated movements with free UEs and speech. In addition, Chiara's uncle is able to observe this method of dressing as a way to assist Chiara at home.

Figure 4.35. Standing independently at the end of her treatment, Chiara's hands are free to model her nail polish and makeup. The posture shows her self-confidence and feelings of success. Her weight is still not distributed evenly between the LEs but is much improved compared to Figure 4.23.

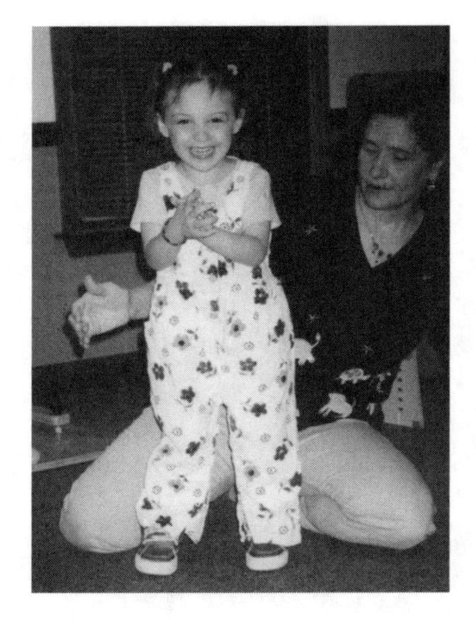

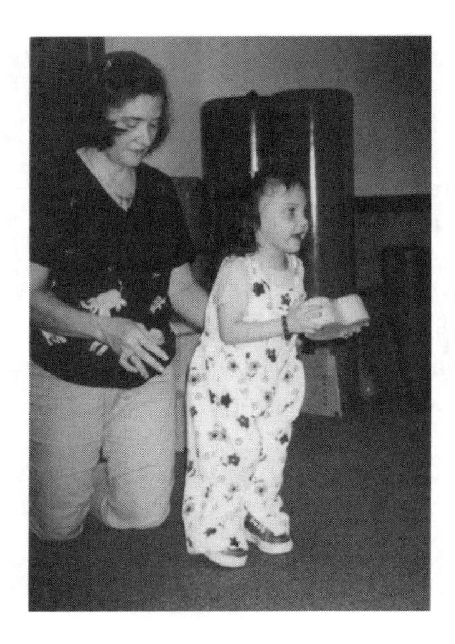

Figure 4.36. To determine whether the outcome for the session has been met, the therapist asks Chiara to carry her makeup kit to her uncle in preparation for going to preschool. Chiara ambulates 12 feet independently, carrying her kit. Her step length is short and cadence is slow, but she is so pleased with herself that she chooses to practice this skill, carrying different items to her uncle and back to the therapist six times. It is during this time that the therapist can establish functional outcomes to be addressed during the next session and begins to outline strategies she will use based on those that were most successful during this session. Although the plan might need to be modified depending on Chiara's energy and interests on another day, a plan is easier to modify than to develop.

Home Activities: The therapist suggests that at home, as time permits, the family encourage Chiara to rise to standing from her chair and walk rather than going to the floor from sitting to crawl. To set up the environment, family members can place play items on tables and bookshelves instead of on the floor. They should place her walker convenient to her seat so that if she chooses, she can stand and walk with this assist. The family will need to understand that walking with the walker will be different from her performance in treatment. The therapist stresses the importance of Chiara choosing to walk as an age-appropriate function. Having observed this treatment session and how capable Chiara is, her uncle suggests that he could play a modified basketball game outdoors with Chiara in her walker, encouraging her to free her hands from the walker to catch, dribble, and perhaps even walk out of her walker when she throws the ball. The therapists who see her in the school setting and the OT in this outpatient center will coordinate these activities.

Case 2: Adult With Stroke

Summary of Data Collection

Note: *The examination of this client is detailed in Chapter 3 and will not be repeated here. This chapter includes only a brief summary of his history and current status to refresh the reader. Please refer to Chapter 3 for additional information.*

Mr. Ron Winkler is a 75-year-old man with right hemiplegia and dysphasia secondary to stroke who lives at home with his wife, Lorraine. Ron was admitted to an acute-care hospital and received medical management for the ischemic infarct. Once he was medically stable, he was transferred to a stroke rehabilitation unit. He remained in the rehab unit for 4 weeks. He received OT, PT, and SLP during his stay. At discharge he was referred to the outpatient intervention program that used an NDT approach to continue OT and PT. SLP was discontinued. The health team, along with Ron and Lorraine, decided that the best way to use his limited number of therapy visits was to focus on OT and PT, with the SLP serving in a consulting role, continuing to see Ron during his visits to the outpatient department to check informally on his progress.

Summary of Impairments and Motor Functions

At the time of admission to the outpatient program, the following system and motor impairments limited function: (a) ineffective postural control, (b) lack of recruitment and activation of the muscles in the right UE, (c) impaired co-activation and interlimb coordination in the LEs, (d) limited and ineffective movement strategies, and (e)impaired balance in sitting and standing. The following photographs and commentary illustrate some of the intervention strategies that addressed these underlying impairments, discuss the problem-solving process and decision-making strategies that the OT and PT used, and show how each strategy related to changing functions at 11, 17, and 27 and 35 weeks post stroke.

Note: *These photos were taken in the outpatient rehab department and show Ron wearing a safety belt during some of the treatment. This was his preference when trying new activities, particularly those that involved walking or moving in a standing position. This was a constraint that the therapists accepted, knowing that as he progressed he would not feel the need for this device.*

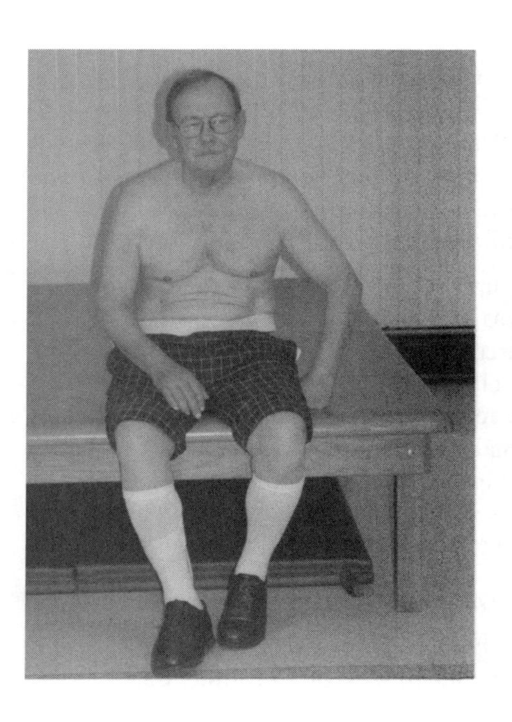

Figure 4.37–11 weeks. Ron's intervention program immediately addressed the mobility functions that he needed to become more independent in daily activities, given that this was one of his stated objectives. Ron was able to get up from his bed or his wheelchair with minimal to moderate assistance. However, this involved his repeated attempts to stand using momentum, incorrect timing of knee extension without correct position of the COM, substitution of trunk flexion for hip flexion to come forward, and pushing with his left hand on the support surface with most of the weight on his left LE.

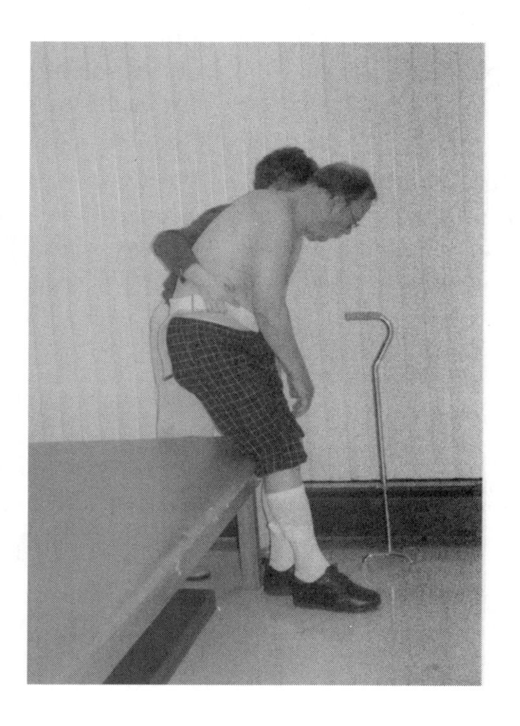

Figure 4.38. As Ron stands, the incorrect timing of hip and knee extension prevents him from bringing his weight forward over his feet. As he rises from sitting, he activates knee extension, which pushes his COM even further backward, causing him to compensate with excessive hip and trunk flexion to prevent himself from falling backward. In addition, his weight is shifted more toward the left because he can activate and support with the left leg more than with the right. The pull of gravity and the weight of the inactive right arm contribute to trunk flexion and difficulties with balance. Here the PT guards Ron, but does not assist, as he demonstrates his ability to stand up independently.

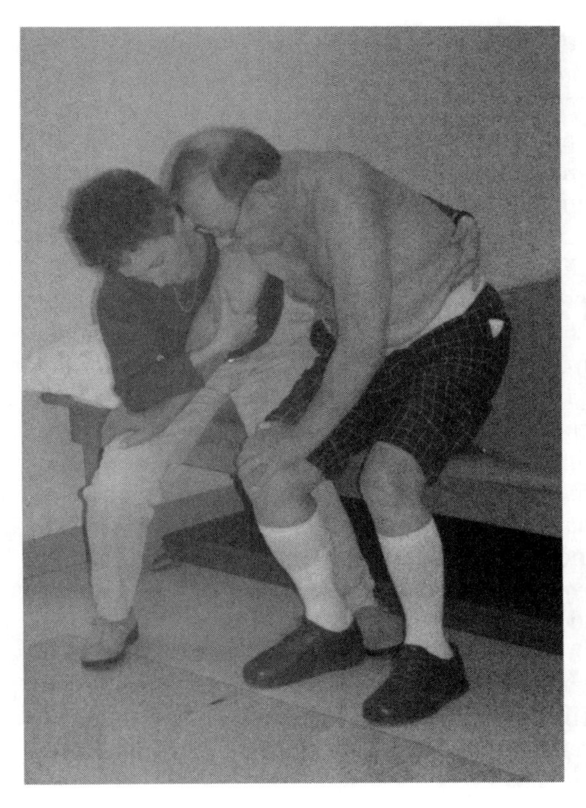

Figure 4. 39. The PT chooses to facilitate sit-to-stand because she feels that this is one way to address many of the underlying impairments effectively *within* a functional activity. Making sit-to-stand easier for Ron will immediately give him a sense of success, reduce his fear of falling when trying new movements, and begin to change the constraints on this task. He will see that if he keeps his COM equally over both feet and keeps his weight forward, he will have better control of his balance, will not fall backward, and will be able to use the power in his legs.

The therapist prepares Ron for standing by asking him to place his feet parallel to each other. The therapist places her left foot behind his right foot to keep his feet aligned, especially during the early part of the movement before he has transferred enough weight to keep it in this position. The therapist then brings both UEs toward the right to assist shifting his COM over the right leg and inhibit the reliance on the left side for stability. His own body mass will facilitate the head and upper body to stay to the right and will facilitate activation of the right LE for support in effective alignment. The PT knows that clients often allow the lower body to shift toward the more affected side while actively leaning the upper body away from that side, preventing the desired weight shift toward the more affected side.

With her right arm and hand, the PT supports the inactive right arm, using compression into the axilla while stabilizing elbow extension with weight bearing through his right hand on her thigh. She uses her left arm around Ron's trunk low enough to facilitate hip flexion during the weight shift forward, but high enough to control the position of his COM as he comes to stand. In addition, by providing a downward and forward pressure on the posterior aspect of the rib cage, the PT can facilitate trunk extension along with hip flexion, a synergy that is very difficult for Ron to achieve and maintain.

Ron works with his prefabricated AFO on the right leg. This was given to him before he left the inpatient rehab program to add stability at the ankle while assisting dorsiflexion and limiting plantar flexion to allow clearance during swing phase of gait. The AFO also provided some minimal but adequate medial-lateral control, because Ron does not have significant structural or control problems in the coronal plane. Ron preferred to wear his AFO when standing and walking, feeling more confident that his right ankle would support him.

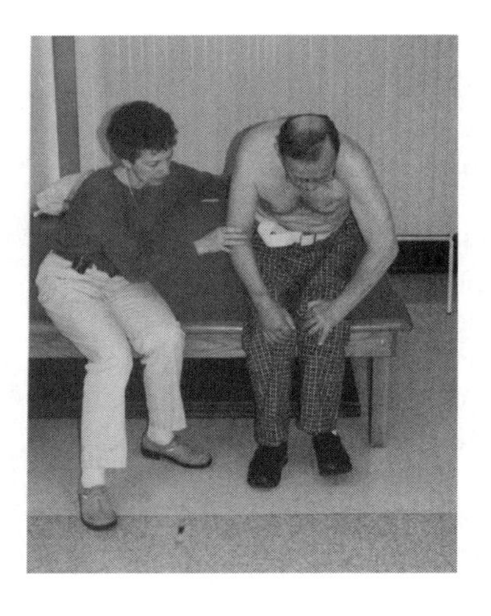

Figure 4.40–17 weeks. The therapist now provides only contact guarding and verbal feedback as Ron comes to standing. The alignment of his body over his feet is more symmetrical in the frontal and sagittal planes. Ron is finding his own solution to getting up more easily, incorporating the components of movement that the PT introduced at 11 weeks. He places his hands forward on his knees to help bring his COM forward. This strategy forces him to use the strength in his LEs rather than depending on his left arm for push and support. Although shown only getting up from the mat-table (in order to have a neutral background for photography), Ron practices getting up from various support surfaces, chairs, and benches during treatment. This skill has improved so that the PT feels comfortable in asking him to practice standing up from a lawn chair, his rocking chair, a recliner, and his kitchen chair with his wife's stand-by assistance. The PT prepares him to generalize to a number of functional situations rather than repeating the practice of one specific activity. Changing the context changes the requirements for posture and movement and provides him with the confidence to perform this task under different environmental constraints. She will discuss with him, on the next visit, which situations were most difficult or easiest, why he thinks there are differences, and what changes in his posture or movement he will still need to get up easily in each situation. The motor control components that are necessary but currently unavailable to him will be addressed in subsequent therapy sessions.

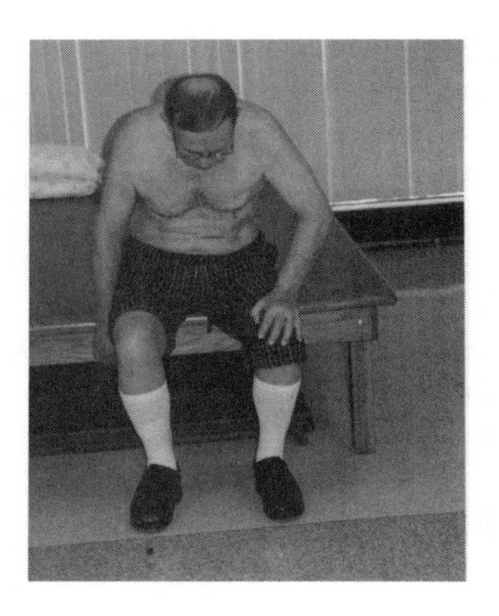

Figure 4.41–27 weeks: Ron is now able to stand up on the first try when sitting on most surfaces, including, he reports, his soft, deep recliner and the seat of the car. His weight is equal on his feet and he can bring his pelvis forward over his femurs rather than flexing his upper trunk to shift his weight forward. He does this task independently, quickly, and safely. Although the function of coming to stand provides the context for gaining many movement components in the LEs (such as activating and timing intra- and interlimb control), Ron still has very little motor ability in the right UE and does not spontaneously use it when standing up.

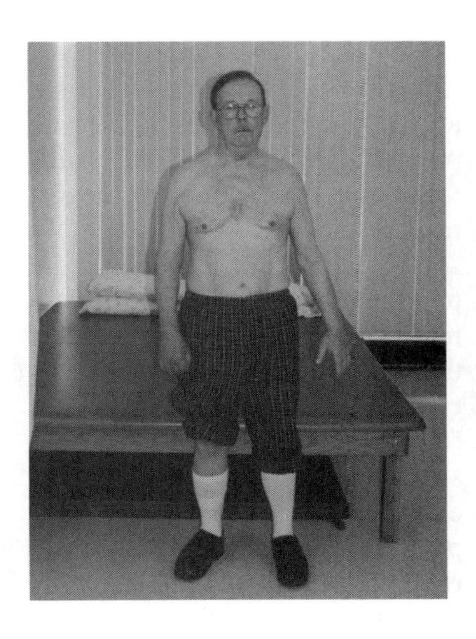

Figure 4.42–27 weeks. From sitting, Ron is able to align himself as needed for the task and stand independently. He has more options for getting to stand, as evidenced here by weight shift to the right and the ability to distribute his weight evenly on both feet. His pelvis is level and balance is adequate, so he does not fear falling. Although the right hand remains inactive during the movement, increased trunk and shoulder girdle activity with improved alignment are evident in standing by observing that the weight of the arm no longer pulls the trunk into flexion.

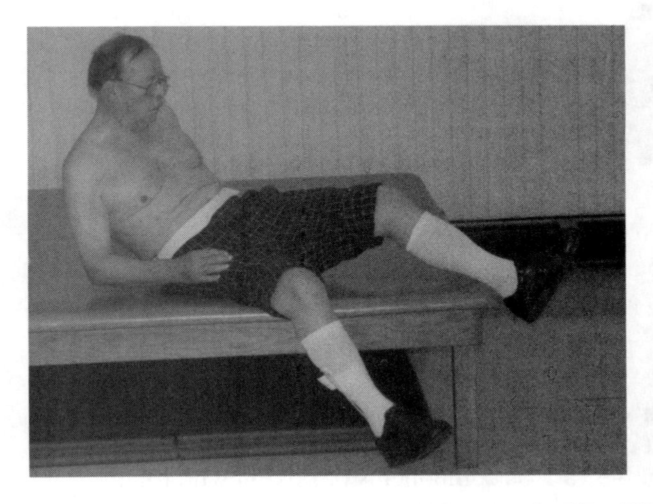

Figure 4.43–week 11. The therapists observe Ron as he moves independently from sitting to a supine position. His right UE appears ready to accept weight, but he avoids a weight shift in that direction because he does not get the somatosensory feedback that his arm is ready to support him during the task. Instead, he uses his abdominals and hooks his legs against the edge of the mat. This compensation pattern reinforces the trunk flexion, forward head, and collapse of the anterior chest wall. The PT, OT, and SLP are all concerned with the head and trunk flexion that occurs frequently. The PT recognizes that excessive use of trunk flexion constrains Ron's ability to time the change from flexion to extension when moving from sitting to standing or to walk with his body aligned over his LEs. The OT is aware that achieving effective scapula stabilization will depend on Ron's increased trunk extension. The SLP is concerned that Ron's trunk flexion and decreased rib cage mobility contribute to inefficient respiration and volume control for speech. Although the movement he has chosen works in this setting and is not undesirable to carry out the function, frequent use of these patterns without variety will limit the movement synergies that are easily accessible for functional movement in other situations. In addition, repeated use of a small number of patterns will increase the imbalance of motor control that already limits his functional abilities.

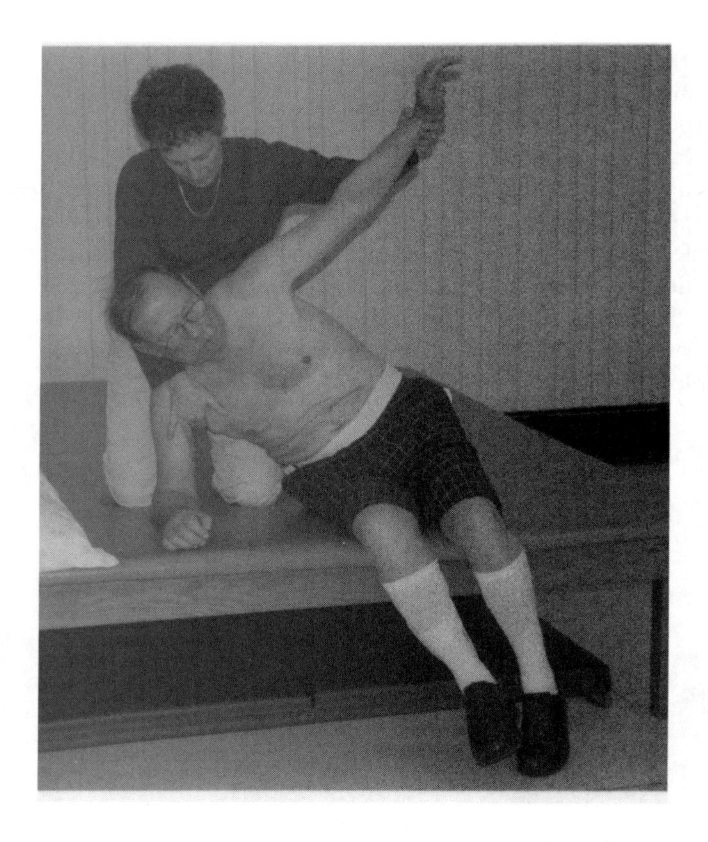

Figure 4.44. To change this pattern of flexion without rotation and to facilitate weight bearing on the right side, the PT facilitates several variations of the sit-to-supine movement; one is shown here. The PT begins the treatment strategy by positioning her own thigh to tuck and support the ribs, which will move Ron's trunk toward extension (with hip flexion) and optimizes alignment so that he can activate his trunk extensors. Her right hand supports the anterior aspect of the right humerus, maintaining correct alignment of the glenohumeral joint. This allows him to increase the weight that he accepts through this arm as he lowers to supine without causing pain due to malaligned structures. As Ron drops the pelvis backward on the left, he activates and controls trunk rotation around the right weight-bearing hip. His pelvis and hips become an active part of his BOS with the legs and upper trunk moving around this base. (All body parts in contact with the support surface are part of the BOS, including his arm and hand.) Change in this movement parameter will improve his ability to move the pelvis forward over his hips when adjusting his sitting posture or rising to stand.

With her left hand, the PT inhibits Ron's tendency to place his left hand on the support surface. She asks him to reach in different directions, which changes the demands on his trunk muscles, requiring that he quickly combine various components of flexion with rotation and extension with rotation. She combines a cognitive approach with facilitation that requires Ron to simultaneously attend to both movement components and cognitive tasks, saying, "Bring your hand down just 4 inches; stop; now, touch just your left index finger to your right knee, touch your left hip, and then bring your arm and hand back to the initial starting position." She can build endurance and facilitate control of movement complexity as he is able to attend to directions, remember, move, and stabilize in order to reach in various directions. The task incorporates manually facilitated movement with tasks that are verbally cued and require him to reproduce the entire pattern. The task of reaching and moving with the left arm requires activation of the muscles of his trunk and right shoulder girdle for positional control in increasingly demanding combinations of patterns of muscle activation.

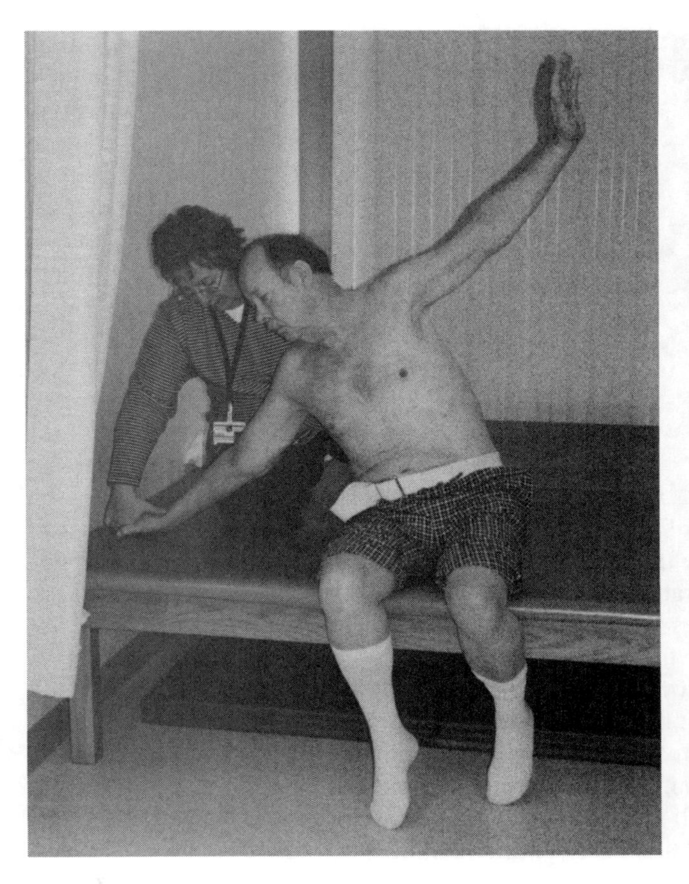

Figure 4.45–week 17. Ron has improved activity in his trunk, providing the postural control to continue the reeducation of active motor control of his right arm and hand. Here the OT uses UE extended-arm weight-bearing to initially gain range and increase co-activation around the elbow and wrist, which will be needed during hand functions. The OT starts by addressing soft tissue length and joint alignment by placing her right hand in Ron's hand. She uses her right thumb and fingers to align the carpals and lengthen tissues to prepare his hand for weight bearing through the heel of his hand. She uses her fingers along his metacarpal joints to maintain the integrity of the palmer arches. With her left hand she can support the scapula as needed, although Ron now can actively control positions and movements through midranges in a closed-loop activity. Her left knee guides the rib cage to achieve active thoracic extension by shifting his COM forward over his ischial tuberosity. With a more active trunk, Ron can now begin to grade the amount of weight taken on the right hand and change the co-activation demands at the scapula, glenohumeral joint, elbow, forearm, and hand as he accepts weight onto the hand. The therapist can feel his ability to respond to directions, such as, "Put a little more weight on your right hand–feel it? Now, push down with your hand, pushing your body away." The OT will feel through her hands whether he is responding to changes in speed and force while actively maintaining elbow extension and an active trunk. Weight bearing far to the side demands that he use the right arm and hand for support and control of the COM, because his COM can no longer be kept safely over his pelvis, and ensures that Ron actively links his trunk and extremity muscles.

Note: In the first case study, it was appropriate for the PT to encourage Chiara to focus on the play aspect of the session. With an adult, the therapist often asks the client to focus not only on the task but also on the posture and movement requirements, using cognition to reinforce the movement and increase the client's responsibility for linking movement with action.

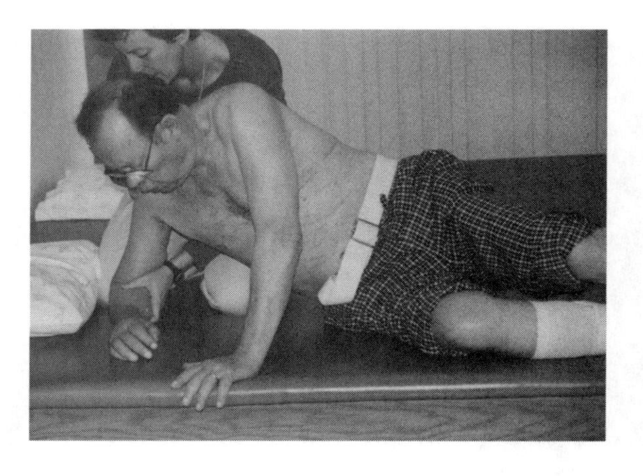

Figure 4.46–17 weeks. At the same point in the program, the PT simulates the task of getting up from bed through sidelying. In a discussion with Ron and Lorraine, the PT has learned that at home, Ron sleeps on the right side of the bed and that prior to his stroke always rolled to his right to get up. Because Ron frequently used this synergy prior to his stroke, the PT assumes that his memory of this method of getting up will aid recovery of similar weight-bearing and movement patterns and will be functional for him at home. Ron needs to relearn how to get out of bed efficiently, and practice of the actual function on a daily basis will strengthen many of the postures and movements he is developing. As Ron moves from sidelying to sitting, the therapist encourages him to use the trunk, shoulder girdle, and pelvic girdle movement strategies that he has been working on in other activities in PT and OT. Here, Ron demonstrates improved alignment of the trunk (notice that the PT is no longer supporting or facilitating trunk alignment with her knee or thigh as she did at 11 weeks). Ron begins to control the translation of his body weight over his right forearm and to combine trunk flexion or extension with rotation for the subtle weight shifts necessary to perform a variety of transitional activities. With her left hand on his right forearm, the therapist can grade the support, direction, timing, and speed of movement as he shifts his weight from the UE to the pelvis and thigh in preparation for sitting up, ensuring that he remains active throughout the range and does not rely on momentum.

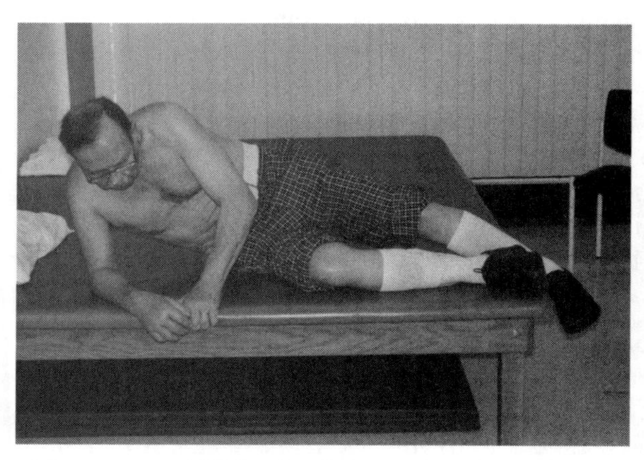

Figure 4.47. Although Ron has not completely regained the movement control that he demonstrated with facilitation (he has more head and trunk flexion here), he does show active muscle control of the right shoulder girdle and more effective coactivation of the trunk so that he does not collapse into trunk flexion or onto the right UE with scapular elevation. He is better able to control his COM and as he shifts more caudally, from weight bearing along his entire right side to a new BOS of pelvis (and perhaps feet) as he moves to sitting.

It is evident that Ron is insecure about relying on his right arm as he grasps the edge of the mat with his left hand. The PT knows that it is important for Ron to take responsibility for using these newly recovered patterns and because he is safe, the PT encourages him to get up from bed each morning without physical assistance or verbal prompts from his wife, being sure to use the method of rolling to the right and pushing up with his right arm and hand. At home he will have to cope with getting his feet and legs from under the bedcovers, which will add additional complexities to the task.

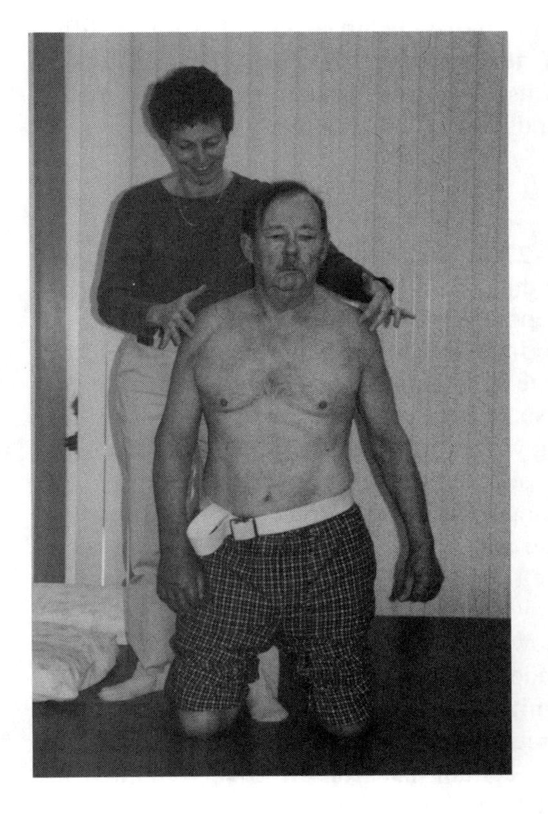

Figure 4.48–17 weeks. As Ron demonstrates improved postural control in sitting and moving from supine to sit, the PT adds activities that challenge him at a higher level of balance against the force of gravity. Work in kneeling and through half-kneeling also serves to establish patterns that Ron will need to get up if he falls. This is a very practical skill and focuses on a concern that Ron's wife has raised. She is a small woman and worries that she will not be able to help him get up. (Ron had fallen during a transfer during his first days at home, and they needed to call their son to help him up.) Once Ron develops the necessary strength and motor control and has practiced the needed patterns for getting up from the floor to standing, neither one of them will feel helpless if he falls at home again.

Kneeling with the ability to weight shift is part of the sequence to move from hands and knees to half-kneel to stand. It is also an activity that places demands on the muscles of the hips to work in patterns of stability while maintaining and regaining balance, synergies that are also needed when walking. The PT uses her left leg against Ron's right hip extensors, facilitating hip extension because Ron continues to use excessive hip and trunk flexion when balance is insecure. While kneeling challenges his stability and balance, it is not an activity that he uses during daily function. Although Ron's balance here is precarious, the therapist facilitates the transition to kneeling with no external support to emphasize the LE and trunk initiated strategy that will assist him in standing and walking. This provides the PT with the opportunity to verbally reinforce Ron's ability to control his balance and posture effectively and build his confidence.

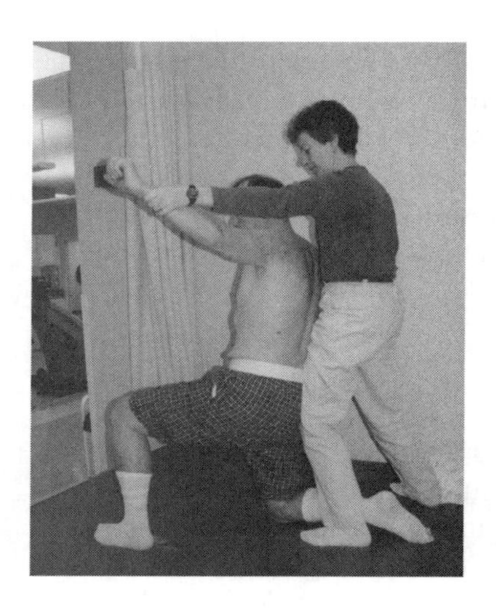

Figure 4.49. Moving into half-kneeling places additional demands on control of the right hip abductors and extensors to stabilize the hip and simulates the movements in the sequence Ron uses when getting up to standing and while walking (stance phase with the right hip stabilized in extension and swing phase on the left as this hip moves into flexion). The PT now facilitates right hip extension with her left knee. Because Ron tends to use a flexion pattern to attempt to control the position of his COM in this high-demand situation, the PT asks Ron to move his left hand and arm into different positions up and behind his body. This inhibits his tendency to use this arm for support and places additional demands on the left shoulder girdle and trunk.

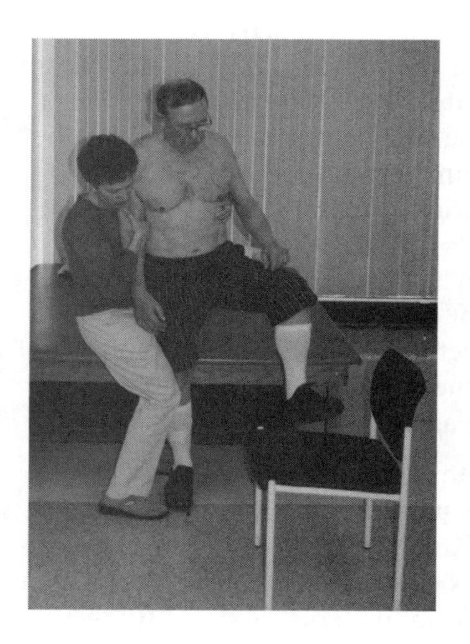

Figure 4.50–27 weeks. As soon as Ron is able, he performs in standing the challenge he first practiced in half-kneeling. Stepping up onto a chair forces Ron to rely on his right side for stability. Although this treatment strategy is extreme (it is unlikely that Ron will step up on a chair to get something off a high shelf), it does provide a challenging way to gain stability of the right hip, knee, and ankle, a skill Ron needs for stepping up from his "sunken" living room or climbing stairs in his home. If he can master this activity, he will have confidence to negotiate one step on his own, or climb the stairs from his basement workshop. The high demand forces Ron to reorganize how he moves. His usual small, quick weight shifts are inadequate for the task; therefore he learns to control a significant, sustained weight shift and to control dissociated movements of his LEs. By her position, the PT makes certain that Ron effectively and actively aligns his COM over his BOS. As needed, the PT can inhibit knee hyperextension, lateral hip displacement, and trunk flexion. This high stepping requires Ron to maintain extension and rotate his body to the left as the left hip flexes so that the foot can reach the chair. The PT's left hand around his rib cage facilitates trunk rotation on a stable right LE as he steps. The PT's right arm and hand support and facilitate Ron's right arm in slight external rotation to bring the scapula into depression on the rib cage. This allows her to control the alignment of the upper body as he shifts his weight onto the right leg.

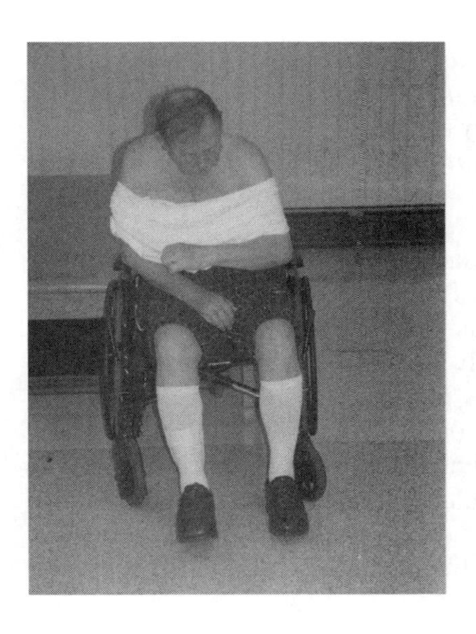

Figure 4.51–11 weeks. At the same time Ron is working on postural control for mobility with the PT, the OT is combining postural control with movements for daily living skills. This photo shows that Ron lacks the postural control and muscle activation to dress or undress even his upper body without excessive effort and increased time. He has insufficient co-activation of the trunk muscles to align his trunk over his base of support. His right UE is inactive and he cannot use it for any daily living skill. All movement is done by the left arm and hand, which is constrained by the lack of postural control to support the action of this less involved arm. He attempts this function in a wheelchair, which is how he attempted to do this activity at home because he could not transfer from the chair or stand without assistance.

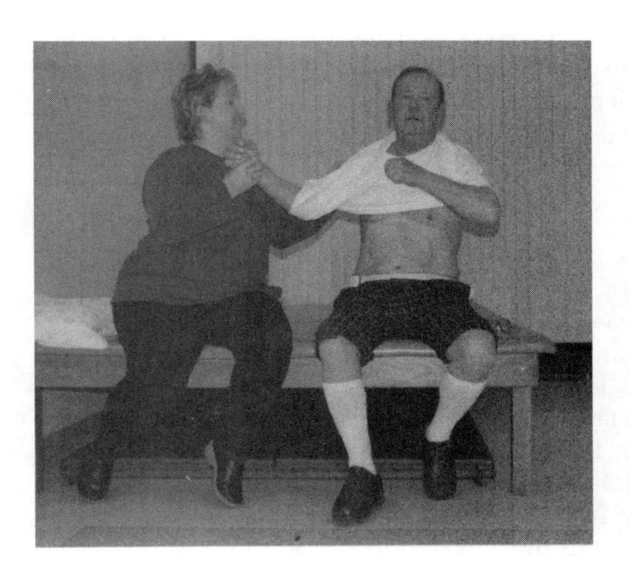

Figure 4.52. The OT begins facilitation of Ron's donning and doffing his shirt from a firm support surface to allow Ron to benefit from the postural control that he is gaining even though he might not be able to simulate this environment at home. The OT suggests that he dress (with the assistance of his wife) while sitting on the side of his bed or in a firm chair. This surface will give him a better base of support for postural control than does his wheelchair. The OT supports his right UE because he does not have functional use of this arm, and when he leaves it at his side, it contributes to his trunk flexion in the frontal and sagittal planes. (This support to the right arm allows the OT to facilitate postural control of the trunk.) With this support, Ron immediately aligns himself, stabilizing his head and trunk to resist the pull from the shirt. The OT will continue to activate the right arm in the appropriate patterns so that Ron will experience and remember the timing of the arm movements with the movements of the head and trunk and not develop compensatory "one-hand" dressing patterns while he works to develop additional motor return. This activity helps Ron to recognize how important gaining active control of his trunk is during many daily living activities.

Note: *The OT does not teach one-hand compensation techniques during OT intervention because she believes that Ron has the potential to eventually use the right arm and hand for functional skills. She has decided that the time in therapy is better spent helping Ron to gain postural control of his body, especially at this early point in his recovery.*

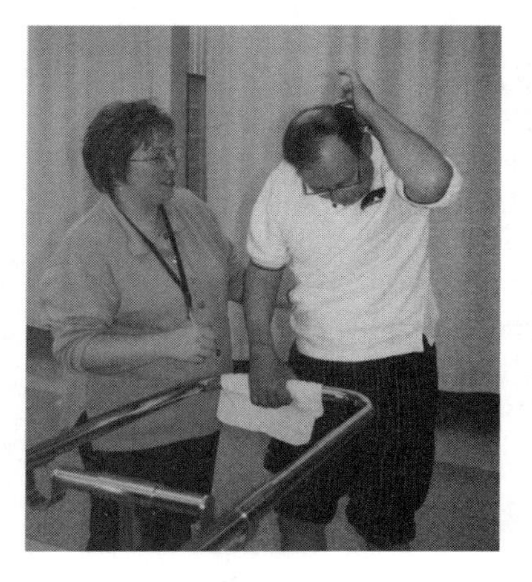

Figure 4.53–27 weeks. Ron now has sufficient stability in standing for the OT to work on dressing skills in this position. These skills require Ron to work at a higher level than he currently does in performing the function at home. There, he sits to put on his shirt and is able to stand with his hand on the dresser or sink in the bathroom to perform activities that involve only small weight shifts. Dressing while standing allocates the postural requirements to the background (as they should be) while he focuses on the movement requirements for the task. The OT provides verbal encouragement and sets up the task to require stabilization from the right arm and hand. Her left hand rests lightly on Ron's back to provide nonverbal assurance of stability and safety. Most clients, including Ron, need reminders or cueing to develop variable ways to perform tasks that were learned early in rehab. Without such reminders, he will continue to dress in sitting, the one way he knows, long after he has developed adequate balance and control to perform part of his dressing while standing.

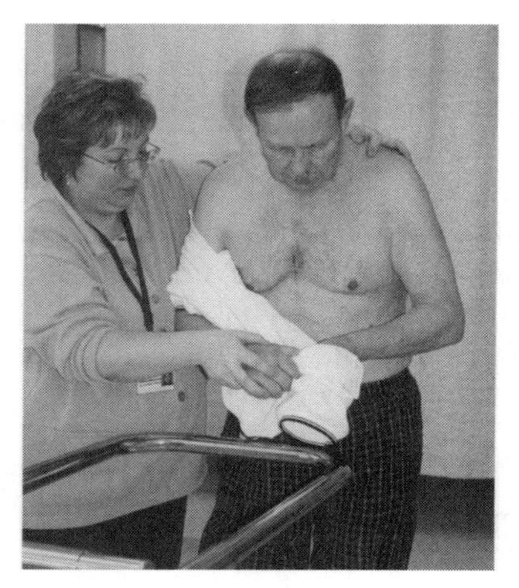

Figure 4.54. At this point, Ron begins to use a compensatory pattern of shaking the left arm to finish getting his shirt off. The OT stops him by placing her hand on his left shoulder, then instructs and facilitates movement in the right arm and hand. Ron needs to be convinced that even if shaking his shirt off is quicker, using his right arm and hand will ultimately lead to overall better function. This can be a difficult lesson at this point in recovery if the client's objective is to be more self-sufficient. It is essential that the therapist explain the reasons for incorporating the use of the more involved side as part of an ongoing educational program for both Ron and his wife. His grasp is still very limited, but this is an opportunity for him to use his limited thumb and finger flexion with elbow flexion to slide the shirt off his left arm. This bilateral midline UE action also reinforces a symmetrical, weight-bearing posture.

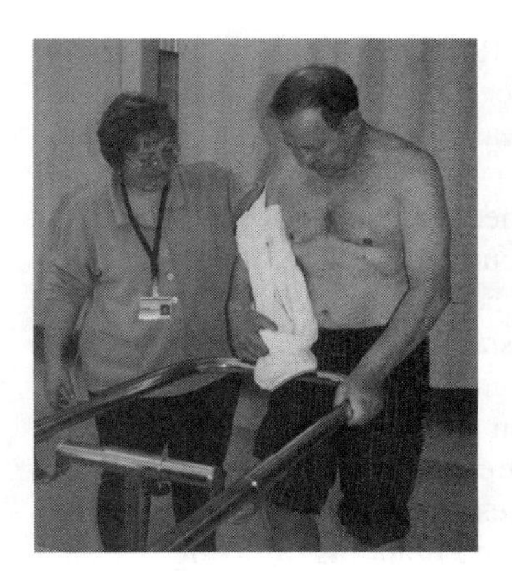

Figure 4.55. To help Ron get his shirt off the right UE, the OT sets up the task so that Ron holds the support with his left arm. This provides support and also occupies the left UE with the stabilizing part of the task. Ron will need to work out a method of using the distal control he is developing in the right arm without help from his left. The OT remains quiet as Ron works out this step of the task.

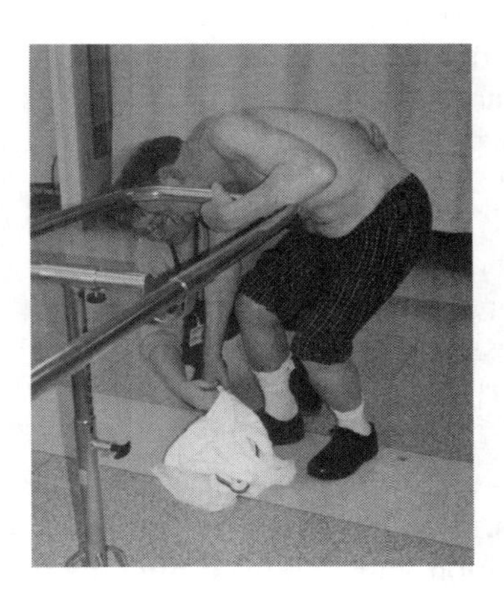

Figure 4.56. During the course of this activity, Ron drops his shirt on the floor–a fairly likely consequence of the task because he does not feel stable enough to lift his left hand from the support quickly to catch his shirt. The OT facilitates orienting, weight shift, and bending (to the shirt) as Ron grasps with the right hand to pick it up. Ron's insecurity in stabilizing himself with his knees bent and the mechanics of the task (holding with the left and reaching down with the right) produces asymmetrical weight bearing with more weight on the left upper and lower extremities.

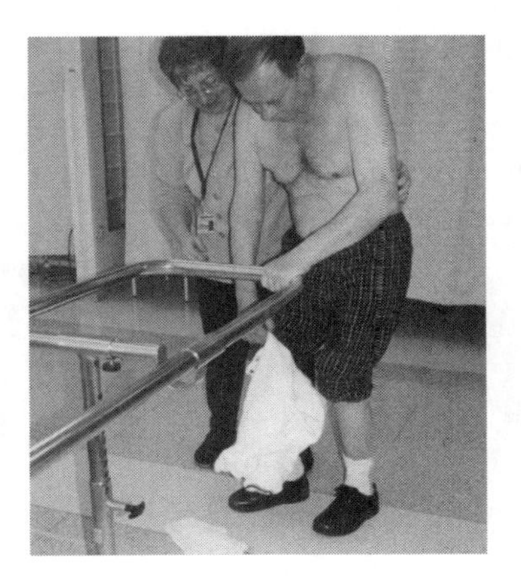

Figure 4.57. Ron is successful in maintaining his grip on the shirt to lift it from the floor while changing his orientation from a stoop to standing position. Although he demonstrates some compensatory patterns (more weight on the left side, excessive trunk flexion), he is successful. The OT does not limit Ron's function in order to have the best quality that she knows Ron can produce. Function needs to be first, and she knows that he can produce better quality of movement when the task parameters are not so demanding. She believes that, with additional recovery and ongoing therapy, he will strengthen the link between postural stability and fine motor control.

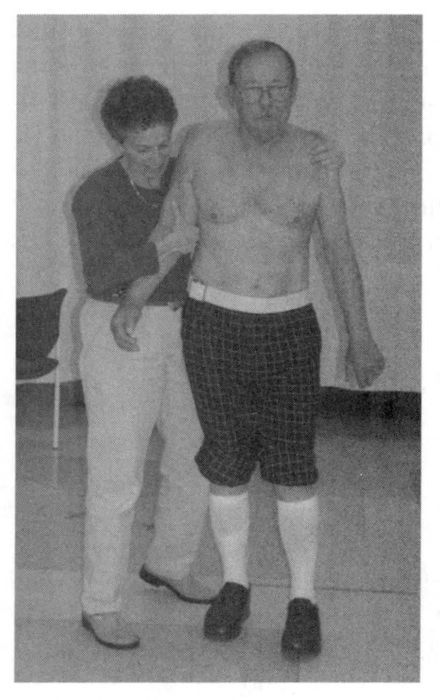

Figure 4.58–11 weeks. Ron had begun walking with a quad cane and assistance before leaving the inpatient stroke rehab unit. He was not able to walk independently with the cane, but it did assist him when standing to transfer from his wheelchair or from the car. Ron was unstable and insecure when attempting to walk without a cane. Already he had begun to use the cane to compensate for lack of stability on the right side, shifting his COM to the left and taking a short step with the right. In this photo, Ron's tendency to shift his upper trunk to the left is apparent even with the PT's efforts to inhibit it. The PT gives strong input, aligning Ron's right UE and shoulder girdle and again using external rotation of the right UE to align the upper trunk. The therapist's left hand prevents the left shoulder from leading the body's progression forward but also provides a diagonal downward pressure toward Ron's right hip to facilitate anterior progression of the pelvis and co-activation of the trunk for stability. This left hand also aligns the upper body behind the pelvis to mechanically facilitate hip extension. She uses her hip posteriorly and laterally to keep Ron's right hip aligned over his BOS and to prevent lateral and posterior displacement of this hip. She cues the timing and direction of the forward, diagonal progression of the pelvis as the COM begins to shift over the left foot to prepare for swing on the right.

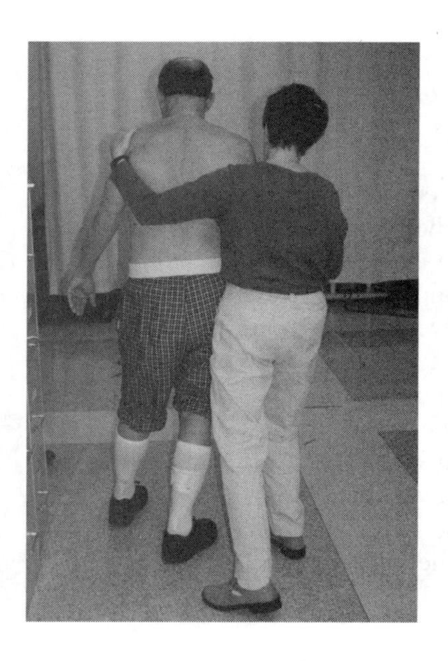

Figure 4.59–17 weeks. Ron now has better trunk extension with co-activation and improved alignment of his head. The PT continues to stabilize the right hip during stance and inhibit his tendency to lead the forward progression with his upper trunk. He is more stable without his cane and has begun to prefer using the standard cane, because he can feel that the quad cane encourages him to lean forward and to the left even more than the standard cane does.

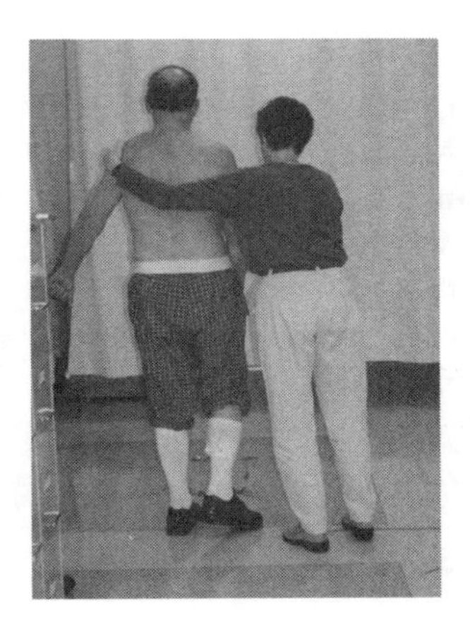

Figure 4.60–17 weeks. During swing phase, Ron activates the right LE to initiate progression forward. The PT withdraws her support at his hip but continues to inhibit the tendency to lead with the upper trunk, which Ron attempts to use to assist right LE swing. The effort and balance required for this isolated control of the right LE are evident in Ron's activation of the left UE for balance.

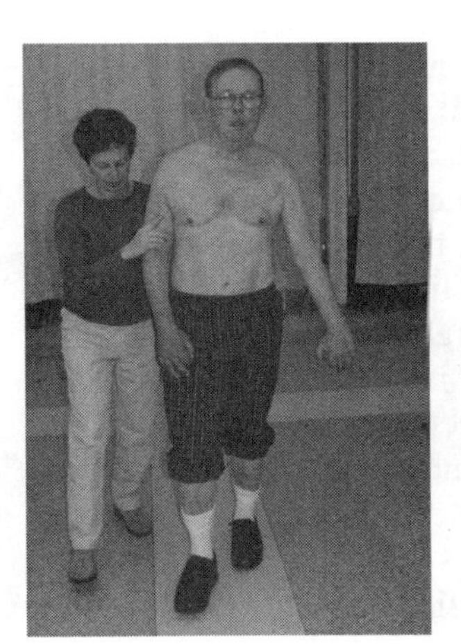

Figure 4.61–27 weeks. Ron can walk functionally with supervision without a cane, using appropriate alignment and longer, more equal stride and step length. During treatment, the PT adds or withdraws facilitation to prepare for Ron's needs in various contexts. Ron practices on a simulated sidewalk, changing speeds to "cross the street" and turning and maneuvering around furniture, all of which are skills he will need in his home and community. Although Ron walks alone at home much of the time, his wife still feels safer if she is standing next to him while he walks.

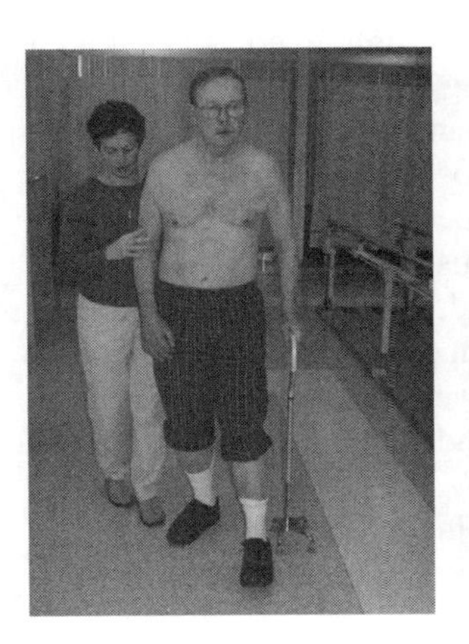

Figure 4.62–27 weeks. Ron has greater confidence with his quad cane, but now is able to keep it close to his body and does not compensate by leaning to the left. His stride is longer and step length more even, but he still tends to have a short stance and swing phase on the right side. Cadence is slow because he cannot activate and time knee flexion during swing or dorsiflexion at late stance phase on the right side quickly enough to increase the speed of his walking. When he tires, he still has instability related to insufficient activation of the right LE during stance, resulting in knee flexion and lateral hip displacement. At this point, Ron is able to get out of the car but does not have the confidence to walk into treatment because he cannot vary his walking speed or cope with obstacles in his path.

In addition, he has difficulty attending to potential dangers in the environment and the movements needed to balance and walk. He still tends to have insufficient foot clearance during swing phase on the right, occasionally dragging his toe. He worries that this will provoke a fall. Fear of falling underlies a secondary impairment of increased muscle stiffness in the right LE such that he occasionally advances this leg forward with minimal joint movement at the hip, knee, or ankle. On the smooth tiled floor, he walks between OT and PT with stand-by assistance and generally accepts walking as his method of mobility indoors. He no longer uses a wheelchair in his house.

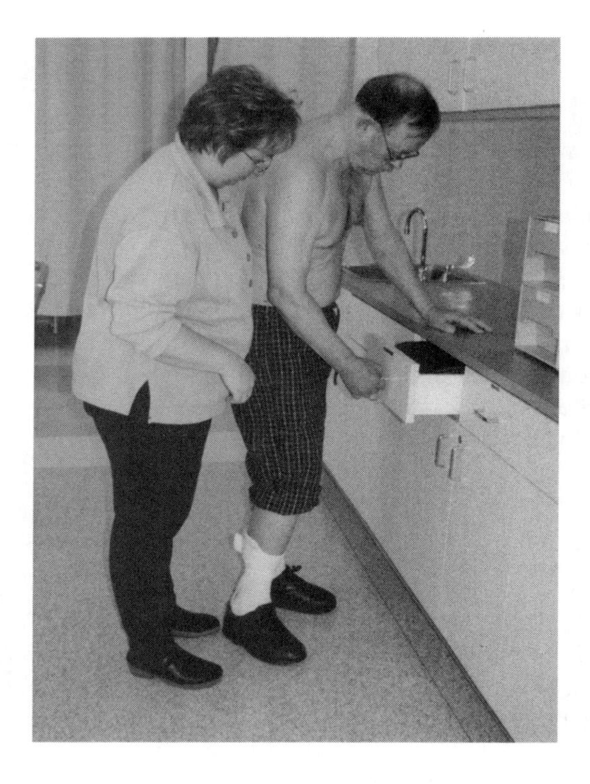

Figure 4.63–27 weeks. At the beginning of the outpatient treatment program, Ron had no active function of the right UE, but based on experience and evidence reports in the OT literature, the therapist was optimistic that he would regain some use of this arm and hand. Among the factors that predicted some return of function in his arm were his ability to initiate muscle contraction in the right UE early in his recovery and his consistent use of the right UE to stabilize objects (even though he could not use his hand independent from his arm), indicating relatively good sensation and perceptual skills. The OT has been helping Ron to find ways to use the right UE during activities, teaching him to use his two hands together and to alternate between using the right hand as the skilled hand or assisting hand, as the requirements of the task demand more or less skill. Now at 27 weeks post stroke, Ron has gained standing balance and postural control and has regained a great deal of motor function of the right UE. This recovery makes it possible for him to do things that require distal function while standing, such as manipulating door and drawer knobs, faucet levers, and light switches. Ron supports with his left hand to make sure that he has adequate postural support to open the drawer with his right. Although Ron still has very limited isolated movements of the fingers and thumb, the OT observes that Ron is able to isolate flexion and extension of his elbow as he opens the drawer. However, the demands for isolated UE control cause him to be inattentive to the activation and stability requirements of the right LE, resulting in hip and knee flexion and causing him to shift his weight almost entirely to the left.

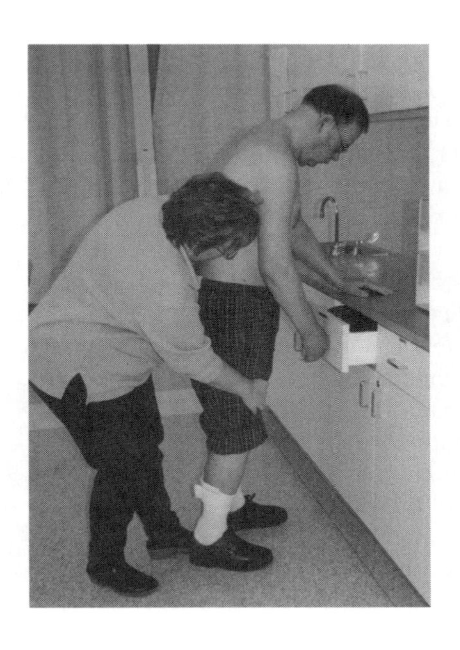

Figure 4.64. In the previous photo, Ron demonstrated his ability "to get the job done," but the OT recognizes the need for Ron to use a variety of movement patterns to open heavy drawers, light drawers, stuck drawers, etc. To do this, he needs to be "connected" from his BOS to his hand in order to have effective use of his hand for all types of functions. The OT facilitates weight shift from left to right, facilitating the link between the postural components with distal movements requiring different orientations of his body to the task, planning and modifying the action as it unfolds: How far will the drawer open? How much force is needed to open it? How big/heavy is the item that will be removed? Will he need to assist with his left hand to remove an item?

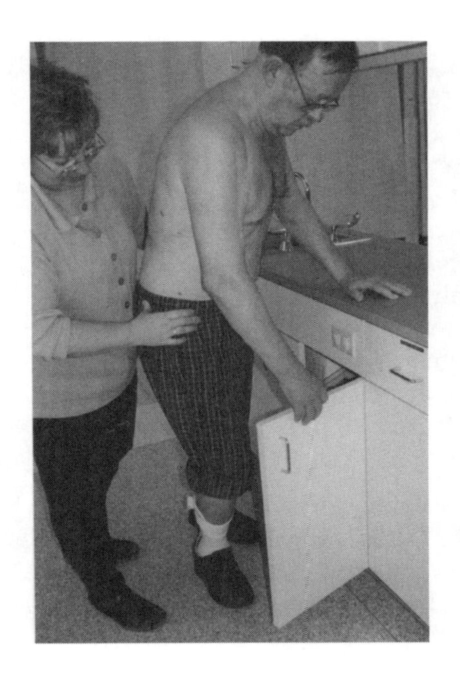

Figure 4.65. Ron experiments with opening and closing the cupboard door while the OT places her hands lightly on his pelvis to feel the activation of anticipatory control and to be ready to facilitate changes in postural alignment as needed during the task. He discovers that the door has resistance and that he needs to get it started by hooking his fingers on the handle, but finds that this strategy does not allow him to open the door completely. After several tries, he discovers that having his hand over the top of the door allows him to use his active thumb and finger flexion to control both opening and closing the door. In this way, he can fine-tune the position of the door without repeatedly changing his hand position, something that remains difficult because it requires speed and timing. Once he accomplishes the task in one way, the OT adds a new challenge by saying, "See if you can keep holding the door open while you squat down and take out a towel." She will structure the context of the task (squat down, look inside, hold the door open, remove an item) but let Ron figure out how to proceed and succeed.

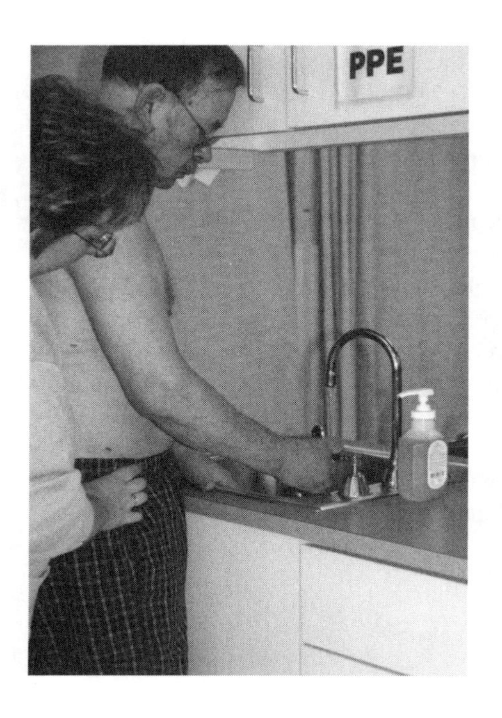

Figure 4.66. With his available shoulder flexion and increasing distal control, Ron is able to turn on the water using lever handles. These are not the faucet controls that he has in his own home, but they allow him to practice using graded, isolated control of the right forearm and hand in the context of hand washing. At this point in recovery, it is important for the therapist to help Ron identify what he is able to do without resorting to using the less involved left UE just because he compensated with one-handed strategies when his movement on the right was more limited. Although he cannot turn on his bathroom faucet yet, he can isolate some active flexion, extension, and supination of the forearm and flexion and extension of the wrist and fingers, timing these distal movements while stabilizing with the appropriate degree of elbow flexion to wash his hands successfully.

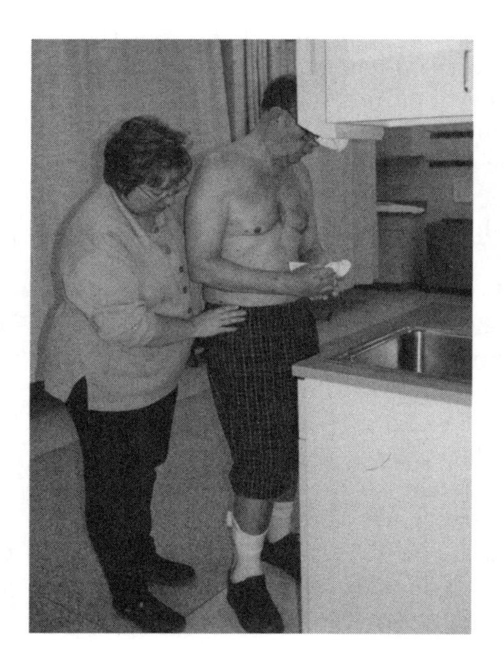

Figure 4.67. The logical follow-up to hand washing is drying. Ron's strategy is to lean into and support against the sink, but the OT facilitates alignment and postural control away from the sink so that Ron uses the standing balance he has developed while drying his hands. Here, he combines symmetrical alignment of the trunk, balance control, and equal weight bearing with bilateral symmetrical placement of the arms, distal manipulation, and visual attention to the task. This is a long way from the lack of all these postures and movements at 11 weeks post stroke.

To combine his ambulation skills with functions of daily living, the OT asks Ron to walk to the wastebasket with the paper towel in his right hand and drop it into the basket, adding a realistic incentive for walking.

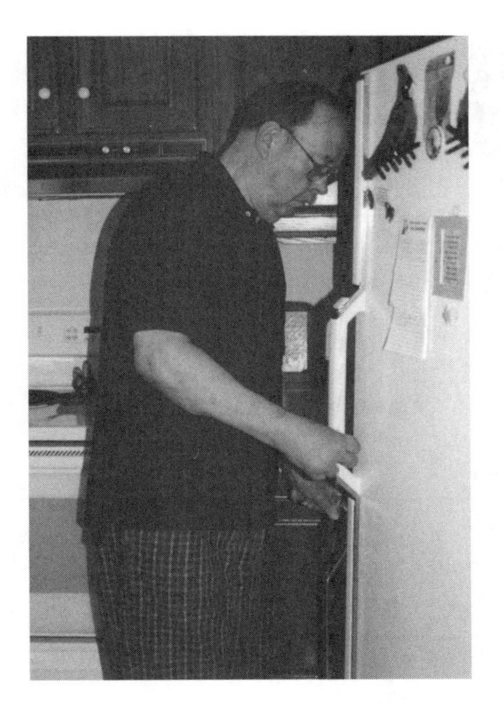

Figure 4.68–35 weeks. At this point, the PT and OT make a joint visit to Ron's home to help him and his wife problem solve how he can incorporate his new abilities into activities he does at home. Even though Lorraine prepared meals, Ron was accustomed to getting himself a snack. The OT realizes that this is an opportunity for him to use his right hand to open the refrigerator, a task with many of the same components that he had worked on in the OT kitchen. A right-opening door, which is common on side-by-side refrigerators, sets up a realistic context and requires the use of finger extension and elbow flexion with precise timing for Ron to place his hand on the handle and use his right UE strength along with his improved postural control to open the door, overcoming the normal resistance of the refrigerator door. Ron is able to do this independently after several attempts.

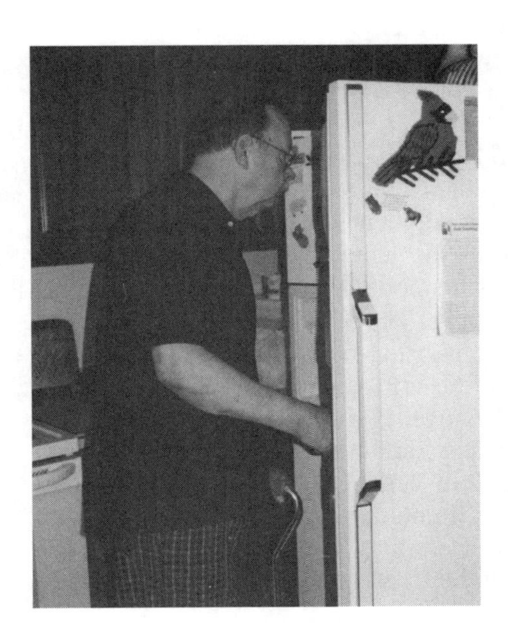

Figure 4.69. Once the door is open, Ron must let go of the handle and move his right hand quickly to the inner side of the door in order to hold it while he looks for an item inside. It takes him several tries to get the door open far enough so that it will stay briefly while he transfers his hand to the inner side. He also has to figure out how to time letting go of the handle before he moves his hand to the inside of the door. This presents quite a timing challenge, but Ron's desire to do things for himself at home is sufficiently motivating. Holding the door open with his right hand also means shifting his weight initially to the left to orient his body to use his right UE to catch the door, then to the right so that he can reach in the refrigerator with his left hand to remove food. All these components of postural control–weight shift, coordinating and timing the movement components of two hands for function–have been part of his rehab program and now come together for function in his home life.

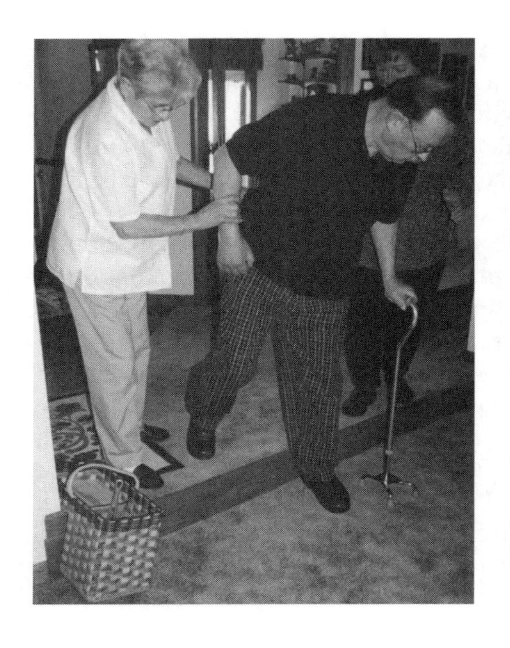

Figure 4.70. At this point in therapy on the smooth floor with no time constraints, Ron walks without his quad cane and only stand-by guarding. On the home visit, the therapists observe that Ron frequently uses his quad cane in his home because it allows him to move more quickly, manage the step into his living room, and walk on the carpet with less concern that he might catch his right foot and fall. However, as he steps down into the living room, the photo shows that his desire to move quickly and his fatigue contribute to his reverting to asymmetrical weight bearing on the left, flexion of the trunk, and leading with the shoulders in front of his hips when stepping down and walking to his chair. The therapists recognize this "reality" and as they encourage Ron to use the alignment and movement synergies he is regaining in therapy (which require more attention and effort), they will learn from the movement patterns he uses when under stress. (Why does he choose this particular pattern? What patterns are difficult, and what does he need in order to incorporate more efficient synergies into his functional repertoire?) They know Ron's capacity for motor learning, have seen more active control while walking, and believe that as the effort to stand and walk diminishes, he will most likely adapt the new movement synergies to all settings in his home.

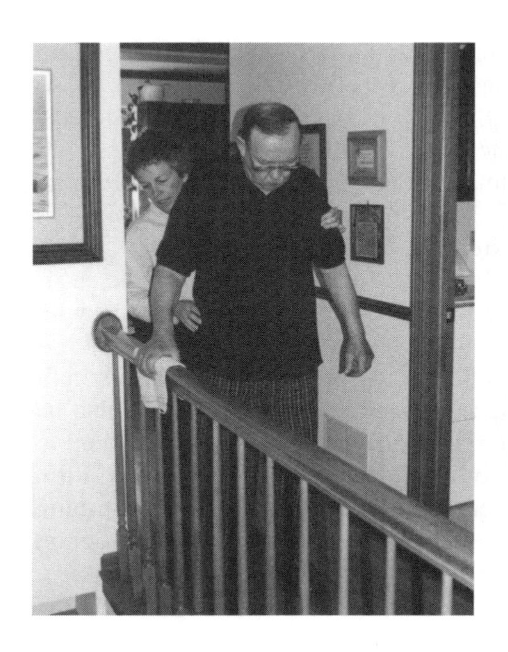

Figure 4.71. Ron is extremely interested in getting downstairs to his recreation room, which has his exercise equipment and his woodcarving shop. The floor in the hallway is hardwood and the basement is a smooth tiled surface, reducing his fear of tripping. The PT demonstrates how Ron can practice assisted right shoulder flexion with activation of his arm against resistance by placing his right hand on a small towel and sliding his hand along the railing. Using the right arm and hand to hold on actively and challenging his balance sets up a natural context to shift his weight to the right. Here the PT uses facilitation to align his trunk in the frontal and sagittal planes.

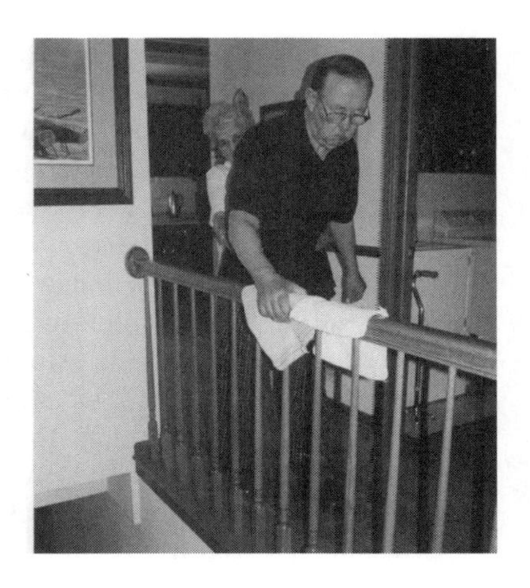

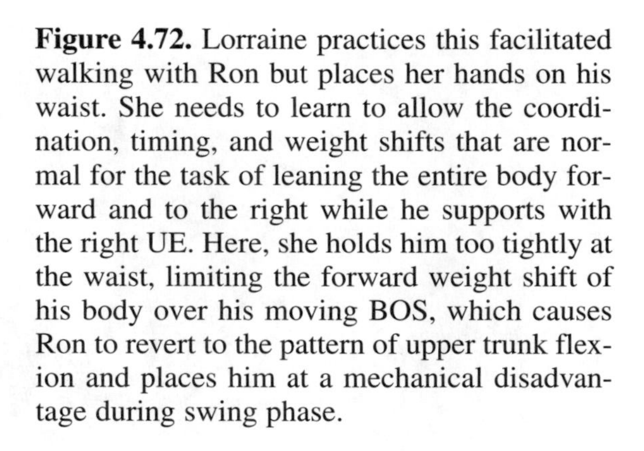

Figure 4.72. Lorraine practices this facilitated walking with Ron but places her hands on his waist. She needs to learn to allow the coordination, timing, and weight shifts that are normal for the task of leaning the entire body forward and to the right while he supports with the right UE. Here, she holds him too tightly at the waist, limiting the forward weight shift of his body over his moving BOS, which causes Ron to revert to the pattern of upper trunk flexion and places him at a mechanical disadvantage during swing phase.

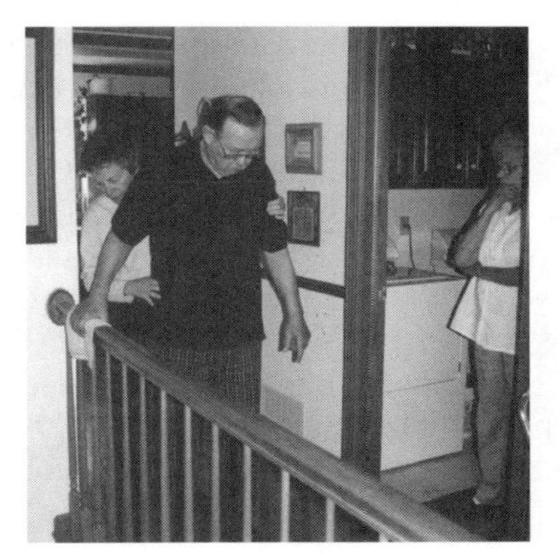

Figure 4.73. The PT demonstrates the appropriate handling, describing what she is doing and why she places her hands on Ron's left arm and right (posterior) pelvis as Lorraine observes the difference in Ron's alignment and walking ability.

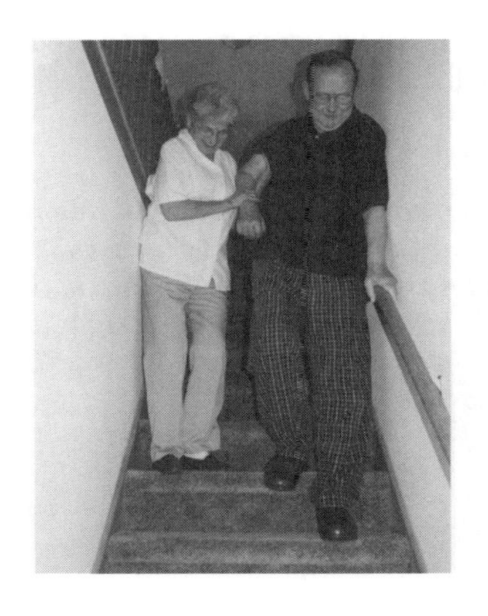

Figure 4.74. Descending the stairs adds additional constraints. The railing is on the left side, but the narrowness of the stairs prevents Ron from leaning his upper trunk too far to the left. Because Ron has active shoulder muscles on the right side, the support that his wife provides encourages him to lean to the right, which helps align his trunk over his hips. Descending stairs also forces him to coordinate interlimb control, timing knee flexion on one side while transferring and accepting weight on the opposite extended leg, alternating flexion and extension throughout a step-over-step descent.

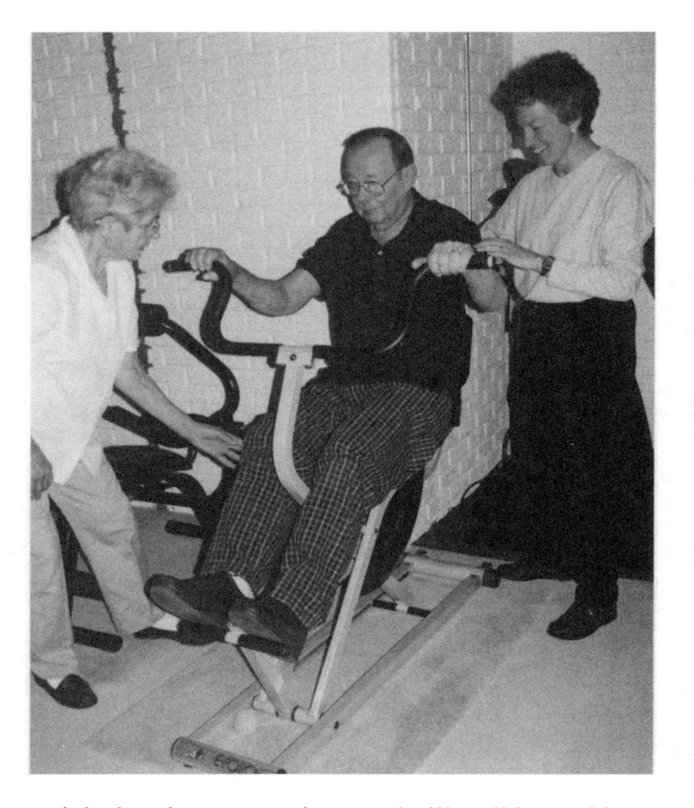

Figure 4.75. Ron has several pieces of exercise equipment in his basement gym that he had used on a regular basis prior to his stroke. One of his goals has been to resume exercising with this equipment in ways that will help his strength and endurance. The home visit makes it possible for the PT to recommend ways to use this exercise equipment that will support his intervention program. He has a treadmill that has a slow speed of 0.5 mph. On this day, he is able to walk for about 1 minute before fatigue and inappropriate muscle timing of reciprocal activation prevents him from swinging the right leg through fast enough. In addition, pain in the left leg interferes with building endurance. Knowing that he has a treadmill, the PT realizes she can add partial-weight-bearing suspension treadmill walking to his outpatient intervention program to practice the components of swing and stance, and he could follow up at home with additional treadmill walking.

Ron is able to mount the exercise device with only his wife's supervision. This device can be used for general strengthening and endurance with simulated weight bearing. On this equipment, Ron pushes down with both legs, which simulates the force needed to produce more ground reaction force as a component of gait. The handgrips provide symmetrical UE posture and movement. Lorraine gives a tactile cue to prevent Ron from allowing the right leg to externally rotate when he releases the pressure on it.

Note: *A secondary impairment of the vascular system now interferes with developing endurance when walking. Ron has claudication and pain in his left leg, which has now become the major limiting factor to his walking. This is an example of an additional impairment in another system that affects the rate of change in function. This was not a significant problem at the time Ron entered the outpatient program because he was walking very little, but it must now be considered as his program progresses.*

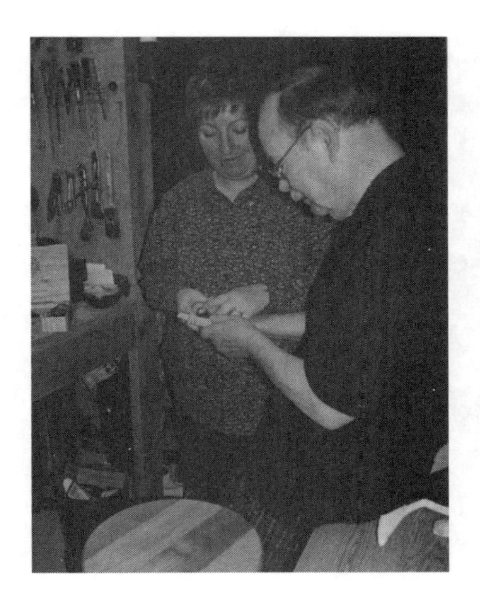

Figure 4.76. Ron's woodworking shop and the various partially finished carvings initiate a discussion about Ron's hobby. Ron is very proud of what he has accomplished and is eager to show the therapists his projects, but he verbalizes the concern that he will be unable to use his right hand for this type of work now. The OT sees this setting as a natural, highly motivating way for Ron to regain many UE postures and movements. She discusses with Ron how she can build up the handles on some of the tools to make them easier to grasp and invites him to bring these in so that she can make these modifications for him. With the OT cueing him, Ron practices timing, sequencing, and changing the stability and mobility between his two hands. When asked if there is anyone who could help him, Ron describes a friend who visits several times a week, who used to go to carving class with him. The OT suggests that he meet with his friend in his shop so that he could sand and paint some of his carvings with assistance from the friend as needed. Ron had broken his right arm some time ago and during that period had become quite skilled with his left, which will now allow him to use his right hand for stabilizing objects and use the left for the fine skills.

Note: *Several days later, Ron relates that he and his friend have scheduled a time to work on their woodworking and that he has decided to try woodburning, a related hobby that he feels will be an easier way to start. He plans to use the right hand to stabilize the wood and the left hand to do the woodburning.*

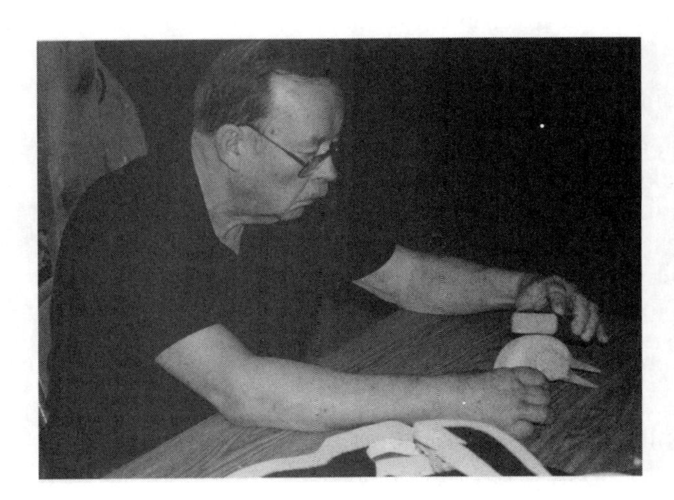

Figure 4.77. Ron holds the duck head with his right hand. The need to change the position of the wood will require precise adjustments of the muscle length and joint alignment and changing placement of his hand and wrist. No specific instructions are given because the table stabilizes his arm with shoulder flexion, and the skill requires timing and sequencing muscle activity. It took only the enthusiasm of the therapists admiring his work, to get Ron back into his hobby, which will provide plenty of practice for his returning UE motor skills.

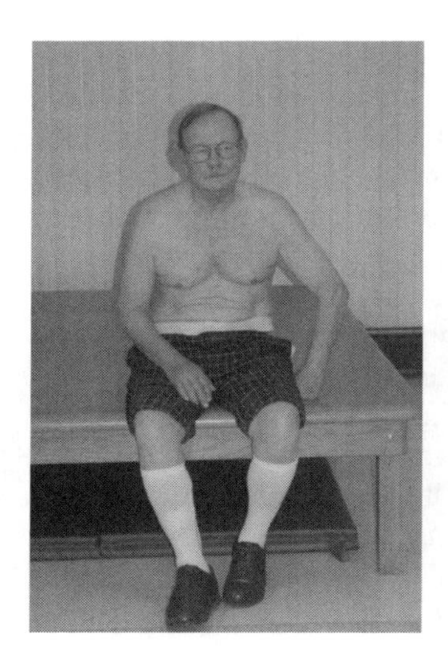

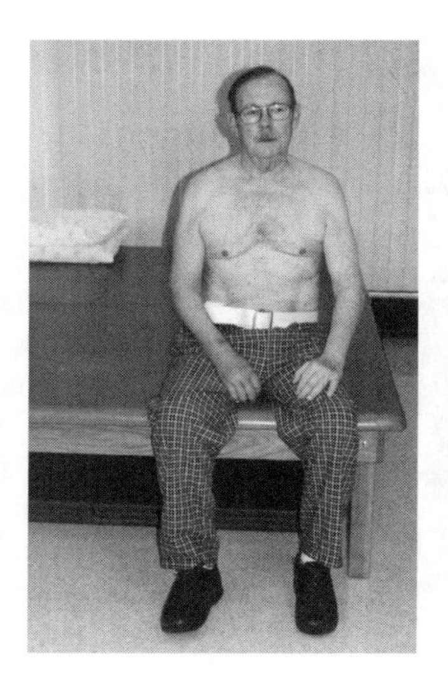

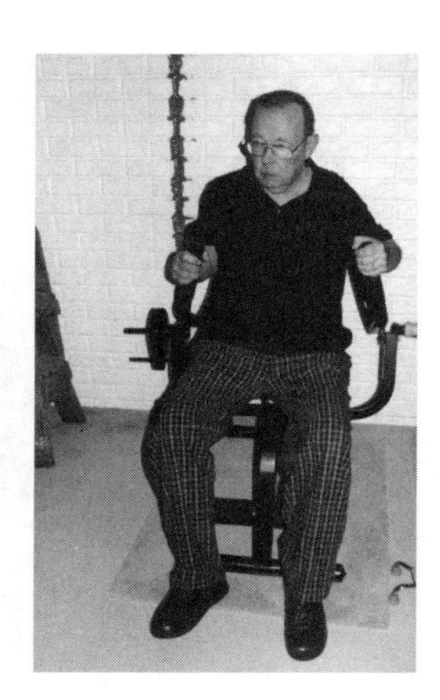

Figures 4.78, 4.79, 4.80. This series of three photos, taken at 11 weeks, 17 weeks, and 35 weeks, shows the changes in one dimension of the neuromuscular and musculoskeletal impairments that limit Ron's function: activation of the muscles for postural control supporting Ron's posture in sitting. The therapists used many strategies in both PT and OT intervention to facilitate change, but Ron's response to the strategies described in this case study are obvious from the changes in alignment and use of the UEs while sitting.

Figure 4.78–11 weeks. Lack of postural control prevents proximal stability to use of the movement available in the left UE. The right UE is completely inactive.

Figure 4.79–17 weeks. Postural muscles are active, the trunk is symmetrical, and the head and trunk are aligned. The left arm is normally active, and movement is returning in the right.

Figure 4.80–35 weeks. Increasing postural control of the trunk allows Ron to use his UEs and LEs simultaneously while exercising in his home gym.

Although Ron has had only consultation and periodic observation from the SLP, his speech production has changed. He now speaks louder due to more active trunk muscles with better extension, which assists his respiratory capacity. He has better coordination of the timing of vocal and respiratory patterns, which also contributes to his increased volume. Functionally, along with improved activity of the oral-motor musculature, his articulation has improved so that he does not have to repeat himself very often and is understood in most social situations. He continues to have difficulty talking while walking and tends to stop talking as he concentrates on motor skills. As he continues to link the timing and sequencing of gross motor control with speech control he will be able to successfully divide his attention as necessary to keep both skills going.

Final Note: *Approximately 9 months after his stroke, Ron walked into therapy from the car with only stand-by assistance from his wife. They decided to take a week away from therapy and are going to their summer cottage for a few days. Both feel confident that they are capable of managing there. Ron is quite excited about the trip, although nervous, because they have not been there since his stroke. His wife feels there will actually be more for Ron to do at the cabin because he has always enjoyed puttering around there. When they return to therapy, he will describe what he was able to do and what he feels he wants to work on. Clearly, Ron demonstrates an understanding of his disability and continues to assume greater responsibility for the direction and goals of his program.*

Chapter Summary

The PT and OT illustrated in these case studies emphasize the problem solving process that is used in all phases of NDT intervention. Immediate posture and movement goals and functional outcomes are set with the client for each treatment session, as described in one day in Chiara's program. Long term goals and objectives, which change as recovery occurs, are shown in Ron's program over 9 months time. In both examples, the NDT clinician focuses on the capabilities and potential of the individual client, employing basic principles of motor learning to keep clients actively working to achieve outcomes that are meaningful in their lives. In both cases, the therapists employ a large variety of treatment strategies that often include preparation of posture and movement components and practice of the whole task to link improvements in impairments with changes in functional outcome. The NDT clinician creates an environment (including objects and persons in it) that is conducive to participation and supports the client's efforts, providing time for the client to plan movement, make mistakes, and solve his or her own problems. This is a difficult, energy consuming approach. Therapist must make informed decisions spontaneously, quickly integrating knowledge, skill and intuition. They must balance the belief that clients need to be responsible for their recovery with the belief that the therapeutic guidance provided by their professional expertise can facilitate the recovery process.

References

Adler, L. (2002). Batter Up! A case study: Playing baseball to develop posture and reaching. *NDT Network, 9* (3), 1, 13, 14.

Bly, L. (1996, September/October). What is the role of sensation in motor learning? What is the role of feedback and feedforward? *NDT Network,* 1-7.

Bobath, B., & Finnie, N. (1958). Re-education of movement patterns for everyday life in the treatment of cerebral palsy. *British Occupational Therapy Journal, 21,* 23-28.

Bobath, K. (1959). The effects of treatment by reflex inhibition and facilitation of movement in cerebral palsy. *Folia Psychiatrica, Neurologica et Neurochirugica Neerlandica, 62* (5), 448-457.

Bobath, K., & Bobath, B. (1964). The facilitation of normal postural reactions and movements in the treatment of cerebral palsy. *Physiotherapy, 50* (8), 246-262.

Bobath, K., & Bobath, B. (1984). The neuro-developmental treatment. In D. Scrutton (Ed.), *Management of the motor disorders of children with cerebral palsy* (pp. 6-18). *Clinics in Developmental Medicine 90.* Philadelphia: J. B. Lippincott.

Boehme, R. (1998, March/April). When children cry in therapy. *NDTA Network,* 7-10.

Campbell, S. K. (1999a). The infant at risk for developmental disability. In S. K. Campbell (Ed.), *Decision making in pediatric neurologic physical therapy* (pp. 260-332). Philadelphia: Churchill Livingstone.

Campbell, S. K. (1999b). Models for decision making in pediatric neurologic physical therapy. In S. K. Campbell (Ed.), *Decision making in pediatric neurologic physical therapy* (pp. 1-22). Philadelphia: Churchill Livingstone.

Curriculum Committee, Neuro-Developmental Treatment Association. (1996, June). *NDTA curriculum guide.* Laguna Beach, CA: Author.

Davis, J. (2002). Bridging the movement and function gap: improving upper-extremity function in adult hemiplegia. *NDT Network*, 9 (4), 1, 11, 14-16.

Diamond, M., & Schenkman, M. (1996). Use of the clinical decision-making process to achieve measurable improvement in function in a patient one year post CVA. *Neurology Report, 20* (2), 72-74.

Effgen, S. K. (2000). The educational environment. In S. K. Campbell (Ed.), *Physical therapy for children* (pp. 910-933). Philadelphia: W. B. Saunders.

Embry, D. G., & Adams, L. (1996). Clinical application of procedural changes by experienced and novice pediatric physical therapists. *Pediatric Physical Therapy, 8,* 122-132.

Fetters, L. (1991). Cerebral palsy: Contemporary treatment concepts. In M. Lister (Ed.), *Contemporary management of motor control problems. Proceedings from II Step Conference. Foundation for Physical Therapy* (pp. 219-224). Alexandria, VA: American Physical Therapy Association.

Finnie, N. (1997). *Handling the young child with cerebral palsy at home* (3rd ed.). Boston: Butterworth and Heinemann.

Gentile, A. M. (2000). Skill acquisition: Action, movement, and the neuromotor processes. In J. Carr & R. Shepherd (Eds.), *Movement science foundations for physical therapy in rehabilitation* (2nd ed., pp. 111-187). Gaithersburg, MD: Aspen Publishing.

Gibson, J. J. (1966). *The senses considered as perceptual systems.* Boston: Houghton Mifflin.

Gibson, J. J. (1979). *The ecological approach to visual perception.* Boston: Houghton Mifflin.

Girolami, G., Ryan, D. F., & Gardner, J. M. (2001). Clinical assessment of the infant. In A. L. Scherzer (Ed.), *Early diagnosis and interventional therapy in cerebral palsy. An interdisciplinary age-focused approach* (3rd ed., pp. 139-184). New York: Marcel Dekker.

Howle, J. (1999). Cerebral palsy. In S. K. Campbell (Ed.), *Decision making in pediatric neurologic physical therapy* (pp. 23-83). Philadelphia: Churchill Livingstone.

Indredavik, B., Bakke, F., Slordahl, S. A., Rokseth, R., & Haheim, L. L. (1999). Treatment in a combined acute and rehabilitation stroke unit: Which aspects are most important? *Stroke, 30* (5), 917-923.

Larin, H. (2000). Motor learning: Theories and strategies for the practitioner. In S. K. Campbell (Ed.), *Physical therapy for children* (pp. 170-197). Philadelphia: W. B. Saunders.

Lawhon, G. (1997). Providing developmentally supportive care in the newborn intensive care unit: An evolving challenge. *Journal of Perinatal and Neonatal Nursing, 10* (4), 48-61.

Magill, R. A. (1998). *Motor learning concepts and applications.* New York: McGraw-Hill International Editions.

Massery, M., & Moerchen, V. (1996, November/December). Coordinating transitional movements and breathing in patients with neuromotor dysfunction. *NDTA Network,* 3-7.

Public Law 102-119 (1990). *Individuals with Disabilities Education Act Amendments of 1997,* 111 Stat. 37-157.

Schmidt, R. A. (1991). Motor learning principles for physical therapy. In M. Lister (Ed.), *Contemporary management of motor control problems. Proceedings from II Step Conference. Foundation for Physical Therapy* (pp. 49-64). Alexandria, VA: American Physical Therapy Association.

Sweeney, J. K. (1994). Assessment of the special care nursery environment: Effects on the high-risk infant. In I. J. Wilhelm (Ed.), *Physical therapy assessment in early infancy* (pp. 13-29). New York: Churchill Livingstone.

Whiteside, A. (1997, September/October). Clinical goals and application of NDT facilitation. *NDT Network,* 1-14.

Chapter 5

Development of the Bobath Approach

"The concept developed here should be considered as no more than a working hypothesis to explain the observed facts." (K. Bobath, 1980, p. 77)

Introduction

Since Dr. and Mrs. Bobath introduced their treatment concept in the 1940s, the concept has undergone many changes, which the previous chapters of this text have described. Dr. Bobath used the term "living concept" to describe the continuous evolution of the approach as he and Mrs. Bobath learned from their clients and the scientific community (B. Bobath, 1948a). The purpose of this chapter is to show the development of the Bobaths' thinking as they built a model for therapeutic intervention, changing their underlying assumptions and clinical concepts to meet the needs of their clients more effectively.

Who Were the Bobaths?

It is not possible to discuss the development of the Bobath Approach and the underlying theories without discussion of the Bobaths themselves. The creation of an approach to aid the recovery of function in adults and children with central nervous system (CNS) impairments was their life work and as such, it developed and changed as they did. Schleichkorn (1992) wrote a biography that makes interesting reading for those students of NDT who wish to know more about the Bobaths. It is not the intent of this text to repeat that information but to theorize about how the adversities the Bobaths faced and the strengths they brought to the process contributed to the development of the clinical concepts that would change the lives of therapists, families, and individuals with neurological or neurodevelopmental disorders.

Berta Busse and Karel Bobath were born in Berlin, Germany, of Jewish parents. Both had inquiring minds and the tenacity to persevere in the face of adversity. They met through mutual school friends in 1924 but went their separate ways to pursue their educations. Karel trained as a physician in Germany but was unable to practice his profession there. This was a difficult time in Germany. Economic conditions had been poor since World War I, the social and political scenes were changing, and anti-Semitism was on the rise (Schleichkorn, 1992). In the hopes of practicing medicine, Dr. Bobath moved to Prague, Czechoslovakia, but had to take his qualifying medical exams again, this time in Czech, which would take another two years while he studied medicine in another language. Finally he qualified as a doctor and accepted a position in pediatrics and pediatric surgery in Brno, Czechoslovakia. His inquisitive mind, professional training, and perseverance brought to the Bobath Approach the medical model and investigative skepticism that sought to answer questions and challenge existing scientific theories.

Berta was raised in Berlin and, contrary to her mother's wishes that she become a secretary, trained as a gymnastics teacher. Her training taught her the analysis of normal movements and various methods of relaxation. In addition, she learned to assess the strength and activity of muscles and their response to relaxation by handling a person in a special way that induced movements in response to being moved. These skills probably formed the basis of her work when, years later, she began to treat clients who had abnormal motor coordination. Her interests and professional background gave her the discipline to observe and appreciate posture as well as movement. In order to understand the various components that contribute to the production of movement, she studied how individuals produce highly skilled movement. She became an expert in imitating and trying out first the components of a total movement, then complete movement sequences. She analyzed movements, then practiced them with variations until she learned how individuals perfected posture and movements. Finally, as she trained in relaxation, her hands developed a great sensitivity to a muscle's tone, its readiness to move, and its responsiveness to change. These five elements–observation, experimentation, analysis, sensitivity of touch, and practice–would become critical components in the teaching methods she developed (as anyone knows who has taken her pediatric or adult courses) as well as in her approach to examining and treating clients with movement disorders.

The commonality of this husband-wife, doctor-therapist team was their analytical, problem-solving ability. They did not have to agree with each other; in fact, they seemed to thrive on challenging each other. Their diversity grew from Karel's belief in scientific inquiry and Berta's belief in clinical observation. He firmly believed that a base of scientific evidence must support clinical practice. She firmly believed that movement could be broken down into components that could be taught in a therapeutic sequence, changed, and improved with practice. They both believed in sharing their findings through exhaustive writings and teachings, publishing many books and articles throughout their careers.

Karel and Berta did not marry until 1941, after they reunited in London as Jewish refugees. Berta had moved to England in 1938 and Karel in 1939 to escape Hitler's politics. Europe was now at war, and England received large numbers of Jews from Germany. However, during these years many of the English were wary of the intent of the German refugees. Both Karel and Berta were challenged as to their motivation, and the threat of "internment camp" was always present. Life was not easy, and access to professional development was limited. Initially, Karel's medical training was not recognized, but in 1941 he finally obtained a position at London's Wilson General Hospital as a "casualty doctor," which permitted him to work as a physician and assist with the war effort. Berta did massage and remedial exercise in a British hospital's physical therapy department. Most likely this is where she became interested in applying her knowledge of movement to individuals with neuropathology.

The driving force to survive the war years, to get on with their lives, and to contribute and share what they learned, shaped the Bobaths' personal and professional lives. There is certainly an interesting parallel between their clients' lives and their own personal lives, with their search for recognition and acceptance. Their clients had to overcome "motor handicaps," which evoked empathy but also rejection, as they strove to gain full recognition as capable, contributing individuals. In the same way, the Bobaths had to overcome their "handicap" of being intelligent Germans in a society that sympathized with their problem of being Jewish refugees but at the same time regarded their German nationality with distrust.

As the Bobaths focused their energy, time, and commitment to the problems of persons with neuropathology, they did not foresee that they would also spend much of their lives trying to convince skeptics of the validity of their findings. Time would be their ally. The number of articles that were written by them and about their approach, the popularity of their courses and lectures, the honors bestowed on them, and the criticism from other professionals are sufficient evidence of the impact of their work. Their contributions to persons with disabilities and to the rehabilitation profession were the culmination of years of learning, questioning, changing, and challenging both themselves and the status quo.

What made this approach so appealing? The Bobath Approach grew out of Berta Bobath's astute observations, practical application, and unrelenting desire to find better solutions to her clients' problems. She was a pragmatic person, more interested in helping her clients than exploring scientific explanations. Although she probed for explanations, she believed that clinical results drove theory, and she accepted as inevitable the lag in obtaining scientific explanations. Mrs. Bobath gathered her data in a systematic manner, closely linking her clinical observations with theoretical assumptions and clinical strategies. She learned from and was influenced by other treatment approaches, including Brunnstrom, Knott, Rood, Peto, Vojta, and Ayres, accepting and expanding on some of these ideas and rejecting others (B. Bobath, 1963; K. Bobath & B. Bobath, 1984). Her systematic writing and teaching style made it possible for therapists to learn her ideas and apply the concepts in clinical practice. She appreciated the complexity of human movement and changed her approach as she gained new information about the application or theoretical basis for her ideas. Only after she was convinced of her findings and could replicate them in the clinic did she ask her husband to help her understand why her methods worked. Dr. Bobath's approach was to read the supporting literature in the neurosciences to provide the theoretical framework for how the CNS controlled movements and what went wrong when there was damage in some part of this system. Dr. Bobath was an analytical thinker, capable of integrating the traditional scientific theories of Sherrington (1947), Magnus (1926), and Jackson (1932/1958) with the contemporary scientific thinking of Bernstein (1967), Martin, (1967), and Ritchie-Russell (1958).

Unfortunately, the Bobaths did not conduct any original research and did not collect clinical data in ways that could offer the medical and scientific community hard evidence for the effectiveness of their treatment approach. They developed their methods during a time when popular acceptance was based on empirical appropriateness. Considering the widespread influence of the NDT approach, this lack of validation from relevant scientific evidence and clinical research continues to plague supporters of this therapeutic approach (Brown & Burns, 2001; Butler, 2001; Butler & Darrah, 2001; Valvano & Long, 1991).

The Bobaths based their approach on a collection of assumptions that reflected the body of motor behavior and neuroscience knowledge of their time. These assumptions provided a framework that defined movement and described how it developed, how it was controlled, and how it changed as a result of specific neurological and developmental intervention strategies. As discussed in earlier chapters, not all of these assumptions and clinical concepts are accepted in current practice. The first section of this chapter describes how Mrs. Bobath's early clinical observations led to the basic operational assumptions of this approach. These assumptions–some of which were clearly stated and others of which must be inferred from Mrs. Bobath's clinical observations and client experience–formed the overall strategic planning for client examination, development of treatment strategies, and evaluation of outcomes.

This therapeutic approach began with clinical observations and operational assumptions and grew into a cohesive concept incorporating acceptable scientific theory of that time. In order to emphasize the cohesiveness of the Bobath Approach, the text notes the relationships between the principles of clinical practices and the observations from which they were derived in **underlined boldface** and the relationships between theoretical concepts and operational assumptions in ***italicized boldface.***

Early Observations and Operational Assumptions

Observation 1:

Spasticity or hypertonus could be reduced in individuals with CNS deficits.

That spasticity could be decreased in individuals with CNS deficits was the first observation Mrs. Bobath made "accidentally" when she began to treat an adult client with hemiplegia following a stroke. This story has several variations, but the underlying observation remains the same (Quinton, personal communication, 2000; Schleichkorn, 1992): Mrs. Bobath was asked to treat just the arm of a 42-year-old man (another physical therapist was already treating his leg) whose stroke had resulted in severe hypertonus with spasticity, no voluntary movement, and shoulder-hand syndrome with pain and swelling. She found that there was resistance when she attempted to straighten his elbow passively. When she flexed his elbow, these same muscles involuntarily assisted the motion of elbow flexion. Because she believed, as did all medical professionals at the time, that she could not change the resistance (spasticity), she focused on the assistance he appeared to give to elbow flexion. She observed that if she stopped passive extension and held his elbow at this point in the movement, she could more easily flex the elbow through a greater range without his unintentional flexion or, as she would later say, "without provoking flexor spasticity." In addition, she found she could extend the elbow and that, in fact, he could voluntarily assist both elbow flexion and extension without the abnormal tonus. She described this observation in a more general way in her first publication (B. Bobath, 1948a), in which she outlined her new treatment for adults with hemiplegia.

NDT Focus: Currently, NDT considers spasticity to be a neural system impairment that is one contribution to abnormally increased tone and skeletal muscle stiffness. NDT attributes excessive muscle tone to a composite of impairments resulting from many interacting systems that can include spasticity (Chapter 2)

Assumption 1:

Muscle tone had a neurophysiological basis and was a dynamic phenomenon that could be influenced negatively by CNS dysfunction or positively by position of the body (or body parts) against the force of gravity and sensory input.

The Bobaths believed that muscle tone was more than the tension produced by elastic properties of the muscles, because this explanation would not account for the dynamic property of tone or the predictable but changeable distribution of hypertonus that they observed in clients with CNS lesions. Mrs. Bobath asserted that spasticity was the greatest impediment to restoration of normal voluntary movement (1948a). She also stated, "The distribution of spasticity is not permanently restricted to certain muscle groups, but influenced, among other factors, by the position of the body in space, the relative position of the head to the body, and by the position of the limbs in relation to the body" (1948a, p. 26). This led to her first treatment methods that included static **reflex-inhibiting postures** designed to reduce hypertonus by controlling the relationship of the limbs, trunk, and head. Bobath treatment emphasized reflex-inhibiting postures in the 1940s (K. Bobath & B. Bobath, 1979). Very quickly, Mrs. Bobath made two additional observations that altered her treatment emphasis and methods. Unfortunately, others taught and used reflex-inhibiting postures in clinical practice long after she had changed her treatment approach.

Observation 2:

Reduction of tone in one part of the body, extremity, or part of an extremity had an influence on tone in other parts of the body.

With the same client with hemiplegia, Mrs. Bobath observed that reduction of spasticity at the elbow resulted in decreased spasticity of the wrist and fingers. Eventually, she found the same thing to be true in the leg. Reduction of tone at one joint produced overall tone changes. She discovered that the state of the muscles of the hip, abdomen, and back determined the behavior of the rest of the lower limb (B. Bobath, 1948b; K. Bobath, 1953). She noted that spasticity affected all the muscles of a limb but that the distribution was selective, with some muscle groups being more severely affected than the others. She believed that it was this selective distribution that led to the characteristic posture of the extremities. This would lead to two additional treatment concepts. The first concept she termed **key points of control,** the use of specific contact points on the muscles and joints to guide movements. The second concept, termed **reflex-inhibiting patterns,** resulted from her discovery of the efficacy of a more limited inhibition, based on the selective distribution of spasticity rather than on attempting to gain total control of the client's body.

> ***NDT Focus: Neither reflex-inhibiting postures nor reflex-inhibiting patterns are current NDT treatment strategies. Clinicians now use localized, limited inhibition of ineffective posture and movement synergies to redirect movement during facilitation of function (Chapter 4).***

Assumption 2:

The abnormality of tone associated with CNS lesions affected the entire muscular system and was expressed in typical patterns of spasticity.

Writing in the 1950s, Dr. Bobath described atypical synergies of flexion and extension involving movement at all the joints of an extremity in clients with abnormal tone. He believed that this lack of selective movements of individual joints and muscles was related directly to the degree of spasticity (K. Bobath & B. Bobath, 1952). Writing about adults with hemiplegia, Mrs. Bobath described the characteristic posture of the limbs when an individual with spasticity and loss of independent muscle action (now classified as a primary, nervous system impairment; see Chapter 2) attempted voluntary movement of a single joint, resulting in activation of all the muscles of the extremity (B. Bobath, 1948b).

Two approaches to managing spasticity were accepted at that time: relaxation and voluntary correction of the faulty movements by conscious effort. The Bobaths dismissed relaxation because they believed, first, that these clients could not successfully relax when spasticity was significant because spasticity was a direct result of neuropathology and was not under the clients' voluntary control. If an individual could produce movement, it was under conditions that required the amount of effort and level of sensory stimulation to be at such a low level that the client could not produce functional movements in everyday life with typical levels of effort and sensory excitation. This relaxation method did improve range of passive motion, but did not change function. The Bobaths also found that the second approach, encouraging active movement with abnormal tone, led to further increased tone and decreased function in other parts of the body because tone affected the whole muscular system. They believed that there had to be a better way.

Observation 3:

Inhibiting abnormal tone did not spontaneously bring about improved movement.

Mrs. Bobath expressed her disappointment in discovering that, even when she was able to alter the client's tone, the individual did not necessarily initiate movement or improve in function (K. Bobath & B. Bobath, 1979). She was certain that her clients had the necessary muscle power and an intact nerve supply, however, they were unable to contract or relax individual muscle groups or move parts of the body independently of others. She found that clients required localized, limited inhibition of tone along with facilitation of active movement sequences before these individuals could produce more normal patterns of posture and coordination. This led to development of **facilitation methods** to address the problem of tone and change the atypical, ineffective synergies.

> ***NDT Focus: Hands-on facilitation continues to be a key NDT intervention strategy to ensure postural alignment, and facilitate effective synergies in functional patterns.***

Assumption 3:

Abnormal tone was only one of the components responsible for the motor control problems in clients with CNS dysfunction.

As early as the 1950s (K. Bobath & B. Bobath, 1952, 1957), Dr. Bobath listed postural tone as one of the three components of the ***postural reflex mechanism*** that together were necessary for performance of skilled movement. The Bobaths maintained that the interaction of these three components–tone, reciprocal innervation, and automatic patterns of postural control–was responsible for normal posture and movement and that an abnormality in any one of these components led to problems of posture and movement. Development and production of normal coordination was turning out to be a very complicated issue.

Observation 4:

The ability to produce skilled voluntary movement was affected by inadequate automatic postural control.

Mrs. Bobath noticed that when adults with hemiplegia tried to make even simple active movements directed toward a goal with the hand and arm that were not directly affected by the CNS lesion, the movements were poorly executed. She observed that there was much more to the control of motor coordination than the "voluntary" part of the movement. She noticed that these individuals did not make the postural adjustments–before or during the task–that would provide them with stability of the trunk and proximal joints to support precise, voluntary actions of the arm, hand, and fingers (B. Bobath, 1959, 1960a, 1969). Her fascination with the role of postural muscles in the production of skilled movement led to the development of intervention methods that stressed control of the **automatic components of posture and movement.** This observation introduced therapists to the importance of postural control before and during all movement and incorporated the roles of righting reactions during movement, anticipatory postural sets, and equilibrium reactions for maintaining or regaining balance. Her emphasis on this automatic component of movement and her effort to find effective strategies to develop postural control unfortunately also led to virtually ignoring the training of specific motor tasks (such as dressing, feeding, grooming, and high-level mobility skills) for many years (K. Bobath & B, Bobath, 1979).

> ***NDT Focus: NDT recognizes that postural control is one element of a motor ensemble that is selected from multiple neuronal maps and organized so that the elements of posture and movement are activated simultaneously in efficient ways for the task conditions (Chapter 1).***

Assumption 4:

Automatic movements made up the fundamental movement patterns and formed the basis of skilled voluntary movements.

The Bobaths contended that the ***postural reflex mechanism*** provided the dynamic background for movement that occurred in constantly changing environmental conditions. These fundamental movement patterns, called ***righting and equilibrium reactions,*** enabled the child to turn over, lift the head, crawl, get into sitting, and balance for standing and walking. The Bobaths followed the maturationist view that these movements were at first automatically produced and then, as the CNS matured and cortical control increased, the child gradually modified, changed, and directed these movements for his or her own purpose (K. Bobath & B. Bobath, 1956; K. Bobath, 1966). The Bobaths acknowledged that these patterns, necessary for attaining and maintaining posture and balance while using the hands freely, were complex. However, they also believed that the highly skilled coordination involved in moving while maintaining balance had its basis in automatic reflexive movement. (This chapter's section entitled The Model of CNS Organization in Bobath Theory continues the discussion of this concept.)

Observation 5:

Clients with CNS dysfunction did not know how to move even when tone was normal.

Clients' inability to move even in the presence of normal tone was most likely a startling observation for Mrs. Bobath. Up to this point, she had assumed that abnormal tone was the cause of inefficient movement and that once tone was controlled, clients should be able to move normally. It was now clear that the problems and solutions were much more complicated. If children with cerebral palsy (CP) had no previous experience with the basic motor patterns of coordination, they were unable to perform developmental skills. In addition, she observed that adults following stroke lost their sense of normal posture at rest as well as the perception and memory of how to produce movement in the affected parts of the body (B. Bobath, 1948a). She observed that children and adults appeared insecure and disorganized, unable to plan or execute even very simple movement sequences, and could not execute movement with either temporal or spatial accuracy. She believed that the difficulty of learning normal movement patterns was due to the abnormal sensory feedback from hyper- or hypotonus, the excessive effort it took to move, and the limited ability to perform selective movement patterns (K. Bobath, 1953).

Assumption 5:

Learning movement was based on prior sensorimotor experiences.

Clients, particularly children who had not experienced normal sensory exploration first of their own bodies and then of the world around them, were incapable of developing variety in motor behaviors and adapting them for complex functions (e.g., adjusting speed, stride, or step length in various environments, or modifying accuracy or force of prehension for skilled tasks) (B. Bobath, 1967). Mrs. Bobath wrote that producing movement that had value to the person was dependent on prior sensorimotor experience. Building a repertoire of posture and movement drew upon previously experienced patterns. She asserted that feedback from very early movements was a key component in producing the appropriate timing, speed, direction, and force for coordinated movements. A client, whether an infant or adult, who experienced atypical sensorimotor patterns, could make use of only those patterns, perpetuating and reinforcing them. Consequently, she asserted that it was not enough to control or change the sensory input and expect more normal output. She stressed the importance of guiding the motor output that then provided more normal feedback on the sensory side. (B. Bobath & Finnie, 1958). She believed that normal movement drove normal sensation, and that clients could then build on these efficient sensorimotor experiences to expand their repertoire of adaptive, functional postures and movements. On the other hand, abnormal posture and movement that persisted over time limited the possibilities for normal sensorimotor expansion. These ideas are consistent with selectionist theory that is currently accepted as part of the NDT theoretical basis.

Observation 6:

Clients' movements were predictable, limited in variety, and stereotypic.

Mrs. Bobath's early clinical experiences were with school-aged children who had severe CP and with adults who had long-standing hemiplegia. She observed that these clients produced limited movement patterns that were predictable and stereotypic even though the individuals could not voluntarily activate the same muscles individually. These patterns usually involved movement at all the joints of an extremity (such as flexion of the hip and knee when dorsiflexing the ankle, or rotation of the head to one side with elbow and finger extension to open the hand or release an object). The muscles functioned, but in atypical patterns of coordination with limited active range of motion (ROM). (For this reason, among others, Mrs. Bobath did not believe that muscle weakness was a problem for these clients.) These individuals could not gain control over these total motor patterns or modify or use them in selective and varied ways with the precision needed for adaptation to the demands of the environment (K. Bobath, 1959b). The Bobaths referred to these abnormal patterns of coordination as ***primitive and tonic reflexes patterns*** because they resembled, particularly in the severely affected individuals, the tonic reflexes described by Magnus (1926) and DeKleijn (K. Bobath, 1971b) in decerebrate animals.

Assumption 6A:

The brain controlled movement, not muscles.

The Bobaths believed that the CNS acted as a coordinating organ for the multitude of incoming sensory stimuli, producing integrated motor responses in which some muscles stabilized, others relaxed, and some moved the limb or body part. The Bobaths followed the work of Hughlings Jackson (1932/1958), frequently quoting, "The cortex knows nothing of muscles, it knows only of movements." Dr. Bobath believed that there was a fundamental and efficient tendency of the brain to repeat patterns of muscle activation, whenever possible, to allow functional, effective movement (K. Bobath, 1980). In the individual who was developing typically, this was an efficient system that allowed frequently occurring patterns of posture and movement consisting of many automatic components to run as programmed responses. Although the Bobaths did not discuss motor programs, they did describe differences in neural levels of control of automatic and willed movements. The "higher centers" directed the action plan (e.g., "Pick up the pencil and write your name," or "Carry that package as you walk to the door and open it."). The subcortical levels of the CNS controlled the details of the execution (muscle selection, speed, timing, direction, force) (K. Bobath, 1960). The CNS was capable of modifying the plan in response to sensory feedback about the correctness of the execution. However, the CNS of the individual with dysfunction was less competent at sorting, selecting, and integrating the large variety of afferent inflow or to adapting motor output for variation in motor actions. Once activated, the movement patterns were of reflex action, outside the control of the client. The individual with CNS dysfunction had great difficulty regulating the amplitude, strength, or variety of responses and retained simple motor responses. Dr. Bobath referred to this as "synaptic chains of typical patterns of abnormal reflex activity" (K. Bobath, 1980, p. 84). He supported this assumption with the theory of ***released abnormal reflex activity***.

Assumption 6B:

The CNS gradually inhibited those parts of a movement that were unnecessary and disturbing to the performance of a specific task.

The Bobaths proposed that a key role of the CNS was the inhibition of early total movement patterns, which they referred to as ***primitive and tonic motor patterns***. They maintained that the retention of total patterns was responsible for the stereotypic characteristics of the movements in children with CP (K. Bobath, 1959b). The persistence of these primitive patterns prevented children from developing the postural reactions (which the Bobaths called ***righting and equilibrium responses***) necessary to move and balance in the upright position. The inhibitory function of the CNS made it possible for children with typical development to combine, time, and direct the motor patterns they already knew in ways that actively brought about new combinations of movements to solve new problems. The Bobaths suggested that the CNS's inhibitory function resulted from its ability to suppress unwanted activity, leaving only the precise grouping of agonists, antagonists, and synergists needed for new combinations. They asserted that the "unlearning" of primitive movements was equal in importance to the learning of new movements (K. Bobath, 1980). The Bobaths theorized that, with CNS pathology, every attempt at a movement resulted in action of many more muscles than were required for the movement (K. Bobath & B. Bobath, 1957). The lack of refinement and selectivity within the CNS produced the stereotypic, grossly organized movements characteristic of individuals with stroke or CP.

> ***NDT Focus: NDT currently recognizes that changes in the biomechanical properties of the musculoskeletal system and the specific requirements of the task in context influence the selection of combinations from various neural maps that contribute to the final posture and movement ensemble.***

Observation 7:

Clients made significant changes in reorganizing their motor patterns when they repeated and practiced guided and controlled movement.

Mrs. Bobath found that when she used physical guidance rather than verbal teaching or visual imitation, she reduced ineffective and compensatory movements and altered the somatosensory input so that the individual could feel, and produce, more normal motor output. She discovered that the effects of her treatment were cumulative and that clients improved continuously with every treatment. She initially claimed that after only a few sessions, individuals with hemiplegia would be able to perform transitional movements (rolling, achieving sitting, and rising to stand) of everyday life, even if the quality of the performance was poor, and that they would be able to resume normal occupation after 6-9 months of treatment (B. Bobath, 1948a). This was, perhaps, an expression of rather ambitious treatment outcomes. She later stated that the clinician is responsible for finding, obtaining, and developing any potential for restoration of function. Treatment could do no more than develop clients' potentialities, but it could help them organize these in the most efficient way (B. Bobath, 1963).

NDT now recognizes from motor learning theory that too much hands-on intervention prevents clients from experimenting and solving motor problems within their own body and neural makeup. The physical guiding of movement, particularly in the early phase of learning or relearning motor control, is a natural interaction between two persons that can assist in establishing efficient movement strategies. This observation led Mrs. Bobath to develop specific clinical concepts of **key points of control** and **facilitation of movement**.

NDT Focus: NDT recognizes that treatment strategies that use physical guidance or handling, applied carefully and precisely during early practice, combined with periods of trial and error and independent movement are all needed to achieve motor learning.

Assumption 7:

The CNS was capable of recovery and development after injury and could be influenced by sensory feedback from the most effective motor output.

That the CNS could recover and continue to develop following injury was and remains an important assumption in the development of the Bobath Approach. If the brain could not recover or develop, then treatment must focus on adaptation and compensation alone, utilizing the functions that remain. The Bobaths believed that their methods of inhibiting unwanted patterns of hypertonus and abnormal synergies while facilitating normal posture and movement encouraged experience-dependent reorganization of the brain to maximize returning and developing functions. The Bobaths asserted that it was possible to influence the state of the CNS from the periphery by handling clients and directing their active responses away from the undesirable spastic patterns. At the same time, this therapeutic technique opened up the higher channels for more normal muscle execution. Dr. Bobath wrote "that when applying this to treatment principles, it means that the permanent carryover of treatment depends largely on the extent to which the higher reactions can be facilitated and their synaptic chains firmly established by repetition" (K. Bobath & B. Bobath, 1984, p. 86).

Observation 8:

Children with CNS dysfunction did not develop movement in an orderly and systematic fashion.

In the 1980s, as the Bobaths described how their treatment approach had changed, they wrote, "Development does not proceed in a definite sequence, . . . children develop many activities simultaneously, which reinforce each other to culminate in a 'milestone'" (K. Bobath & B. Bobath, 1984, p. 99). With the evolution of this premise, the framework of treatment shifted. Rather than focusing on the sequential development of motor milestones, therapists began analyzing the components underlying **movement sequences** in adults and children. This shift represented a significant change in the Bobaths' thinking and in their treatment approach from the early years. In 1952, Mrs. Bobath had written, "The normal child develops his motor patterns in a regular sequence. He progresses from one motor activity to the next in definite steps, preparing for the next stage by vigorous exercise and constant practice. . . . The more difficult task is only undertaken after the less difficult one is fully mastered," and, "In the spastic child development is not simply arrested, but, owing to the child's effort to overcome the handicap, [the developmental] sequence is interfered with and it becomes patchy and uneven" (K. Bobath & B. Bobath, 1952, p.

112). The maturationist theories of McGraw (1945/1963) and Gessell et al. (1940) supported their view. Unfortunately, long after the Bobaths abandoned this early hypothesis, adherence to the developmental sequence as a framework for treatment was frequently cited as defining the Bobath Approach (Bleck, 1987; Lunnen, 1999; Mayston, 1992). Even in the 1950s, when the Bobaths did adhere to the importance of developmental milestones, they also emphasized the development of *patterns of movement*, which resulted in the achievement of motor milestones.

NDT Focus: NDT emphasizes that motor development emerges from the cooperation of many body systems in a task-specific context including, but not limited to, elements of posture and movement. Motor milestones are viewed as age-appropriate motor behaviors based not on a linear acquisition in which one milestone develops as the foundation for the next, but on an expansion of movement repertoires established by experience and selection.

Assumption 8:

Problems in motor control were the expression of either damage to the centers that control these movements, or excessive action of other centers preventing the inhibitory function of the higher control centers.

Dr. Bobath wrote that the various parts of the brain interacted harmoniously to direct and regulate movement patterns (K. Bobath, 1953). Damage to any part of the neural mechanism, particularly to the higher centers in the cortex, affected the orderly progression of motor behavior that occurred as the infant developed. Initially, this normal progression involved movements that had little variety, involved large parts of the body, and were primarily automatic. As the infant developed, maturation of the higher neural centers caused movements to become more selective and diverse, directed toward purposeful movements for daily-life skills. Damage either before birth or at the time of birth prevented this development and the resulting motor behavior was dominated by excessive action of the lower neural centers, which consisted of automatic reflexive synergies characterized by a lack of variability and adaptability.

Observation 9:

Clients were unable to maintain balance within a position or protect themselves from falling.

Mrs. Bobath observed that, in addition to problems of tone and movement, clients also had primary impairments in balance. She attributed problems with balance to fear of falling or of being moved. Early on she believed that ineffective balance reactions were a secondary impairment caused by hyper- or hypotonus that interfered with the timing and speed of muscle action, which hindered the ability to (a) adjust posture prior to a movement or (b) move quickly enough to maintain or regain balance (B. Bobath, 1948b; B. Bobath & Finnie, 1958). Initially, she facilitated righting and equilibrium responses as a means to inhibit abnormal reflex patterns. However, she later observed that even when she was able to inhibit abnormal tone and facilitate movement, many of these clients were still unable to adjust their posture in anticipation of changes within their base of support (BOS) or to recover if they were displaced outside their BOS (K. Bobath & B. Bobath, 1964). She noted, for example, that when children with CP used their arms for support in sitting and then lifted an arm to reach out for an object, they would lose their balance and fall sideways or backward. As she observed that ineffective balance prevented some clients from developing skilled movement, she acknowledged that balance was a part of an overall movement synergy that included postural control and that developing or perfecting balance was, in itself, an appropriate treatment goal (K. Bobath & B. Bobath, 1979).

Assumption 9:

Damage in one part of the CNS affected the function of other parts of the CNS.

Clients who had lesions in the CNS, but not necessarily in the cerebellum, showed deficits in the onset and quality of equilibrium reactions, a function that was generally attributed to the cerebellum. Dr. Bobath hypothesized that in a damaged nervous system, afferent input from vestibular and somatosensors was "shunted" away from the specific pathways that controlled and produced responses to a displacement of the center of mass (COM) over the BOS, to a more primitive synaptic chain of abnormal reflex patterns even when the specific pathway was undamaged (K. Bobath, 1960). The Bobaths postulated that equilibrium reactions were inhibited for two reasons: the presence of abnormal tone prevented the normal movement responses of the trunk and extremities, and overactivity of tonic reflexes, controlled at lower neural levels, prevented the appearance of these automatic movements.

Observation 10:

Clients' muscles became stiffer and movements less effective when the individuals put forth excess effort during functional activities.

Mrs. Bobath often described the negative effects on the tone and isolated movement of extremities or body segments when adults with hemiplegia attempted to perform a task that they were not capable of doing easily (B. Bobath, 1990). She asserted that this inability to produce isolated muscle control was caused by irradiation or overflow of contractile activity in multiple muscles, both in the same segment and in muscles far removed from the prime mover. These associated reactions, first described by Walshe (1921), interfered with the coordinated responses of agonists and antagonists and led to deterioration of postural alignment and precise movement when the client was encouraged to make great effort to accomplish a task. She also noted this atypical characteristic in children with CP (B.

Bobath, 1953). Since she observed a correlation between exertion and an increase in tone, she prohibited the use of strengthening exercises and forceful movements in treatment.

Assumption 10:

Tone, posture, and movement were linked through the postural reflex mechanism such that increasing tone produced a deterioration in posture and movement.

As Assumption 3 proposed, the Bobaths believed that tone was part of the postural reflex mechanism and that abnormality of tone led to abnormalities in posture and movement. From her earliest observations, Mrs. Bobath concluded that if tone could be controlled, then the client could move more easily. This assumption was based on a hierarchical model of CNS organization (see the following section of this chapter) and was an important premise in the development of the Bobath theory and treatment principles. Recent clinical and scientific findings have shown that this link is not so direct and that strengthening and forceful exertion do not necessarily influence movement negatively (Carr & Shepherd, 1998; Woll & Utley, 2001).

Observation 11:

Movement problems affected every domain of the client's life.

Anyone who has been taught by Berta Bobath remembers her words, "You must treat the whole child," which meant that, for example, one could not treat the hands without understanding the tasks one wanted the hands to do and under what circumstances, and without appreciating the interdependence of the function of the arms and hands with the rest of the body (B. Bobath & Finnie, 1958). This tenet stemmed from Mrs. Bobath's understanding of the effects of neuromotor impairment on all domains of function, including the ability to perceive, plan, execute, and react to tasks in various environments. In the first article that Mrs. Bobath published in 1948 describing treatment for adults with hemiplegia, she said, "There is a reversion to the faulty movement under certain psychological stimuli. This reversion is produced under the stress of fear, insecurity, old environment and self-consciousness and associations connected with the recent acquisition of new movements" (B. Bobath, 1948a, p. 29). Describing children with CP, she wrote, "The sensori-motor problem of the child is the one that embraces all other problems, which include the emotional, mental and social difficulties. . . . Sensori-motor development is the basis for all our experiences, for all our learning, for our ability to adjust ourselves to the environment, to the people we live with and to the objects we have to handle. If we want to treat the whole child, we have to start from there" (B. Bobath, 1960b, p. 248). The Bobaths did not develop their concepts based on theories that described the contributions of multiple systems to movement control and development, nor on motor learning theories that stressed the importance of the context of the motor task. Their writings, however, indicated appreciation for and understanding of these ideas. If they had had access to theories of motor learning or systems approaches to motor control problems, they might have explored these ideas more thoroughly.

Assumption 11:

The CNS absorbed multiple stimuli and reacted with variable responses based on conditions of the environment.

The Bobaths recognized that CP resulted from damage of the immature brain, which interfered with the child's growth and development. They believed that children learn first about themselves and their environment through movement. They smile and evoke a response from others. They explore their own bodies and develop a concept of self. They reach out and explore space and the objects and people in that space. Without the ability to move normally, children are affected in domains of development without any damage to these areas. The Bobaths believed that the various associated sensory and perceptual problems were secondary to the physical handicap that prevented the child from exploring. Dr. Bobath wrote, "It is difficult to decide whether a child with CP suffers from primary or secondary retardation, due to lack of experience caused by his enforced immobility" (K. Bobath, 1980, p. 2). The inability and inexperience of the parents as they managed their infant with a sensorimotor handicap could compound this problem if they misinterpreted the infant's movements. Insufficient or inappropriate feedback to the child from the environment and the people in it added to the primary impairment. The Bobaths used this argument to support **early identification and management** of neuromotor impairments, such as CP (K. Bobath & B. Bobath, 1984).

These eleven observations and their underlying assumptions comprised the beginnings of the Bobath Approach in the 1940s and 1950s. The emphasis of the approach changed over the years as the Bobaths gained experience and increased their understanding of the development of movement and movement control. Dr. Bobath sought to provide a rational explanation of these initial concepts based on the neurophysiological evidence available at that time. He did not conduct any research studies to examine their beliefs and assumptions, but attempted to provide a consolidated theoretical foundation by researching the neuroscientific literature, interpreting and applying this information to their concepts of managing clients. In the 1940s and 1950s, the common theory held that the nervous system was organized and functioned in a hierarchical fashion. It was in this theoretical framework that Dr. Bobath constructed a working hypothesis for the clinical observations and their underlying assumptions. As with any theory, the hierarchical/reflex-based model of neural organization both expanded and limited the development of the Bobath Approach.

Theoretical Basis: What Evidence Was There That These Assumptions Were Correct?

Dr. Bobath offered theoretical explanations for their empirical observations and assumptions based on a reflex/hierarchical model of the nervous system that was a combination of the various acceptable neural control theories in existence at the time they developed their treatment concepts. In the hierarchical model, described by Jackson (1932/1958), four successively higher levels of neural integration exerted control over the preceding levels.

Consequently, a lesion in the higher centers permitted expression of normally suppressed patterns of movement, which would then dominate the person's posture and movement. In the reflex model based on animal brain transection studies by Magnus (1926) and Sherrington (1906, 1913), movement was driven by sensory stimuli. Reflex movements were initiated by sensory stimuli, and there was a fixed relationship between the form and intensity of the stimuli and the form and intensity of the response. This rigid model, combining these two concepts, has generally been discarded today in favor of more flexible models that distribute neural functions throughout brain structures. Dr. Bobath found this popular hierarchical model to be useful in correlating the structure of the brain and nervous system with the organization, development, and control of movement in individuals of typical ability and in those with neuropathology (see Figure 5.1).

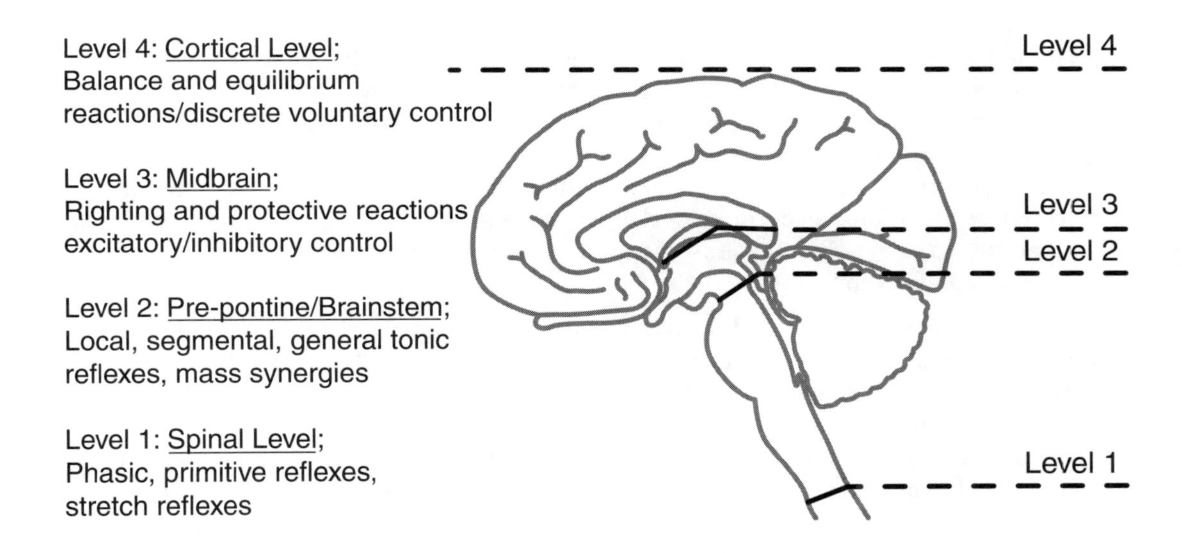

Figure 5.1. The concept of hierarchical levels of CNS integration of motor function. (Illustration by Claire Wenstrom.)

The Model of CNS Organization in Bobath Theory

The Bobaths believed and taught that the CNS was organized as a hierarchy and divided the control of movement into four levels of integration: spinal, prepontine brainstem, midbrain or thalamic, and cortical. Each level made use of centrally controlled inhibition so that, finally, the higher centers had the ability to suppress all but the required part of any intended movement. The resultant self-determined movements were discrete, selective, and variable, combining the necessary postural support with the ability to move any part of the body independently from others in the most varied ways, for the sole purpose of accomplishing a specific task in a specific situation at a specific time.

For example, the eyes can move separately from the head in relationship with the arm and hand to locate, reach for, and pick up coins from a table. The fingers and thumb on the radial side of the hand can move separately at each joint in relation to each other and in relation to the wrist and forearm to grasp, manipulate, and hold the coins within the palm with the ulnar fingers as the task is completed. Posture is secure in the upright position to support the visual attention and movement. All other potential movements of other body parts are silent.

Dr. Bobath described an active process of inhibition, beginning at the spinal level and reaching culmination at the cortical level, in which only those automatic (reflex) movements that aided and assisted willed movement remained a part of the movement synergy (K. Bobath & B. Bobath, 1950). Dr. Bobath stated, however, that this information from animal studies could not simply be translated in terms of human neurophysiology. He agreed that the levels of motor control were valid in humans but stated that the evolution of motor patterns in humans was more complicated than just an elaboration or recombination of simple reflexes (K. Bobath & B. Bobath, 1950). He asserted that the lower levels of integration had surrendered their autonomy and independent function to higher levels during humankind's phylogenetic development such that a lesion anywhere in the CNS would not produce the clear clinical picture seen in experimental animals (K. Bobath, 1959a). He hypothesized that there was an ordered pattern of overlapping representations at the various levels of the CNS that governed the combinations of muscular action and resulted in a vast diversity of increasingly complex movements.

Dr. Bobath identified posture and movements in clients with CNS dysfunction that related to the four distinct levels of neural integration. He stated that although the lesions in children (or adults) might be extensive, scattered, or localized and did not produce the total disruption of the neuraxis that occurred in animal studies, "This scheme did present an idea of the type of motor response to be expected from a lesion which interrupts the afferent inflow at any of these four levels and disturbs the interaction of the whole central nervous system" (K. Bobath, 1959a, p. 452). This neural organization is not part of NDT theory today but is presented here to describe the theoretical explanations that supported the clinical concepts developed by the Bobaths. Additional information is available from the Bobaths' extensive writings, particularly those articles and books from the 1950s and 1960s (see the list of references at the end of this chapter).

NDT Focus: The model of organization of movement that NDT currently uses has changed. Posture and movement are viewed as elements of an action that is achieved through the interactions of many neuronal networks widely distributed throughout the brain, combined with information from various body systems, previous experiences in specific environmental contexts, and driven by the desire to accomplish a task.

First Level of Integration: The Spinal Level

Sherrington (1906, 1913, 1947) found that a transection at the upper cervical level of the spinal cord left the remaining nervous system capable of producing various spinal reflexes. These animal preparations produced spinal reflexes that were purely phasic movements in response to sensory stimulation. The reflexes coordinated the muscles of the limbs in patterns of either total flexion or extension. Sherrington (1947) made two points in his study of these patterns of movement that Dr. Bobath found useful when explaining the control of movement. First, Sherrington believed that these experiments provided evidence of spinal reciprocal inhibition, that inhibition of antagonistic muscle groups was an active process exerted by the CNS at the spinal level. (Reciprocal inhibition does not exist in the intact nervous system.) Second, he demonstrated that it was the release of control, or as Dr. Bobath often called it, "release of inhibition by higher centers," that produced synergies of movement in mass patterns of flexion or extension. (This concept of CNS inhibition is discussed in detail in a separate section of this chapter entitled Neural Inhibition.)

In general, with the exception of withdrawal of a limb due to pain, the continued influence of these spinal reflexes is not useful to the maturing infant or child because the movements are phasic and cannot sustain the child's posture against the force of gravity. The Bobaths recognized the limitations of these reflexes in serving the upright posture and believed that the continued presence of these spinal reflexes was responsible for the inability to move one joint selectively while the neighboring joints remain motionless (K. Bobath, 1954). Dr. Bobath proposed that three reflexes originally described by Sherrington–the *flexor withdrawal*, the *extensor thrust*, and the *phasic crossed extension reflexes*–were responsible for the mass, phasic movements of the entire lower extremities (LEs) that occurred in clients with hypertonus or athetosis (with intermittent hypertonus). That clients with spasticity generally did not exhibit these phasic reflex movements, which Dr. Bobath attributed to the stronger influence of the tonic reflexes in humans that dominated the posture and movement at the second level of integration.

Second Level of Integration: Prepontine Level of the Brainstem

The Bobaths placed a great deal of importance on dysfunction at the prepontine level of neural integration because it affected posture. Sherrington (1913), Magnus (1926), and Rademaker (K. Bobath, 1971b) demonstrated that transection at the prepontine level of the brainstem, just below the level of the red nucleus, produced decerebrate animals that could generate only limited and ineffective muscle synergies that were unlike those of the spinal animal preparations. They called these stereotypic movements *tonic reflexes,* sustained contractions characterized by an increase in postural tone of the antigravity muscles and often co-contraction (co-activation) rather than reciprocal innervation patterns of muscle activation. This explanation accounted for the presence of and changes in abnormal tone and the typical but abnormal patterns of movements the Bobaths saw in adults and children with CNS dysfunction. The findings regarding released tonic reflexes supported two fundamental concepts of their approach. First, the Bobaths hypothesized that hypertonus was an abnormal, patterned response of the damaged CNS and second, predicable changes in hypertonus seen with changes of position resulted from release of tonic reflex activity following brain damage. These ideas were the most basic aspects of the Bobath Approach and were initially given great significance. Dr. Bobath later stated, "I feel that in the past I may have overrated the significance of the 'tonic reflexes,' probably to the detriment of credibility in this approach to treatment" (K. Bobath, 1980, p. 34). Long after they abandoned this emphasis, the therapeutic community continued to view these ideas as basic assumptions in NDT (Horak, 1991; Lunnen, 1999).

The Bobaths asserted that patterns of tonic reflex activity could be recognized in the client's posture and movements. They acknowledged that isolated reflexes were rare, except perhaps in individuals with the most severe involvement, because the motor patterns resulted from a *combination* of reflexes acting simultaneously that reinforced, inhibited, or canceled the influence of others. Magnus classified tonic reflexes into local, segmental, and general static reactions, according to whether they involved one limb, both upper or lower limbs, or the whole body (Jackson, 1932/1958).

In their early writings, the Bobaths used the terms *reflex* and *reaction* interchangeably, taking their interpretation of these movement patterns from animal research in which various investigators used one or the other term. Later, Dr. Bobath said it was unfortunate that they had used the term *reflex* because the motor patterns of the child with CP were the result of the interplay of various abnormal patterns, compensatory activities, and other factors resulting from the injured brain, and the interaction of all of these elements with postural control, balance, and functional activity (K. Bobath, 1980).

Local Static Reactions

According to Dr. Bobath, the important local static reaction was the *positive supporting reaction,* characterized by simultaneous contraction of flexors and extensors. This reaction was a modification of the extensor thrust, a spinal reflex originally identified by Sherrington (1913). The stimulus for the positive supporting reactions was either proprioceptive stretch of muscles produced by weight bearing or exteroceptive stimulus evoked by contact of the foot with the ground. When the foot contacted the ground and the intrinsic muscles of the foot stretched, the antagonists did not relax, as was ordinarily the situation, but instead contracted simultaneously with the agonists. This exerted a synergic function that resulted in the fixation of the joints, and the leg became a stiff pillar. Under normal circumstances, the positive supporting reaction occurred only in a very modified form to increase the tone in the support leg when a person shifted from two-foot to one-foot standing. This reaction produced co-contraction of the muscles of that limb to support the additional weight; however, the limb remained mobile and the person was able to flex any one joint in the supporting leg without collapsing.

Mrs. Bobath wrote that this reaction occurred to some degree in all clients with spasticity who attempted to stand and walk (B. Bobath, 1954). These individuals touched the ground with the ball of the foot, evoking the positive supporting reaction. The ball of the foot took the weight of the body, which added proprioceptive stretch as well. The entire extremity became stiff with simultaneous contraction of flexors and extensors. The rigid limb carried the weight of the body but actually interfered with balance reactions that needed mobility of the joints and constantly changing fine postural adjustments to cope with displacement of the COM over a constantly changing BOS.

Segmental Static Reactions

The *crossed extension reflex* was considered a modification of the phasic spinal crossed extension reflex that combined with the positive support reaction to produce flexion of the ipsilateral leg and extension of the contralateral leg (Magnus, 1926). The *crossed extension reflex* was considered a segmental static reaction because it involved both LEs. Mrs. Bobath contended that this reflex augmented the positive support reaction and accounted for the hyperextension of the knee in the adult with hemiplegia. She hypothesized that this combination produced a compensation pattern allowing the adult with hemiplegia to advance the leg forward to take a step. As the person shifted weight to the involved side, the contact of the foot provoked the positive support reaction. If this reaction was strong, the spastic leg remained a pillar with extension, adduction, and foot inversion, and the individual was unable to step. If, however, the crossed extension competed with the positive support reaction, the client might have been able to overcome the strong extension (produced by the augmentation of these two reflex patterns) sufficiently to flex the trunk and hip and bring the entire extremity forward in a pattern of circumduction that allowed advancement of the entire extremity to step.

General Static Reactions

General static reactions affected the tone, posture, and movement of the trunk and limbs. These reactions were of great importance to the Bobaths when they offered an explanation for the changes and distribution of tone, as well as an explanation of the stereotypic patterns of movement that occur in CNS dysfunction (B. Bobath, 1985; K. Bobath & B. Bobath, 1955, 1956). They believed that the consistent appearance of these reflexes in response to the appropriate stimulus indicated the severity of the CNS pathology, and that the ability to overcome these patterns of movement was a good predictor of the treatment approach's success. The Bobaths divided these reactions into three groups:

1. *tonic neck reflexes*, including the *asymmetrical and symmetric tonic neck reflexes,* evoked by change in the position of the head in relation to the body
2. *tonic labyrinthine reflexes*, evoked by change of orientation of the head in space
3. *associated reactions*, induced by the effort to move or balance (or the fear to do so)

Tonic Neck Reflexes

Asymmetric Tonic Neck Reflex (ATNR). The typical, predictable movements of the ATNR were induced by rotation of the head, which produced an increase in extensor tone or extensor movement of those limbs toward which the face side of the head rotated, and a decrease in extensor tone or flexor movements of those limbs toward which the skull side of the head rotated. The Bobaths believed that these changes in tone in clients with CNS dysfunction followed the same laws as those observed by Magnus (1926) in decerebrate animals. The Bobaths observed that the strength of the reaction varied with individual cases. In severe cases, the reaction to passive rotation was quick and strong, producing movement of at least both upper extremities (UEs). In individuals with lesser degrees of involvement, the reaction might occur only after the head was rotated and held for a second or two and produced only partial extension or flexion of the more distal joints. The observable movement varied, with the greatest occurrence in the UEs. In premature infants, the reaction was often seen more strongly in the legs. Walshe (1921) and other investigators (Gesell, 1938; Hellebrandt, Schade, & Carns, 1962) found that the reaction was more pronounced if the individual turned the head actively, particularly if the rotation occurred against resistance. Even in children with diplegic CP, the change in tone in the UEs was perceptible even when the pattern of movement was not evident (B. Bobath, 1975).

In infants developing normally, investigators described the ATNR pattern as most pronounced between 2 and 4 months, contributing to visual discovery and attending to the hand on the face side. In children with CP, this reflex was thought to interfere with visual regard because the extensor component was so strong that the head not only rotated but extended as well, and as a consequence the hand did not come into visual range. The Bobaths also noted that this reflex movement affected the way in which some clients reached for an object. The child turned the head to find the object, which caused the arm to extend on that side. However, to flex the fingers and thumb to grasp the object, the individual turned the head away and attempted to bring the object close to the body without visual regard. The Bobaths believed that this asymmetric pattern prevented a child from bringing the fingers to the mouth. The child was not able to flex the elbow when the head was turned toward the hand, nor would the child be able to keep the head in the midline while attempting to bring the hand to the mouth. If the child succeeded in getting the hand to the mouth, the hand was fisted, and the early exploration of fingers in the mouth did not occur. In addition, the Bobaths believed that the retention of the ATNR interfered with the development of symmetry, preventing the use of both hands together in front of the body for examining and transferring objects and for skills of dressing and feeding.

The Bobaths emphasized the impact of the ATNR in children with CP and adults with stroke. They hypothesized that the persistent, strong asymmetrical postures and movements that resulted from the ATNR contributed to the development of such deformities as scoliosis and subluxation or dislocation of the hip (on the skull side). In addition, they believed that many abnormal compensatory movements and postures resulted as the client attempted to override or use the influence of this tonic reaction for function.

Symmetrical Tonic Neck Reflex (STNR). Extending or flexing the neck evoked the STNR. The stimulus arose from the proprioceptors in the muscles of the neck. Extending the head led to an increase of extensor tone or to extensor movements in the UEs, with a relative increase of flexor tone in the LEs. Flexing the head had the opposite effect on the limbs.

The Bobaths found that most often clients who showed the effects of the STNR exhibited the effects of the ATNR as well. The persistence of this reaction in individuals with CNS dysfunction limited their movements in prone and four-point crawling. For example, the child was able to maintain weight on the extended arms only with the head extended. However, the child was not able to distribute the weight evenly between the hands and knees but sat back on dorsiflexed feet. (Because this was an uncomfortable and unstable position, the child externally rotated the tibias and W-sat between the legs.) If the child tried to look at toys placed on the floor near the hands, the arms collapsed as the hips extended, and the child fell onto his or her face. The Bobaths hypothesized that distribution of tone in arms and legs that was dependent on the position of the head could be a serious obstacle to learning to crawl. They proposed that the familiar "bunny-hopping" pattern frequently displayed by children with athetosis, or spastic quadriplegic CP, was the outcome of attempting to move in the hands-knees position while under the influence of the STNR. These children progressed forward by keeping the head and arms extended, pulling symmetrically with the arms, and "hopping" forward with the legs held in a symmetrical flexed posture (B. Bobath, 1975). The Bobaths classified this pattern as one of the abnormal patterns of movement that developed compensatorily when a child attempted to overcome the STNR. Even when the STNR produced only slight changes of tone, as in children with spastic diplegia, these changes limited the ROM at the hips and produced short excursions of flexion and extension as well as abnormal interlimb coordination.

Tonic Labyrinthine Reflexes (TLR). The TLR could be studied separately only by excluding the tonic neck reflexes. Because this was not possible in humans, therapists determined the influence of the TLR by observing the reaction of the extremities when the head was moved in space because stimulus to the labyrinths initiated these reflexes. If, when the head was moved, all four limbs responded with similar changes in tone, then the TLR was considered dominant. The Bobaths found that when the TLR dominated the child's posture, the child exhibited rigid extension and adduction when placed in supine and was unable to bring the hands to the mouth, flex the knees, or place the soles of the feet on the floor in a "hook-lying" position. The same client in prone showed increased flexor tone such that the hips could not contact the floor and the knees would not fully extend. The arms were flexed under the chest in a way that prevented the child from pushing up on extended arms or even fully extending the head. Trying to bring the child to a sitting position from supine produced strong extension across the hips, particularly if the head fell into extension, preventing the child from flexing the hips and trunk and assuming a sitting position. If the head fell into flexion when the child was placed in sitting, the entire trunk flexed forward and the child was unable to regain a position with erect trunk and head due to the increase in flexor tone. The Bobaths believed that the tone changes influenced by the TLR severely restricted the client's ability to move in either prone or supine or roll from one position to another.

The Bobaths tried to determine the influence of the individual tonic reflexes for a theoretical understanding of the posture and movement problems in CNS dysfunction. However, they did not evaluate individual reflexes as part of the examination of a client, but rather evaluated the strength and distribution of the postural tone and the association with the normal and abnormal motor patterns linked to these reflexes (B. Bobath, 1990; K. Bobath & B. Bobath, 1958). As early as 1953, they described the difficulty in determining which reflex(es) played a dominant role at any particular moment in producing a particular distribution of tone or posture (B. Bobath, 1953). They presumed that the resulting reaction was most often due to the interaction of a number of reflexes that reinforced, neutralized, or inhibited each other.

Associated Reactions. Walshe (1921) first described associated reactions as tonic reflexes arising in and acting on the limb muscles. Associated reactions resulted from proprioceptive stretch in a muscle group that irradiated into muscles that often were very distant from the prime mover. This irradiation prevented intralimb or interlimb coordination by making it impossible for the individual to move the muscles of one joint while keeping other muscles silent. Walshe found that tonic and sustained contractions of the muscles of the sound limbs produced an increase in the tone of the spastic muscles in adults with hemiplegia. However, other stimuli, such as clenching the jaw, yawning, and stiffening the neck also produced associated contractions in spastic limbs. Mrs. Bobath observed that associated reactions could result from any difficulty the individual experienced that produced a change in tone, such as fear of falling or difficulties in speech in clients with dysarthria. These reactions also occurred when the client put forth great effort to perform even simple movements, such as grasping an object or making a step. Mrs. Bobath believed that associated reactions were particularly problematic in adults with hemiplegia. In such adults, as well as children with hemiplegia CP, flexing the joints of the LE to take a step produced greater flexor tone in the UE. The more the client tried to walk, the more the flexor tone increased in the UE. For example, an individual walking with the support of a walker or quad cane would begin to take steps with fairly good alignment. An increase in effort or speed (e.g., to keep up with nondisabled friends or family) would produce increased flexor tone in the arm. Because the arm was stabilized by the handgrip, the trunk was pulled forward (or sideways) into flexion (or lateral flexion), and alignment deteriorated as the person walked. Mrs. Bobath maintained that in clients with CNS dysfunction, excitation and effort resulted in stereotyped, associated reactions with long-lasting hypertonus due to after-contraction. The gradual deterioration of repetitive movements stemming from after-contraction arose from the lack of inhibition between movements (B. Bobath, 1990). Therefore, to reduce the detrimental effect of associated reactions in treatment, the Bobaths taught that clients should move slowly, with adequate time for inhibition between repetitions. They also urged that excitation and effort be kept to a minimum at the beginning of each treatment session, then increased gradually as the client learned to move without evoking associated reactions (B. Bobath, 1990).

NDT Focus: Currently, NDT considers tonic and primitive reflex movements to be examples of linkages among biomechanical aspects of the musculoskeletal and neural systems that attempt to simplify movement requirements, reducing the degrees of freedom as the individual develops or recovers function. These sensory-elicited movements exhibit abnormal qualities when neuropathology limits movement experiences, reinforcing these linkages even when they no longer have value to the individual and actually limit the individual's options to adapt movement synergies to various objects and events.

Third Level of Integration: The Midbrain Level

Magnus (1926) showed that transection of the neuraxis at the level of the midbrain led to very different motor behavior in animals. The remaining nervous system evidenced normal distribution of tone and active righting reflexes. The animal could now "right" itself, that is, bring the head and body into alignment with respect to gravity by its own movements, and could maintain balance against disturbing influences. Although the animals that were studied (cats and dogs) could function nearly normally, humans need an intact CNS to adapt to changing circumstances and to form flexible chains of synaptic connections in response to various demands of the environment.

The Bobaths recognized five groups of righting reactions that Magnus had described:

Righting Reactions

The **Labyrinthine Righting Reaction** is stimulated by the labyrinths and produces orientation of the head in space to assume the "normal" position, with face vertical and mouth horizontal. This reaction occurs in infants from the second month onward and allows the head to maintain a normal position in space without the aid of vision.

The **Neck Righting Reaction** is stimulated by the proprioceptors in the neck and occurs in the newborn. If the head rotates, the entire body turns to align the body with the head. This reaction supports the infant's ability to turn from supine to sidelying.

Body Righting Reactions. It is impossible to separate the body righting reaction on the head from the body righting reaction on the body. These rotations of the body are evoked by asymmetrical stimulation of the sensory receptors on the surface of the body. Together they are responsible for the rotation between the pelvis and the shoulder girdle, and between the shoulder girdle and the head as the infant rolls over, gets to sitting, or moves into standing. If the infant is placed in supine and the shoulder girdle lifts from the surface when the arm moves or is brought across the body, the pelvis will follow, as will the head, bringing the child to the sidelying position. The same movement occurs if the head or pelvis rotates first. The end goal is to align the head with the body.

In the last quarter of the first year, children who are developing typically use these reactions linked with self-initiated actions to gain the sitting position from supine. As they try to sit up, they roll onto one arm, and the head follows with rotation and flexion, as do the pelvis and leg. These shifts in position allow the child to move into sitting.

Optical Righting Reaction. Researchers did not identify the optical righting reactions in the midbrain animal preparation because these reactions depended on the integrity of the optical cortex. These reactions are included here to complete the descriptions of all reactions of righting in children and adults. Through the optical righting reaction, the eyes contribute to postural orientation in space. A moving visual stimulus will produce rolling to the side or righting of the head in space in very young infants, movements that are considered part of the primary repertoire. Infants with typical development initially rely more heavily on the labyrinthine righting reactions than on visual righting, but over time visual righting becomes the dominant means of spatial orientation.

The Bobaths believed that the sequential appearance of the righting reactions during the course of typical development supported the infant's drive to changing postures (K. Bobath & B. Bobath, 1954, 1964). They hypothesized that these reactions were the foundation for the rotational component of normal transitions. Whether the first stimulus was head turning or pelvic or shoulder girdle turning, the other body parts and the head moved in a rotational manner in response to asymmetrical body contact, visual or labyrinthine stimulation. In addition, the Bobaths hypothesized that these reactions accounted for much of the similarity of motor patterns in different children at the same stage of their development. They believed that the absence of these reactions in clients with CNS dysfunction directly contributed to stereotypic movements by allowing the tonic reflexes to have a more dominant influence (i.e., the tonic reflexes are not inhibited by the presence of the righting reactions). Finally, because the patterns of rotation that resulted from these righting reactions originated at the third level of CNS integration, the Bobaths used these movements in treatment to inhibit the tonic reflexes associated with the second level of integration.

Protective Extension of the Arms. Schaltenbrand (1928), describing this reaction in children when the COM was displaced outside the BOS, referred to it as the "Sprungbereitschalt," or readiness to jump. He asserted that this reaction was similar to the movement and posture that an animal assumes as it jumps and safely lands at the end of a jump. Berta Bobath included this reaction in her thesis (1954) as a midbrain reaction but gave little significance to it. She described the reaction of extension and abduction of the arms with extension of the fingers when the child was quickly pushed forward from a kneeling position or held in space around the body and moved quickly downward. By the time she published this thesis as "Abnormal Postural Reflex Activity Caused by Brain Lesions" in 1965, Mrs. Bobath detailed the development of these reactions, first forward, then sideways, and finally backward in the child of typical development. She hypothesized that protective extension consisted of two phases, (a) the phasic extension of the arm, wrist, and fingers reaching for the support, and (b) tonic weight bearing on the supporting arm and hand to protect the face in case of sudden displacement of the body outside the BOS. She proposed that the purpose of these reactions was to protect against falling and to serve as a backup to equilibrium responses. The importance of these reactions became clearer to her as she realized that stiffness when walking or moving the body through space correlated with a fear of falling and lack of protective reactions rather than to the primary impairment of tone. Developing protective reactions of the arms gave clients a sense of security against falling and promoted greater confidence when attempting new movement.

Fourth Level of Integration: The Cortical Level

At this level of integration in the hierarchical model, the CNS acquired its most fundamental and important capacity, instantaneously adjusting to changing circumstances as demanded by the purpose of the movements and the environment. Movement synergies were initiated at will with specific goals in mind and manifested in infinite varieties depending on the purpose of the movement. Postural control and tone were perfected. The righting reactions were integrated with the equilibrium reactions resulting in perfect balance while moving within a posture and smooth transitions from one position to another. Weisz (1938) attributed the integration of automatic reactions that served the function of balance to the cortical level. He described a mechanism, which he called "equilibrium reactions," that was responsible for maintaining balance in standing and walking. The level of integration of these reactions was not known at this time, but he hypothesized that these reactions needed cortical control for their function because they were of a more complex nature than the righting reactions and occurred only when muscle tone was normal.

The Bobaths hypothesized that the equilibrium reactions were compensatory or reactive movements that occurred automatically, making balance possible when there was a change in the BOS or in the COM as movement occurs. These reactions allowed the body, head, and extremities to maintain alignment relative to gravity and to regain alignment when the body was displaced within the BOS. The stimulus that elicited the equilibrium reactions was a displacement of the body away from the COM but within the BOS. The reaction followed immediately, but first usually appeared in the trunk and head and then the extremities when the person reached the point where balance was severely threatened. The movements were an attempt to equilibrate the body mass around the COM with an equal and opposite reaction to the mass displaced. Clinicians could best evaluate these reactions if they induced the displacement gently, gradually increasing the speed and range of movement, keeping the displacement within the BOS (K. Bobath & B. Bobath, 1964).

The Bobaths linked the client's limitations in demonstrating equilibrium responses to abnormalities of tone, that is, the more abnormal the tone, the less developed and useful the equilibrium response. They also speculated that these reactions were the underlying postural basis for skilled movements and that the reactions must be present in any given developmental position for a child to function within that position. For example, a child must demonstrate equilibrium reactions in sitting before that child could move easily within sitting, turning, reaching, bending, and recovering.

The Bobaths tested equilibrium reactions by noting the reactions of clients following disturbance of their balance by displacement of the COM in sitting, kneeling, and standing (K. Bobath & B. Bobath, 1964). Although they described these same responses in supine and prone, they did not test these positions.

The reactions are as follows:

1. Displacement of the trunk forward of the COM causes a compensatory extensor movement of the head and trunk with adduction of the scapula and extension of the shoulders, elbows, and wrists. When an individual is sitting on a bench, this response can include hip and knee flexion as well. In standing, the response includes ankle plantar flexion.
2. Displacement of the trunk backward of the COM causes the head and trunk to flex, scapulae to abduct, shoulders to flex, and elbows and wrists to extend. When the individual is sitting on a bench, the knees extend; in standing, the ankles dorsiflex.
3. Lateral displacement of the trunk produces curvature of the head and trunk in the direction of the stimulus and abduction of the arm on the upward side with elbow and wrist extension. The arm on the downward side may horizontally adduct with elbow extension.

4. A displacement forward and to the side produces head, trunk, and shoulder rotation with extension toward the displacement. If the legs are free (as in sitting on a table), the pelvis also rotates and on the upward side, the hip extends and adducts.
5. Displacement backward and to the side results in head, trunk, and shoulder rotation with flexion. The rotation is toward the displacement, bringing the shoulder on the downward side forward of the shoulder on the upward side. The shoulders flex, the elbows extend. If the legs are free, the pelvis also rotates, and the hip and knee on the upward side flex and abduct.

In all positions, the movements of equilibrium are a compensation to the displacement of the COM. The Bobaths noted that in subjects of typical ability, these movements were brisk, immediate, and regulated in timing, speed, and direction exactly with the amount, speed, and direction of the displacement. These movements are constantly modified throughout the course of their execution to maintain equilibrium during active movement.

The hierarchical model of motor control first articulated by Jackson (1932/1958) and the reflex model of movement progression from Sherrington (1906, 1947) provided the framework for the neurophysiological basis of the Bobath Approach. Both Mrs. and Dr. Bobath encouraged others to seek additional answers to explain their rationale for treatment, but they never abandoned this model. It was the basis for additional theoretical concepts underlying the treatment rationale.

The Importance of Motor Development

The Bobaths believed that the motor milestones developed in a predictable sequence based on the maturation of the structures of the CNS. They held that motor behavior correlated to the hierarchical levels of the nervous system. Primitive reflexive movements of the neonate originated from the lower levels (spinal and brain stem) of the CNS. As the infant developed, deliberate, voluntary skills emerged from the newly maturing subcortical and cortical levels. Function could only follow development of structure, and changes in function depended primarily on structural changes in the CNS, which was the driving force for developmental changes.

The Bobaths based these concepts on maturational theories of motor development that were consistent with their model of hierarchical organization of the CNS. These concepts, predominately from Gesell et al. (1940) and McGraw (1945/1963), dominated the field of motor development in the 1940s and 1950s (Heriza, 1991). In addition, the Bobaths observed, as did Gesell et al., that there was a direction to development: control of movement developed from cephalic to caudal and from proximal to distal. Movement patterns of flexion and extension developed before rotation. Primitive and tonic reflexes were inhibited before righting and equilibrium reactions developed. Higher-level skills, such as walking, talking, and skilled use of the hands, depended on perfection of lower skills.

The progressive development of automatic postural reactions provided the foundation for skilled movements. For these reasons, the Bobaths initially wrote that it was important to teach control of movement by closely following the typical developmental sequence of motor behavior (B.

Bobath, 1953). They later discarded this concept as they observed that many skills develop at the same time because they have similar components (i.e., alignment, weight bearing, base of support, ROM, and movement combinations). This shift brought about a significant change in the applied therapeutic concepts, focusing on the importance of treating in many positions at the same time rather than following a sequence of motor milestones (K. Bobath & B. Bobath, 1984).

In addition, the Bobaths believed that observing and describing the quality of posture and movement, rather than the achievement of motor milestones, provided the means for recognizing differences between typical movement and movement pathology. Early on, the Bobaths focused on perfecting the quality of performance before moving on to higher developmental skills, but they soon recognized that if a child worked too long in one position, deformities could result because of the unequal development of various muscle groups. Mrs. Bobath (1967) used the example of a child who worked to perfect crawling (which demands activity of the hip flexors in their shortened range) and was not placed in standing to elongate the flexors and develop the hip extensors. This child would be at significant risk for developing hip flexor contractures.

Explanation of Tone in the Bobath Approach

According to Dr. Bobath, tone was a neurophysiological phenomenon that, under normal circumstances, served to regulate the degree of readiness of muscles to maintain posture against gravity and simultaneously adapt the tension of the muscles to alter posture for immediate execution of movement (K. Bobath & B. Bobath, 1952). The Bobaths accepted the findings from studies of decerebrate animals that hypertonus was abnormal activity of the gamma system released from cortical and subcortical inhibitory control that attempted to serve posture but at the expense of movement (K. Bobath, 1980). Sherrington (1913) found that the prepontine transection of the brainstem induced a state of exaggerated posture characterized by continuous contraction of the extensor skeletal muscles. He referred to this as a "caricature of standing" resulting from the interruption of projection fibers from higher centers. (Recall that he had found earlier that transection of the cervical cord produced only phasic extensor tone.) Magnus (1926) suggested that this state of sustained muscular contraction was significant in maintaining posture against gravity because the animal could support its body weight against gravity indefinitely, even though it was unable to maintain balance.

Mrs. Bobath found a comparable condition in clients with severe degrees of spasticity: they could support their body weight when put on their feet but were unable to maintain their balance (B. Bobath, 1985). This led Dr. Bobath to conclude that *spasticity was a state of exaggerated, abnormal distribution of postural tone and excessive co-contraction of antagonistic muscle groups expressed in atypical patterns of posture and movement* (K. Bobath, 1980). This was consistent with Mrs. Bobath's clinical observations and the findings of the animal research at that time. The Bobaths viewed tone on a continuum, from low to normal postural tone to hypertonus. *Spasticity* and *rigidity* were the terms they used to describe the most severe degree of abnormal tone. They did not discriminate between severe hypertonus and spasticity because they viewed the CNS as fully responsible for problems of tone rather than considering abnormal conditions of elasticity of the muscle fibers being responsible for this finding.

In her thesis (1965), Mrs. Bobath described three aspects of tone that were the early foundations for explaining the interconnection of tone and movement:

1. Tone was an ongoing physiological condition of readiness of the motor periphery to prepare for support and movement.
2. Tone was a condition of the entire neuromuscular apparatus, including the final spinal synapse and final common pathway.
3. Tone was related to muscle coordination and served to maintain posture and prepare movement.

This understanding of the correlation between tone and movement led the Bobaths to conclude that any case of neuropathology would demonstrate pathology of tone and of motor coordination, that these two neuromuscular phenomena were interrelated, and that the disorder was alterable and could be influenced by facilitating movements related to higher centers of control.

The importance of abnormal tone in clients with CNS dysfunction was not unique to the Bobath Approach (Payton, Hirt, & Newton, 1977; White, 1984). However, the Bobaths believed that of equal importance was the idea that spasticity showed itself in typical patterns involving all the affected parts, or even the whole body. They hypothesized that spasticity resulted from the release of abnormal postural reflexes (tonic or static reflexes). This was an important idea because it explained why a client could show abnormally strong extension in supine such that the individual could not dorsiflex the ankles or flex the head, trunk or knees, yet in prone, the same individual could not raise the head, fully extend the hips and knees, or plantar flex the feet due to extensive flexor tone. The Bobaths proposed that the release of a facilitory activity within the brainstem acting on the spinal gamma system not only produced spasticity but also resulted in the typical patterns of spasticity (B. Bobath, 1985). They wrote that spasticity was not permanently present in any one muscle group but shifted in predictable patterns as a result of changes of position of the body in space or alterations in the relative position of the head to body. Moreover, they contended that the distribution of the tone in a limb was dependent on the position of the proximal joint (K. Bobath & B. Bobath, 1950). This idea is an important aspect of the development of handling from **key points of control**.

Viewing tone as a CNS occurrence was a great change in thinking, given that hypertonus had been considered a muscle phenomenon due to an alteration of the elastic properties of the muscle fibers themselves. This concept was consistent with problems in skeletal muscles, either muscle contracture (which shortened the muscle fibers) or muscle weakness (which lengthened the fibers). Either of these situations produced a change of tone, but the idea that abnormal tone originated from muscle alone restricted the concept of tone to a more or less unalterable state given the permanent physical problem inherent in the muscle. The Bobaths, on the other hand, hypothesized that tone could be altered by influencing the higher inhibitory centers, presumably in the midbrain and cortex, which would *inhibit* the facilitory mechanism within the reticular formation of the brainstem. Without the normally functioning inhibitory mechanism, the facilitory function of the reticular formation enhanced the sensitivity of the gamma system. The gamma system became hyperexcitable and reacted to a normal stretch in a maximal manner, resulting in a synchronized total discharge of all anterior horn cells to a given muscle group, which produced hypertonus in those muscles.

> ***NDT Focus: NDT recognizes that both neural and musculoskeletal mechanisms contribute to abnormalities in muscle tone. Spasticity is only one factor that causes the abnormalities in muscle and postural tone in individuals with CNS pathology.***

Neural Inhibition

The Bobaths recognized that inhibition was an active CNS process and, in accordance with the hierarchical model, they asserted that the higher levels of the CNS (midbrain and cortex) had the capacity to inhibit unnecessary direction, force, and timing of the primary muscles, their synergists, and antagonists so that which remained was the precise movement needed for the task of the moment and nothing more (B. Bobath, 1990; K. Bobath & B. Bobath, 1954). The Bobaths wrote that inhibition was both a positive and negative force in movement control. Following the studies of Sherrington (1913), they agreed that inhibition was present at every level of the CNS, from spinal reciprocal inhibition (which produced mass synergies of flexion or extension) to the cerebral cortex (which drove the inhibitory reticular formation). They believed that the balance of inhibition and excitation during a movement controlled the speed, range, and direction of selective and graded movements for function (Mayston, 1992).

They also hypothesized that *lack* of neural inhibition explained the presence of abnormal tone and abnormal movement. They believed that the lack of inhibition by the cerebral cortex to the reticular formation allowed increased gamma motor activity on the final common pathway and abnormally high tone. They viewed abnormal movement patterns as a lack of inhibition from the higher levels of integration (midbrain and cortex), allowing the tonic reflex patterns of the subthalamic and spinal levels to dominate. The importance of neural inhibition formed the basis for many of their early treatment methods which began with **reflex-inhibiting postures** and **reflex-inhibiting patterns.**

Release Phenomena

The concept of release phenomena parallels the concept of neural inhibition. The Bobaths wrote that the mass patterns of abnormal coordination in individuals with CNS dysfunction occurred because of the release of lower (reflex), more primitive movement patterns from higher control of the brain. Current theory describes both "positive" and "negative" impairments in CNS pathology. Negative signs manifest themselves in the absence of function, such as weakness or loss of movement. Dr. Bobath placed more importance on the "positive" signs, which were produced by the hyperactivity of those lower level parts of the CNS that had lost the controlling influence (because of injury) of higher-level structures in the CNS.

He referred to these impairments as "release symptoms." The patterns of released reflex activity were those of the spinal and midbrain (tonic) reflexes that limited the coordination of the muscles of the limbs to synergies of inter- and intra-limb flexion or extension. The tonic postural reflexes produced sustained tonic contractions of the antigravity muscles, which caused stiffness in the individual and prevented movement. The Bobaths did acknowledge paucity of movement and apparent weakness, but considered these to be secondary to the presence of hypertonus and excessive co-contraction (K. Bobath & B. Bobath, 1956).

Automatic Basis of Movement

The Bobaths described a series of automatic (reflex) movements arranged in a hierarchy of complexity and which, in normal conditions, explained the synergies or muscle sets common in human behavior. They hypothesized that the CNS utilized the lower centers of the CNS (the brain stem, cerebellum, and basal ganglia) with their older, more primitive patterns of coordination, to provide an automatic base for maintenance of posture and equilibrium. Consistent with the peripheralist view of Sherrington (1906, 1947), they held that these automatic patterns were linked initially to specific sensory stimuli but that with repetitive use, these automatic patterns provided the fundamental temporal and spatial coordination of muscle activation such that the higher centers executed the precision demanded by the moment. The Bobaths' contention that reflexes formed the base for voluntary movements was supported by the maturationist theories of McGraw (1945/1963) and Gesell et al. (1940). These investigators maintained, as did the Bobaths, that primitive and developmental reflexes were the building blocks of complex skills. The Bobaths believed that these primitive and tonic reflexes contained many of the primary movement synergies that helped very young infants to initiate and sustain posture and movement as they learned to meet postural requirements in the postnatal environment. The normally occurring, genetically determined maturation of the nervous system inhibited these early reflexes so that children developed righting and equilibrium reactions to support self-initiated, task-oriented movements.

Although the Bobaths' treatment focused on inhibition of these reflexes that, in their view, persisted and produced functional limitations, it appeared that at least some "reflex" behaviors were useful and unique in this early developmental phase and could be called upon to enhance movement performance if certain contextual elements were present to trigger or sustain them (without peripheral sensory initiation). Early practitioners believed that reflexes assisted overall motor action when increased force or speed was required (Easton, 1972; Fukuda, 1961). Fukuda illustrated the presence of these movement patterns in sports and dance. The inclusion of the contextual element helped to explain why a reflex pattern occurred, or why one reflex overrode another in given circumstances. While not obligatory, these patterns might be preferred in certain contexts. This view broadened the concept of developmental and tonic reflexes first described by the Bobaths and offered an explanation for the presence of these movement patterns in children and adults of typical ability, as well as in individuals with CNS pathology. The Bobaths asserted that persistent tonic reflexes were particularly problematic for clients with CNS pathology and that these reflexes were responsible for many of the stereotypic movements in children with CP and adults following stroke (B. Bobath, 1954, 1977).

NDT Focus: NDT currently accepts that all movement synergies are examples of coordinative structures constraining the number of independent parts to reduce the complexity of motor control that must be adapted to the functional requirements of the individual.

The Bobaths held the view that major portions of motor actions (including righting and equilibrium reactions) that produced complex postural and movements plans were recruited automatically "not because of a hypothetical memory center, but because of the firmly established chains of synaptic connections" (K. Bobath & B. Bobath, 1972, p. 119). They maintained, based on Ritchie-Russell's work (1958), that if, in the past, a certain response had followed a given experience, there would be every likelihood that the same stimulus would continue to evoke the same response in the future. They offered this reflex/hierarchical model as a solution to the problem of how the CNS could control the multitude of possible combinations of muscles and joints in the constantly changing demands of movement coordination.

The Bobaths believed that the person of typical ability made use of the large store of automatic righting and equilibrium movement patterns gained in early infancy and childhood. They proposed that these automatic movements developed in a definite sequence from birth onwards and that their appearance coincided with the recognized milestones (K. Bobath & B. Bobath, 1956). They further postulated that skilled movement depended on the presence and orderly development of automatic righting and equilibrium reactions. Without this foundation, the highly skilled movements needed for speech, manipulation, balance, and movement of the body through space would not be available and execution would be inefficient and energy-consuming.

The Bobaths also hypothesized that all adults exhibited a sameness of posture and movement as they changed position, reacted to disturbances in balance and gait, and protected against falling, because each individual relied on the same set of automatic protective, righting, and equilibrium reactions, which were available under stress or emergency. For example, to brace against a fall, an individual would spontaneously extend an arm due to the persistent protective extension reaction, land with wrist extended, and end up with the typical "Colles' fracture." Whereas this is the typical response to a sudden perturbation, an individual with a normal CNS can overcome this automatic tendency, as evidenced by football players who must hold onto the football when tackled. However, the protective extension reaction is so strong that to overcome this tendency takes repeated practice.

The Bobaths further hypothesized, supported by Schaltenbrand's (1928) findings, that in individuals with a CNS lesion, retention of these primitive, automatic movement patterns contributed to hypertonus. The abnormal tone inhibited the movements of higher organization so that the higher centers did not develop the variability and selectivity in movement combinations that gave the individual more options for movement execution (B. Bobath, 1953). The person was left with the dominance of primitive reflex patterns that were stereotyped and widespread and involved the whole body in predictable synergies of muscle action. As a result, children and adults with CNS dysfunction demonstrated stereotypic motor behavior, exhibiting similar atypical, limited postures and movement. The repetition of the automatic patterns regulated and determined the individual's activities and interfered with the development of selective, refined movement. As an example, the Bobaths described a client who showed the influence of the tonic labyrinthine reflex as he attempted to sit. The individual would exhibit excessive extensor muscle activity, insufficient hip flexion, and compensatory, excessive thoracic and cervical flexion. He could not maintain balance in sitting, which directly affected skilled hand use. An ATNR that dominated posture when his head was turned, interfered with visual contact and maintenance of grasp when bringing his hand, and objects in it, toward his body (K. Bobath & B. Bobath, 1955).

Plasticity

The first observation Mrs. Bobath made (see Observation 1) was that she could modify the muscle tone in the arm of a man with hemiplegia. She assumed, based on changes in this client's function, that even in the adult brain, modification was possible to the extent that it could lead to at least some recovery of function. This was a very exciting and controversial idea in the 1940s, given that the leading models of motor behavior–the reflex/hierarchical model of Sherrington and Jackson and the neuro-maturational model of Gesell and McGraw–supported the concept that function of the CNS depended on maturation of the structures (Van Sant, 1993). Loss of structure, as a result of lesions in the CNS, produced loss of function. The belief that the CNS was unalterable encouraged clients to make the best use of their remaining function by compensating with less-affected parts (K. Bobath, 1980; Craik, 1991). Dr. Bobath later wrote, "The outstanding quality of the higher CNS activity is its plasticity, its ability to learn and perhaps one should also add the 'gift of forgetting,' the ability of forming temporary and constantly changing chains of synaptic connections in response to the many and various demands of the environment" (K. Bobath, 1980, p. 81).

The Bobaths believed that this concept of plasticity supported their treatment methods of "facilitating" patterns of movement that they wanted the CNS to "learn" while at the same time "inhibiting" those patterns that they wanted the CNS to "forget." The Bobath Approach did not allow the client to use abnormal motor patterns for function and did not accept splinting and bracing as methods of preventing deformities. Dr. Bobath used the findings of Ritchie-Russell to support his ideas. Ritchie-Russell (1958) wrote that although there was evidence of a neural mechanism that favored repetition, this same mechanism was extremely sensitive to afferent influences. The neuronal pool could be influenced to make new responses that, if repeated, could take priority over earlier well-established patterns. Dr. Bobath maintained that this change was even more likely if the newly facilitated responses belonged to phylogenetically inherent patterns, such as the righting and equilibrium reactions. Applied in treatment, the concept of neural plasticity suggested that it was possible to establish synaptic bonds of higher-level postural reactions. Once the higher postural reactions were firmly established, treatment could progress to linking patterns of normal movements to this automatic postural component, producing efficient broad global maps, currently hypothesized by Edelman (Hadders-Algra, 2000).

The concept of plasticity also formed the basis for early intervention with children and adults. The Bobaths contended that it was very difficult to eradicate long standing, abnormal patterns because the CNS had a strong tendency to strengthen arrangements that have been repeated frequently. Because it was impossible to prevent older children or adults with long-standing dysfunction from using the compensatory strategies they had achieved, normal or not, the Bobaths considered these strongly linked "habit patterns" to be a powerful feature of the CNS and extremely resistant to change.

Principle of Shunting

Shunting, according to the Bobaths, explained the efficacy of reflex-inhibiting postures as a treatment method. Dr. Bobath took the information from Sherrington's (1906) studies on spinal frogs and Magnus's (1926) work on spinal cats. Each found that the same stimulus applied to the same place could produce directly opposite reflex responses, depending on the position of the animal (and muscles). Analyzing these observations, Magnus found that the afferent inflow favored the contraction of the elongated muscles, leaving the shortened muscles in a state of inhibition. From this, Magnus formulated the "Law of Shunting," which proposed that at any moment, the CNS mirrored the state of the body musculature. In other words, the state of contraction and elongation of the muscles determined the distribution of excitatory and inhibitory processes within the nervous system and the subsequent outflow of excitation to the periphery (K. Bobath, 1980; Magnus, 1926). In addition, Magnus also found that the greatest determinant of shunting was the position of the proximal joints of the body, spine, shoulder, and hips. The Bobaths viewed this law of shunting as strong support for the ability to influence the state of the CNS from the periphery. They developed techniques of handling clients from proximal joints, which they called **key points of control,** as ways of directly influencing the output of the nervous systems. They maintained that, by changing the position of the limb, particularly the proximal joints, they could stop the outflow of excitation into undesirable channels of muscular activity and direct the excitatory and inhibitory processes into new synaptic chains of normal muscular activity reflected in appropriate levels of reciprocal innervation (K. Bobath, 1959a; K. Bobath & B. Bobath, 1950).

Postural Reflex Mechanism

The Bobaths asserted that posture consisted of subtle automatic fluctuations of muscle tone and compensatory movements in response to perturbations (K. Bobath & B. Bobath, 1964). They proposed a theoretical, highly complex neural mechanism that they called the "postural reflex mechanism" to explain the constantly changing tone and automatic activation of coordination patterns necessary for conducting any skilled activity while maintaining balance. From the 1960s onward, they presented this mechanism as a viable scheme to explain the interrelationship between posture and movement. They proposed that the postural reflex mechanism consisted of three components that must always be expressed together:

1. **Normal postural tone:** For the purposes of postural and movement control, muscles are activated in patterns in which single muscles lost their identity (hence

the term "postural tone" rather than "muscle tone"). The adaptations of tone in anticipation of change in posture and during the movement involve the total body musculature and occur automatically to respond to the constant need to maintain or change balance at any give moment.

2. **Multiple degrees of reciprocal innervation:** Reciprocal innervation results in (a) co-contraction of agonists and antagonists, especially around proximal parts of the body (such as hips and shoulders) for stability prior to movement, (b) rapid reciprocal movement for selective, highly fractionated movements to respond to perturbations in the most efficient way, and (c) precise degrees of action of agonists, antagonists, and synergists to provide power and strength to stabilize posture while simultaneously allowing accurate, coordinated movement, both directed toward the intended functional goal.

3. **Normal automatic patterns of postural control, which were the common heritage of humans:** Children display common patterns as they develop movements for turning over, sitting up, standing, and walking due to the systematic development of the righting and equilibrium reactions during maturation in infancy. All persons exhibit a similarity in the expression of defense under stress because of the development of the protective extension reaction against falling or the flexor withdrawal reflex from pain. Once upright, individuals display a similarity of posture (head vertical, "normal" alignment of the trunk and limbs) and movement (which uniquely involves rotation within the body axis due to the righting reactions). With the development of the equilibrium reactions, small, invisible, compensatory shifts of tone or noticeable countermovements restore disturbed balance. Finally, recognizable facial gesture and body language automatically communicates such concepts as cold, hot, tired, excited, and afraid, in nearly every culture.

The Bobaths contended that posture and movement are inseparable, and that analysis of the normal reflex mechanism or any deviation in it is particularly valuable in early recognition, examination, and treatment of individuals with CNS dysfunction (K. Bobath, 1971a). Focusing on these automatic components of posture and movement made it possible to examine and treat very young babies and individuals who could not cooperate or perform when given verbal directions. The Bobaths also held that, because normal coordination requires development of all three components, damage to any one component alters all aspects of posture and movement, resulting in abnormal degrees of tone, abnormal reciprocal innervation, and abnormal automatic patterns of muscular coordination that negatively affect execution of functional skills.

Sensorimotor Connections

The Bobaths asserted that motor output occurred in response to various types of sensory input but that, in addition, movement was a powerful stimulus for excitation of the sensory subsystems. Movement was initiated by the exteroceptors (eyes, ears, and touch) and was guided by the proprioceptors of the muscles, tendons, joints, and labyrinths. A child or adult would move and, in moving, activate feedback through the various sensory receptors, which would provide the brain with the correct sense of position, range, timing, and direction of movement (B. Bobath, 1953). The normal nervous system had the ability to absorb a large quantity of this afferent inflow and reacted to it with a unitary response that was variable and adaptable to changing demands. (K. Bobath, 1959a). The resultant motor response provided feedback to the proprioceptors and exteroceptors that then corrected any discrepancy between the intended movement and the actual movement. The Bobaths considered this sensory feedback to play a major role in the acquisition and regulation of existing movements and the creation of new movement combinations (Bly, 1996). Repetition caused motor performance to be quicker and more automatic, and to require less effort by the individual (B. Bobath, 1975). This sensory-motor-sensory feedback paradigm was based on Sherrington's reflex theory of motor control (1906, 1947).

CNS dysfunction interrupted this normal sensorimotor connection. The Bobaths theorized that the CNS of the child with CP or the adult with stroke was less competent to deal with the afferent inflow. They did not believe that the injury consisted of a primary impairment in the sensory systems but rather that a lesion in the CNS resulted in limited, stereotyped reflex movements. The CNS could respond to any sensory input only through the existing patterns of abnormal reflex activity. These abnormal reflexes formed the primary motor patterns that, with their feedback through the exteroceptors and somatoreceptors, provided abnormal sensory input to the CNS and produced additional abnormal motor output (B. Bobath & Finnie, 1958). With continued use, this dysfunctional cycle reinforced only abnormal motor patterns. If this disordered process was not interrupted, what was abnormal would simply become more so. This concept was the basis for many of the Bobaths' therapeutic methods that prevented clients from using (and thereby reinforcing) their abnormal movement patterns while facilitating the pattern of movement that would drive normal sensory input.

These concepts, described within the reflex/hierarchical model of motor control, comprised the theoretical basis of the Bobath Approach. The Bobaths placed great emphasis on the importance of various neural components of movement and the central influences when describing normal and abnormal posture and movement. Mrs. Bobath developed her clinical concepts directly from her clinical observations. However, changes in her treatment methods during the many years she taught and treated came about not only from her own observations and feedback from her clients but from the theoretical evidence that Dr. Bobath provided to support her findings. Clinical assumptions and theoretical foundations developed simultaneously and became the basis for clinical practice.

What Principles of Clinical Practice Were Supported by this Theory?

The goal of all Bobath treatment strategies was to help the client produce active, automatic adaptations in response to the therapist's handling. The Bobaths believed that in this way they could reduce, increase, or stabilize tone and regulate the coordination of agonists, antagonists, and synergists to improve function. Through handling, the therapist could inhibit ineffective movements and atypical postural patterns and facilitate automatic and voluntary movement. In addition, the Bobaths believed that active response to being moved imitated the development and learning of movement in infants who were developing typically (K. Bobath & B. Bobath, 1964).

Treat the Whole Person

CP or stroke affects the entire individual in life roles. All of the problems–posture, movement, communication, hearing, vision, perception, and socializing–are related (B. Bobath, 1971, 1977). As early as 1958, the Bobaths stated, "In considering these problems, one must remember that one deals with a . . . total personality with special needs, emotional, intellectual and social. An evaluation . . . requires the study of his place in the family as well as the . . . extent and quality of his physical handicap, both sensory and motor" (K. Bobath & B. Bobath, 1958, p. 19). The Bobaths believed that physical development and motor performance had a direct bearing on mental development and success in educational programs (B. Bobath, 1975). This relationship between movement and general development began as the infant adapted to the movements of the mother's handling for nursing, comforting, and general care. The interrelationship continued as the child moved the body and hands and discovered him- or herself and then the surroundings, seeking novelty and experimenting all the while. This early learning through movement gradually affected perceptual and visual-motor development, speech and language, and even the child's emotional and social development. The link between motor development and mental abilities further developed as the child became independent through the ability to move, satisfying his or her curiosity and solving problems.

In describing the adult with stroke, Mrs. Bobath (1977) also stressed that the sudden changes in sensation and movement caused confusion, disorientation, and fear, as well as direct confrontation of a physical disability. She emphasized that, for treatment to be effective, everyone concerned with the client's program–family, teachers, and therapists–must provide opportunities for treatment in daily life situations (B. Bobath, 1977). This basic clinical concept continues today.

NDT Focus: Beginning with the teachings of Mrs. Bobath, NDT emphasizes the individual as a whole person with competencies and limitations. The current enablement model addresses these competencies and limitations in Body, Motor, Individual, and Social Dimensions.

Examination Process

Mrs. Bobath stated, "The assessment should enable the therapist to make a systematic treatment plan related to the individual patient's main difficulties and needs" (B. Bobath, 1977, p. 313). She wrote and taught that clinicians must not regard examination and treatment as separate entities. She often said that each treatment should be an evaluation of what works and what does not. She also stated, that systematic treatment could not be done without a general examination of the individual client that would allow for comparisons at future times. The actual examination changed over time, reflecting the changes in treatment methods, but the process continued to focus on what the client could or could not do, the quality and effectiveness of posture and movement, and the potential for change (B. Bobath, 1990; K. Bobath & B. Bobath, 1958; Mayston, 1992). Mrs. Bobath listed the components of examination for children with CP (K. Bobath & B. Bobath, 1979):

1. Observe the child and mother (or other family members accompanying the child). What expectations does the parent have for the child? The child for the parent? Is the relationship supportive, caring, overprotective, fearful, impatient?
2. Observe the child's functions, beginning as the child comes in for the examination–how the child walks, interacts with family and assessor, talks, and plays. Ask yourself why the child functions this way.
3. Start at the functional level, then hypothesize reasons for the child's limitations.
4. Observe first the child's abilities, then the limitations.
5. Observe the quality and effectiveness of the child's posture and movement.
6. Observe the child's balance and ability to regain balance.
7. Investigate the child's potential. Encourage the child to stand up if sitting, walk if crawling, and use hands alternately if using both together. Find out what additional skills the child can do with physical assistance, and compare that to what the child can do when unassisted.
8. Put your hands on the child to find out how he or she reacts to being moved and how posture, tone, and movement change, for either better or worse.
9. Determine how various levels and combinations of sensory stimuli affect posture, movement, tone, and function.
10. Feel the tone and changes in tone as the child moves or is moved.
11. Observe the child's movements in as many positions as possible and how he or she makes transitions between one position and another.
12. Decide on the main functional limitations and the possible causes for these limitations. Always ask "Why?"
13. Decide on the aims of treatment, what to inhibit or facilitate to improve movement needed for function.

Mrs. Bobath's guidelines for examination of adults with hemiplegia included many of these same ideas, beginning with observing the client with the family (B. Bobath, 1977, 1990). She began with a general examination of the status of the individual that included the person's state of health (including mental and emotional state), understanding and expression of language which are areas of particular concern for adults who have had a stroke. Specific problem areas for the person with stroke (that were not part of her CP examination) included:

1. Loss of memory of former movement patterns
2. Sensory deficits and their impact on posture and movement, particularly their effect on the upper-extremity functions
3. Compensation with the less involved side
4. Pain and edema
5. Cardiopulmonary status
6. Energy and endurance for physical activity and intervention

The examination was a narrative description that left much to the individual therapist, his or her level of skill, and the therapist's interpretation of movement disorders. Although this method of examination was useful for planning treatment and noting changes for an individual client, evaluation or comparison of treatment outcomes in groups of clients was impossible.

Early Intervention

The Bobaths asserted that early identification and treatment was important for individuals with CP or stroke. They believed that normal movement started with normal perception of movement. The longer a client attempted to move with abnormal tone, posture and abnormal patterns of movement and perceived this as "normal," the more ingrained these patterns became and the harder they were to change. On the other hand, the Bobaths also believed in the adaptability and plasticity of the brain and asserted that it was important to capitalize on this capacity for change. They recognized that the problems of tone and movement were affected by effort against the force of gravity. Treating clients with stroke and children with CP before they tried to move and function in the upright position had greater potential for producing normal movement sequences, and there were no "bad habits" to overcome (B. Bobath, 1960a, 1960b, 1967).

Motor Development in Treatment

Motor development in treatment was another clinical concept that changed as the Bobaths developed their approach. Initially, the Bobaths used as their framework for treatment the development of motor milestones described by Gesell and McGraw in infants who were developing typically (B. Bobath & Finnie, 1958). Their commitment to the sequence of motor milestones as the organizing principle for intervention was so strong that in 1952, they stated that deformities often developed because a child was treated in standing and walking before treatment had prepared the child for this stage of motor skill. Borrowing from normal development, the Bobaths wrote that it was important to teach control over movement in the proper sequence (K. Bobath & B. Bobath, 1952). Originally, they taught that the therapist needed to guide adults through the motor milestone sequence so that they could relearn control of posture and movement in the same way that children did (Bly, 1991).

As the Bobaths acquired more experience with babies and infants and their treatment methods evolved, they realized that using the sequence of motor milestones as a framework was not appropriate and they discarded the concept. They benefited from the work of Milani-Comparetti (1967), who described the importance of competition among motor patterns as infants developed. They recognized that children developed many different motor skills simultaneously, practicing a large variety of combinations of postures and movements against the force of gravity, given different goals for these movements. The Bobaths found that every new activity built on previous sensorimotor experiences, which were gradually elaborated and modified for new purposes.

By the 1960s, the Bobaths' writing described the development of basic motor patterns and the acquisition and gradual perfection of the postural reflex mechanism as the basis for motor development (B. Bobath, 1967; K. Bobath & B. Bobath, 1967). They believed that posture and movement developed in overlapping patterns that made possible the complex functional skills referred to as motor milestones. They realized that it was not necessary, in fact in some situations was harmful, to perfect one motor milestone before continuing to the next. Rather, it was more useful to facilitate the basic motor patterns that the child or adult could use for an entire group of functional activities. The process by which posture and movement developed, and **not** the development of motor milestones, became and remains the "developmental framework" in the Bobath Approach and in NDT intervention.

Functional Carryover and Home Programs

In 1956, in an article on motor function in CP, the Bobaths concluded with, "The fundamental automatic movement patterns which the patient acquires in treatment can then be used by him for voluntary skilled movements" (K. Bobath & B. Bobath, 1956, p. 303). At this point in time, they maintained that the strength of their treatment was successful inhibition of abnormal tone and facilitation of normal movement. The successful development of automatic movement patterns alone, would allow the client to develop normal functional movements. As their approach evolved, the Bobaths realized that preparing normal movement by developing the automatic components was not sufficient, and they included systematic preparation for specific functions as part of treatment. In 1977, writing about adult hemiplegia, Mrs. Bobath stated,

> It cannot be expected that a reduction of spasticity and the activation of certain muscle groups during treatment . . . will lead directly to more normal use of arm and hand or an improved gait. Even if the muscles can function well in such "developmental" exercises, it will be impossible for the patient to carry over the obtained movement patterns into the activities of daily life, or use the newly acquired but not established movements in different functional situations. Everything done in treatment, therefore, should serve as a *direct* preparation for specific functional use. The sequences of movement chosen for such preparation should be as similar as possible to those movements needed in daily life. This means the . . . therapist should treat the patient in situations of daily life. (B. Bobath, 1977, p. 312)

Mrs. Bobath recounted that what she did in these functional situations was actually what she had always done–using inhibition and facilitation to elicit the most normal posture and movement possible–but she did this now in situations that as nearly as possible matched the client's life at home, in the community, or at school (K. Bobath & B. Bobath, 1979).

The Bobaths (K. Bobath, 1960) further asserted that the role of families and teachers of children with CP was to provide opportunities for the children to practice those postures and movements that they did fairly normally, to make them as independent as possible and take advantage of their readiness and initiative for advanced activities. Because of these beliefs, Mrs. Bobath stressed that mothers and, as often as possible, fathers must be an active part of each therapy session. The therapist must make time to explain what is being done and why, because only in this way would the family be able to adapt the goals to the home setting (K. Bobath & B. Bobath, 1968).

NDT Focus: NDT has taken the clinical concept of functional carryover even further, using information on motor learning combined with information on motor control to directly address functional limitations by including practice of the specific parts and entire functions in simulated or real-life settings as an active part of the treatment approach.

Treatment Strategies

It is important to note that the Bobaths worked initially with older children with severe degrees of CP who had not been treated successfully with other methods, and with adults with long-standing symptoms of stroke. The most obvious problems the Bobaths saw were hypertonus and clients' inability to move actively and purposefully. It was a logical step to draw a causal relationship between these two characteristics and, as a result, they first focused their primary treatment strategy on inhibiting tone as a means to gain movement.

Reflex-Inhibiting Postures

Mrs. Bobath felt that clients could not, by their own effort or even when directed and prompted verbally, overcome the abnormal tone or influence of abnormal postures and movement as they attempted functional activities. Based on her understanding of the "law of shunting," she developed a special type of handling and manipulation to break through the abnormal motor patterns (B. Bobath, 1948b). The client was placed in postures that were roughly the opposite of those the person assumed when sitting, standing, or lying on the back or stomach. These postures, which inhibited the abnormal tone normally exhibited by the client, she called "reflex-inhibiting postures." She described reflex-inhibiting postures not as static postures, but as parts of a movement (K. Bobath, 1953). The therapist selected a position and controlled the client's posture so that the muscles could adjust to normal tension. As the person learned to tolerate the reflex-inhibiting posture, he or she would learn to move from one posture to another without the interference from abnormal stiffness or movement.

Early in the development of the Bobath Approach, the Bobaths wrote, "Once the patient learns to tolerate and take up a group of reflex-inhibiting postures, he will only have to connect them by moving from one posture to the next in order to perform the whole movement in a normal way" (K. Bobath, 1953, p. 5). They later found that the early reflex-inhibiting postures reduced spasticity by changing its patterns, but they acknowledged that the problem of producing active movement for these individuals was more complicated. Passive positioning in reflex-inhibiting postures did change tone but did not carry over into movement and function (K. Bobath & B. Bobath, 1984).

Reflex-Inhibiting Patterns

The next step beyond reflex-inhibiting postures was to develop reflex-inhibiting patterns. Dr. Bobath wrote, "For functional activity both the spastic extension patterns *and* the total flexion patterns have to be modified and elements of one pattern must be combined with elements of the other. . . . For the purpose of combining elements of both total patterns, various 'reflex-inhibiting patterns' have been devised" (K. Bobath, 1980, p. 84).

Reflex-inhibiting patterns evolved as Mrs. Bobath realized the importance of using active movement to reduce tone and improve function. This method combined elements of the total reflex-inhibiting postures and handling the client in such a way as to use only parts of the total reflex-inhibiting posture, which would lead more quickly to function. The Bobaths called these patterns of inhibition *reflex-inhibiting patterns*, to focus on movement rather than the static postures. This change in treatment came about gradually but reflected a shift in the responsibility for movement between the therapist and the client. The therapist had to become more sensitive to controlling only those elements of the abnormal posture that needed to be controlled and at the same time allow the client active adaptations to these reflex-inhibiting movements. Inhibition was now used only to limit the client's atypical postures and movements that were preventing more selective muscle activation. The therapist needed to discover at what point during movement the client might begin to react abnormally, then prevent the hypertonus with its abnormal patterns from asserting itself. This point in a movement execution, different for every individual and often different for the same client on different days, gave the client the possibility of developing his or her own active control over the abnormal movements. Dr. Bobath wrote, "These reflex-inhibiting patterns must not be looked upon as static postures, but as phases of movement away from the total patterns. . . These patterns by themselves achieve nothing; the child will learn nothing from being moved passively. What is of decisive importance is his reaction to these movements away from his established pathological patterns and his active adaptation" (K. Bobath, 1980, p. 85).

Mrs. Bobath presented five considerations for the therapist to keep in mind when using reflex-inhibiting patterns (K. Bobath & B. Bobath, 1972):

1. The aim was to reduce hypertonus, spasticity, rigidity, or intermittent increases of postural tone.
2. The patterns were introduced gradually, beginning proximally from the head, shoulder girdle, spine, or pelvis.
3. Handling must not start at the place on the body where hypertonus was strongest and most obvious.

4. The goal was for clients to gain their own control of abnormal postural reactions so that they could attain independence from therapists' control.
5. It was important to give clients a great variety of postural patterns and to use similar combinations in different positions at certain stages of treatment.

More changes were yet to come. At this stage in the development of the Bobath Approach, the therapist still controlled treatment, initiating and directing movement by maintaining physical control of the client, and the focus was still on controlling tone and reflex movement.

Key Points of Control

The concept of key points of control was and remains a critical treatment strategy in NDT. Other therapeutic approaches use physical handling of clients to encourage movement, but facilitation from specific points on the body began with Mrs. Bobath and remains unique in NDT. Mrs. Bobath developed this concept as she changed the method of applying reflex-inhibiting postures. She observed that, often, the less severely involved clients (and, at some points, severely involved individuals as well) did not need total control to inhibit their tone or control movement, and that she could influence tone in the distal muscles by controlling the tone in the muscles of the proximal joints.

This concept, modifying the tone in distal muscles by controlling the tone of the proximal muscles, was supported by Dr. Bobath's interpretation of Magnus's research. Because the abnormal postural reflexes (tonic neck and labyrinthine reflexes) originated from the head and neck, clinicians could control the strength and distribution of the abnormal muscle tone of the extremities most successfully from these locations (K. Bobath & B. Bobath, 1964, 1972). Changing the client's position from these key points inhibited abnormal postural movement patterns while maintaining the person's freedom to move the limbs. Handling from key points on the body permitted the therapist to use the techniques of inhibition and facilitation simultaneously, retaining control from the key points and preventing deterioration of movement and any increase in tone. All the while, the client had much more freedom for active movement. The therapist had to be aware that active movement could not take place at or near the point on the body at which the person was held or supported, and that the best active reactions took place in muscles and joints distal from the key point of control.

The therapist places his or her hands purposefully and specifically on the client's body to produce changes in alignment before a movement sequence, or to control the speed, direction, or effort the client uses during a movement. The therapist can position his or her hands on muscles to monitor the speed, timing, or direction of an ongoing movement execution, or across a joint to gain alignment, initiate a weight shift, or stabilize that body part. The therapist must plan and monitor the location of his or her hands on the client and the amount of pressure used on the joint or muscle group to prevent distracting tactile or somatosensory stimulation in order to direct the client's attention and movement toward the action. To obtain sequences of active automatic movements with the desired parts of the body leading the appropriate movement pattern, the clinician must select the key points of control carefully and change them constantly during treatment as the client adapts his or her response to this input (Manning, 1972). Each hand can shift from one key point to another several times during a long movement sequence as the therapist senses the best way to assist the client's posture and movement.

Therapists choose proximal or distal key points of control depending on the goal of handling. Proximal key points are the trunk and spine with its connections to the head, shoulder girdle, and pelvic girdle. Handling from proximal key points has a strong influence on introducing the patterns of rotation that play an important role in all human movement. Proximal key points give the therapist much stronger control and are often useful when new movement patterns are being introduced or combined in new activities. Distal key points are parts of a limb: elbows, knees, hands, and feet. Control from distal key points allows movement of the trunk and head for righting, balance, and precise, selective grading of the proximal parts of the body. Because of the overlap in the effects of proximal and distal key points on movement, the clinician can interchange and combine them, making adjustments according to the client's reactions. The therapist can control movement sequences by changing key points as the client moves, according to which patterns are to be inhibited or facilitated during the movement. Obviously, no one key point is responsible for, or will be effective in, obtaining whole sequences of movements.

Facilitation of Automatic Movement

In the early 1950s, treatment consisted primarily of inhibition *followed* by facilitation. As the Bobaths realized that the reflex-inhibiting postures created only the precondition for the use of facilitation, the emphasis and application of these methods changed. They wrote, "The permanent reduction and stabilization of muscle tone depends on the degree to which the normal postural reflex mechanism and normal sequences of movement can be developed by techniques of facilitation. A permanent carryover of treatment into activities of daily life will depend . . . on the extent to which active normal sequences of movement can be facilitated and their patterns firmly established" (K. Bobath & B. Bobath, 1964, p. 7). In any individual case, inhibition of abnormal reflex activity and facilitation of movement could follow each other or be used alternately or simultaneously, but the important factor was that the client be given a chance to move actively. With this change, treatment became more dynamic.

The Bobaths defined facilitation as "techniques of obtaining inherent automatic movement patterns in response to handling, in contrast to movements performed at request" (K. Bobath & B. Bobath, 1964, p. 250). With facilitation techniques, therapists can obtain active movement through the automatic component of any movement available to the client. Because the Bobaths believed that stress or excessive effort increased tone (which inhibited normal movement), facilitation of righting and equilibrium reactions afforded a means by which, without excessive effort, the client could produce entire sequences of movement (such as rolling over, sitting up, standing up, and even walking). Righting reactions provide the ability to initiate activity against gravity and utilize the patterns of rotation within the body axis, two components that are fundamental to every human activity. Equilibrium reactions contain the postural sets and relationships among antagonists, agonists, and synergists that produce countermovements to maintain or restore balance (K. Bobath, 1970). Therefore, facilitation of these automatic movements supplies the selective movement patterns and postural basis underlying all skilled movement (B. Bobath, 1955; K. Bobath & B. Bobath, 1956). The Bobaths used a combination of tactile and proprioceptive stimulation to elicit the spontaneous production of these automatic reactions (B. Bobath, 1953).

Although the following quotation concerns children with CP, these remarks are appropriate for all clients. The Bobaths described facilitation in treatment this way:

> While treating the child, the therapist must carefully watch the child's reaction to her handling. She must be able to appreciate changes of muscle tone and constantly adjust her handling to them. Treatment is an unending interchange between the therapist's actions and the child's response to them. The therapist must be guided by the child's reactions. They tell her when and where to hold him, how much or how little to support and guide him, which directions and ranges of movement to avoid and at what speed to move him. She must be able to judge the quality . . . at any moment and to anticipate the child's ability or inability to respond to her techniques of facilitation with normal movements. Only by observing the child's response will she know whether her handling has been of value, useless, or even detrimental to his progress. In advancing treatment the therapist's guidance and control must be withdrawn gradually and systematically. In this way the child will . . . learn to move more normally and independently. (K. Bobath & B. Bobath, 1964, p. 249)

The Bobaths stressed that the therapist must carefully choose the techniques of facilitation according to the client's needs and the ability to respond satisfactorily. Once the therapist gains an active movement from the client, the therapist must then aim at making these movements reliable, immediate, and adequate in strength and ROM (K. Bobath & B. Bobath, 1972).

Facilitation with specific attention to key points for handling remains the key to the NDT approach. Any therapist who has struggled through an NDT course will attest that NDT facilitation methods are very difficult to master. Developing skill with these techniques requires practice, experience, training, and observation (K. Bobath & B. Bobath, 1964). It is an energy-consuming task, both physically and mentally. Finding the balance between control and freedom–for therapist and client–and responding to the constant change in this relationship requires skill and intuition. Mrs. Bobath and, more recently, other NDT Instructors (Bly, 1999; Bly & Whiteside, 1997; Boehme, 1988, 1993; Bohman, 1998; Davies, 1985, 1990; Girolami, Ryan, & Gardner, 2001; Howle, 1999; Ryerson & Levit, 1997; Stamer, 2000, Quinton, 2002) have described specific facilitation sequences for children and adults. In addition, the Neuro-Developmental Treatment Association (www.ndta.org) maintains a large library of videotapes. These videos, books, and articles are primarily illustrations, because the movement techniques cannot be described adequately in sentences (which make multidimensional ideas appear to follow a linear sequence). For this reason NDT courses teach these methods in supervised practice sessions with both peers and clients.

Techniques of Tactile and Proprioceptive Facilitation

In the words of Mary Quinton, all the techniques of tactile and proprioceptive facilitation "paint the picture of the body image" (Bly, 2001). In some cases, once spasticity is inhibited, the resultant postural tone is too low, or the therapist discovers that the client has real weakness. The Bobaths developed specific facilitation methods to stabilize muscle tone and regulate reciprocal muscle function. They described the following methods of proprioceptive and tactile stimulation (B. Bobath, 1960a; K. Bobath & B. Bobath, 1964, 1972).

Tapping

1. **Inhibitory Tapping** is a facilitation technique that follows inhibition. Once spasticity or hypertonus has been reduced, the underlying muscle tone may be too low to support co-activation for stabilization or to allow the normal balance of antagonistic muscles for reciprocal interaction. Inhibitory tapping is applied directly to muscles and must be done with great care so that hypertonus does not recur.
2. **Sweep Tapping** employs a strong tactile stimulation, "sweeping" over the muscles in the direction of the movement. This technique is particularly useful in situations where, once tone has decreased, the client does not seem to know how to produce a posture or movement to activate synergic patterns of muscle function.
3. **Alternate Tapping** is useful for obtaining proper grading of reciprocal innervation. Therapists frequently use this method to stimulate balance responses. The therapist alternately taps the agonist and antagonist, allowing little or no movement, to make the muscles work in patterns of co-activation. Alternate tapping often precedes pressure tapping. There is a moment in which the therapist's hands are completely off the client, which allows the individual to hold a posture.
4. **Pressure Tapping** is a combination of weight bearing and compression through the joint to build up co-activation of the agonists and antagonists. Despite the name, pressure tapping does not involve tapping on muscles. This type of stimulation adds strong, somatosensory input and increases postural tone for the maintenance of a posture.

Weight Bearing, Pressure, and Resistance

Clinicians can assist the client's weight bearing in relationship with the support surface prior to and during a movement sequence by using small weight shifts with pressure, requiring the client to adapt to the changes in the COM, BOS and the effects of gravitational forces. Combining weight shifts with pressure is useful to build postural tone, aid alignment between the COM and BOS, and help the client develop strategies that will link weight bearing with movement. This must be done carefully so that the therapist does not produce conflicting sensory information as the client begins a movement. Combining weight shifts with pressure is useful to aid alignment and link appropriate weight bearing with a movement sequence. Often these techniques are done with the client on a mobile surface, such as an inflatable ball, roll or bolster. The therapist can either require the client to respond to movement of the surface or, time the movement of the surface with the client's weight shift to link initiation of active movement with a strong postural component.

Resistance is used as a client activates movement to give the client a stronger sense of direction or timing or to make the client work harder to produce a successful action.

Pressure is used to reinforce posture and alignment. Pressure is given through the joint(s) to reinforce the client's sense of position prior to movement initiation. For example, a therapist might add pressure down through the shoulders to a child while in the prone position on a ball, prior to facilitating the weight shift needed as the child actively reaches for a toy.

Placing and Holding

Placing is the ability to hold body segments in a precise alignment relative to a place or object in the environment. The ability to place (an arm, hand, fingers, thumb, leg or foot) is necessary for steady state control throughout the range of motion during every voluntary movement. For example, to practice the posture and movements needed for dressing, an adult with hemiplegia might be asked to hold a hoop with both hands, stand on one foot and place the other through the hoop, simulating putting on pants. This requires placing and holding the arms at the precise distance from the body, while adapting the length of reach, then timing the direction of the LE for stepping through the hoop, placing and holding the leg as necessary as the task progresses.

The Bobaths developed these special tactile and proprioceptive facilitation techniques to assist clients as they developed active coordinated movement. These specific methods all served to add strong tactile or somatosenory input to posture and thereby link the postural requirements to the movement components.

Chapter Summary

Table 5.1 compares the emphases in the 1950s to the emphases in the 2000s. This approach evolved during the Bobaths' lifetime and continues its evolution today. In November, 1990, the Bobaths summed up their feelings about their work in the foreword to their biography.

> We are very proud of the fact that the concept in its long development has remained a living thing, based on and modified by clinical observation and practical experience. . . . We enjoyed every minute of it and are happy at the end of our career to look upon an eventful and fulfilling task, requiring our total absorption which we considered an adventure, the result of an accidental discovery, impossible to judge at first, and only proved through long experience of evaluation and treatment. (Schleichkorn, 1992, p. ix)

The Bobaths died in January, 1991.

Comparison and Ideas From the 1950s to the 2000s.

The Bobath Approach: Where we began	The NDT Approach: Where we are now
1. Analytic problem-solving approach based on reflex/hierarchical models	1. Analytic problem-solving approach based on a systems/selectionist model
2. Hierarchical model of CNS structure and function	2. Distributed model of CNS structures and function
3. CNS viewed as the "controller". Automatic postural control mechanism simplified the responsibility of the CNS in control of movement.	3. The CNS determines the pattern of neural activity based on input from the multiple intrinsic systems and extrinsic variables that establish the context for movement initiation and execution.
4. Skilled movement is determined by maturation of reflexive movement.	4. Skilled movement is determined by the specific functional goal.
5. Muscle and postural tone determine the quality of the patterns of posture and movement used in functional activities.	5. Task goal, experience, individual learning strategies, movement synergies, energy, and interest all affect the quality of the final action.
6. Sensory feedback is important for the correction of movement errors.	6. Sensory feed-forward and feedback are equally important for different aspects of movement control.
7. "Positive signs", including spasticity and abnormal coordination of movement, are the most important aspects of the sensorimotor impairment.	7. The "negative signs," including weakness, impaired postural control, and paucity of movement, are recognized as equally important as the "positive signs" in limitations of function.
8. The CNS is not "hard-wired." Spasticity and abnormal coordination are changeable, but limitations occur if abnormal movement patterns are repeated and practiced.	8. The CNS is capable of recovery and remains plastic throughout the lifetime. Functional changes are limited by structural damage to the CNS, secondary changes in the body systems, and the inability to adapt to environmental conditions.
9. Neurological and developmental aspects of the CNS pathology are the most important considerations during examination and treatment planning.	9. Interactions of neural and body systems and environmental context are all part of examination and treatment planning.
10. Clinicians must always ask "why" when examining and treating clients.	10. Clinicians must always ask "why" when examining and treating clients.
11. Clinicians can most strongly influence movement through the peripheral sensory system.	11. Clinicians can use the body systems and the environment to influence movement outcome.
12. Treatment methods involve primarily inhibition and facilitation through "hands-on" control of the client.	12. Motor learning concepts, including changing the environment, verbal reinforcement, self-initiated movement, and trial and error, have expanded treatment options. NDT recognizes limitations in physical guidance as a treatment strategy.
13. Functional movement develops from automatic components of movement.	13. The need to teach and practice functions is as important as facilitating components of movement.
14. Family and others in programs ensure carryover in life settings.	14. Direct teaching of functional activities in community settings adds to carryover.
15. Successful outcomes are measured in subjective, descriptive terms based on the individual's response to intervention strategies.	15. Outcomes must include collecting clinical data to provide efficacy of NDT intervention.

Table 5.1. The evolution of the Bobath Approach.

Where Will We Go from Here?

The NDT approach will continue to change and be enriched by the emergence of new theories, new models, and new information in the movement sciences. Clearer classification systems, such as the NDT enablement model, serve as a framework within which to describe the dimensions of disabilities and clarify communication among professionals, clients, and their families. Our understanding of motor control and motor learning has expanded treatment options while maintaining the basic concepts of NDT, whose aim is for an optimal match between the client's needs, the therapeutic process, and the goal of achieving the best possible functional abilities for each client to pursue a full and meaningful life.

NDT is still evolving. Therapists who believe that intervention is effective and essential must accept the challenge presented by new theories and integrate these ideas with current standards of practice. This is an exciting time. We must be willing to recognize and separate what we *know* from what we *believe,* and integrate art and science in making clinical decisions. We must provide the clinical data, generate testable hypotheses, blend therapists' intuition and art with current scientific knowledge, and submit our beliefs to the rigors of experimental research. This will develop the evidence base for our clinical practice that will advance the care of our clients and strengthen our professions.

References

Bernstein, N. A. (1967). *The co-ordination and regulation of movements.* Oxford, England: Pergamon Press.

Bleck, E. E. (1987). Orthopaedic management in cerebral palsy. *Clinics in Developmental Medicine,* #99/100.

Bly, L. (1991). A historical and current view of the basis of NDT. *Pediatric Physical Therapy, 3* (3), 131-135.

Bly, L. (1996, September/October). What is the role of sensation in motor learning? What is the role of feedback and feedforward? *NDTA Network,* 1, 3, 5, 7.

Bly, L. (1999). *Baby treatment based on NDT principles.* Tucson, AZ: Therapy Skill Builders.

Bly, L. L. (2001). A tribute to Mary Quinton. *NDTA Network, 8* (2), 1, 7.

Bly, L., & Whiteside, A. (1997). *Facilitation techniques based on NDT principles.* San Antonio, TX: Therapy Skill Builders.

Bobath, B. (1948a, January/February). A new treatment of lesions of the upper motor neurone. *British Journal of Physical Medicine,* 26-30.

Bobath, B. (1948b). The importance of the reduction of muscle tone and the control of mass reflex action in the treatment of spasticity. *Occupational Therapy and Rehabilitation, 27* (5), 371-383.

Bobath, B. (1953). Control of postures and movements in the treatment of cerebral palsy. *Physiotherapy, 39* (5), 99-104.

Bobath, B. (1954, September-December). A study of abnormal postural reflex activities in patients with lesions of the central nervous system. *Physiotherapy, 40* (9), 259-267, (10), 295-300, (11) 326-334, (12) 368-373.

Bobath, B. (1955). The treatment of motor disorders of pyramidal and extra-pyramidal origin by reflex inhibition and by facilitation of movements. *Physiotherapy, 41* (5), 146-153.

Bobath, B. (1959). Observations on adult hemiplegia and suggestions for treatment. Part I. *Physiotherapy, 45,* 279-289.

Bobath, B. (1960a). Observations on adult hemiplegia and suggestions for treatment. Part II. *Physiotherapy,* 46, 5-14.

Bobath, B. (1960b). Opening address and principles of treatment. In G. Beinart (Ed.), *Proceedings of a conference on cerebral palsy. Medical Proceedings, 6* (11), 234-248.

Bobath, B. (1963, April). Treatment principles and planning in cerebral palsy. *British Journal of Physical Medicine,* 1-3.

Bobath, B. (1965). *Abnormal postural reflex activity caused by brain lesions* (1st ed.). London: William Heinemann.

Bobath, B. (1967). The very early treatment of cerebral palsy. *Developmental Medicine and Child Neurology, 9* (4), 373-390.

Bobath, B. (1969). The treatment of neuromuscular disorders by improving patterns of coordination. *Physiotherapy, 55,* 18-22.

Bobath, B. (1971). Motor development, its effect on general development and application to treatment of cerebral palsy. *Physiotherapy, 57,* 526-532.

Bobath, B. (1975). Sensorimotor development. *NDT Newsletter, 7,* 1-5.

Bobath, B. (1977). Treatment of adult hemiplegia. *Physiotherapy, 63* (10), 310-313.

Bobath, B. (1985). *Abnormal postural reflex activity caused by brain lesions* (3rd ed.). Rockville, MD: Aspen Publications.

Bobath, B. (1990). *Adult hemiplegia: Evaluation and treatment* (3rd ed.). London: William Heinemann.

Bobath, B., & Finnie, N. (1958). Re-education of movement patterns for everyday life in the treatment of cerebral palsy. *British Journal of Occupational Therapy, 21,* 23-28.

Bobath, K. (1953). The treatment of cerebral palsy. *Spastic's Quarterly, 2* (2), 3-6.

Bobath, K. (1954, September). The treatment of cerebral palsy by reflex inhibition and the facilitation of automatic movements. *British Council for Welfare of Spastics,* 76-85.

Bobath, K. (1959a). The effects of treatment by reflex inhibition and facilitation of movement in cerebral palsy. *Folia Psychiatrica, Neurologica et Neurochirugica Neerlandica, 62* (5), 448-457.

Bobath, K. (1959b). The neuropathology of cerebral palsy and its importance in treatment and diagnosis. *CP Bulletin, 1* (8), 13-33.

Bobath, K. (1960). The nature of paresis in cerebral palsy. *Developmental Medicine and Child Neurology, 22,* 88-93.

Bobath, K. (1966). The motor deficits in patients with cerebral palsy. *Clinics in Developmental Medicine,* #23. London: William Heinemann Books.

Bobath, K. (1970). The problem of spasticity in the treatment of patients with lesions of the upper motor neurone. *Proceedings of the 6th International Congress of the WCPT, Netherlands,* 459-464.

Bobath, K. (1971a). The normal postural reflex mechanism and its deviation in children with cerebral palsy. *Physiotherapy, 57,* 515-525.

Bobath, K. (1971b). The work of Magnus and his collaborators on the nervous regulation of posture, and its bearing on some modern neurological problems. Unpublished NDT course lecture notes.

Bobath, K. (1980). *A neurophysiological basis for the treatment of cerebral palsy.* Philadelphia: J. B. Lippincott.

Bobath, K., & Bobath, B. (1950). Spastic paralysis: Treatment by the use of reflex inhibition. *British Journal of Physical Medicine, 13,* 121-127.

Bobath, K., & Bobath, B. (1952). A treatment of cerebral palsy based on the analysis of the patient's motor behavior. *British Journal of Physical Medicine, 15,* 107-117.

Bobath, K., & Bobath, B. (1954). The treatment of cerebral palsy by inhibition of abnormal reflex action. *British Orthopedics Journal, 11* (1), 88-98.

Bobath, K., & Bobath, B. (1955). Tonic reflexes and righting reflexes in the diagnosis and assessment of cerebral palsy. *CP Review, 16* (4), 4-11.

Bobath, K., & Bobath, B. (1956). Control of motor function in the treatment of cerebral palsy. *Australian Journal of Physiotherapy, 2* (2), 295-303.

Bobath, K., & Bobath, B. (1957). Control of motor function in the treatment of cerebral palsy. *Physiotherapy, 43* (10), 295-303.

Bobath, K., & Bobath, B. (1958). An assessment of the motor handicap of children with cerebral palsy and of their response to treatment. *British Occupational Therapy Journal, 21* (5), 19-34.

Bobath, K., & Bobath, B. (1964). The facilitation of normal postural reactions and movements in the treatment of cerebral palsy. *Physiotherapy, 50* (8), 246-262.

Bobath, K., & Bobath, B. (1967). The neuro-developmental treatment of cerebral palsy. *Physical Therapy, 47* (11), 1039-1041.

Bobath, K., & Bobath, B. (1968). Foreword to N. Finnie, *Handling the young CP at home.* London: William Heinemann Medical Books.

Bobath, K., & Bobath, B. (1972). Cerebral palsy. Part II. In P. H. Pearson & C. E. Williams (Eds.), *Physical therapy services in the developmental disabilities* (pp. 114-185). Springfield, IL: Charles Thomas Publishers.

Bobath, K., & Bobath, B. (1979). Acceptance Speech (audiotape transcription), First Currative Foundation Awards Dinner, Milwaukee, WI.

Bobath, K., & Bobath, B. (1984). The neurodevelopmental treatment. In D. Scrutton (Ed.), *Management of the motor disorders of children with cerebral palsy* (pp. 6-18). Philadelphia: J. B. Lippincott.

Boehme, R. (1988). *Improving upper body control: An approach to assessment and treatment of tonal dysfunction.* Tucson, AZ: Therapy Skill Builders.

Boehme, R. (1993). Developing hand function. In B. H. Connelly & P. C. Montgomery (Eds.), *Therapeutic exercise in developmental disabilities* (2nd ed., pp. 155-166). Hixson, TN: Chattanooga Group.

Bohman, I. M. (1998). *Handling skills used in the management of adult hemiplegia: A lab manual.* Albuquerque, NM: Clinician's View.

Brown, G. T., & Burns, S. A. (2001) The efficacy of neurodevelopmental treatment in paediatrics: A systematic review. *British Journal of Occupational Therapy, 64,* 235-244.

Butler, C. (2001). Evidence tables and reviews of treatment outcome. In A. L. Scherzer (Ed.), *Early diagnosis and interventional therapy in cerebral palsy. An interdisciplinary age-focused approach* (3rd ed., pp. 183-330). New York: Marcel Dekker.

Butler, C., & Darrah, J. (2001). Effects of neurodevelopmental treatment (NDT) for cerebral palsy. An AACPDM evidence report. *Developmental Medicine and Child Neurology, 43* (11), 778-790.

Carr, J. H., & Shepherd, R. B. (1998). *Neurologic rehabilitation: Optimizing motor performance.* Oxford, England: Butterworth and Heinemann.

Craik, R. L. (1991). Recovery process: Maximizing function. In M. Lister (Ed.), *Contemporary management of motor control problems. Proceedings From II Step Conference. Foundation for Physical Therapy* (pp. 165-174). Alexandria, VA: American Physical Therapy Association.

Davies, J. (1985). Steps to follow. *A guide to treatment of adult hemiplegia based on the concept of K and B. Bobath.* New York: Springer-Verlag.

Davies, J. (1990). *Right in the middle. Selective trunk activity in the treatment of adult hemiplegia.* New York: Springer-Verlag.

Easton, T. A. (1972). On the normal use of reflexes. *American Scientist, 60* (5), 591-99.

Fukuda, T. (1961). Human dynamic postures from the viewpoint of postural reflexes. *Acta Oto-laryngologica. Supplementum, 101,* 1-52.

Gesell, A. (1938). The tonic reflex in the human infant. *Journal of Pediatrics, 13* (4), 455-464.

Gesell, A., Halverson, H. M., Thompson, H., Ilg, F. L., Castner, B. M., Ames, L. B., & Amatruda, C. S. (1940). *The first five years of life.* New York: Harper and Row.

Girolami, G., Ryan, F., & Gardner, J. (2001). Assessment and treatment planning. In A. Scherzer (Ed.), *Early diagnosis and interventional therapy. An interdisciplinary age-focused approach* (3rd ed., pp. 15-205). New York: Marcel Dekker.

Hadders-Algra, M. (2000). The neuronal group selection theory: Promising principles for understanding and treating developmental motor disorders. *Developmental Medicine and Child Neurology, 24* (10), 707-715.

Hellebrandt, F. A., Schade, M., & Carns, M. L. (1962). Methods of evoking the tonic neck reflexes in normal human subjects. *American Journal of Physical Medicine, 41,* 90-139.

Heriza, C. (1991). Motor development: Traditional and contemporary theories. In M. Lister (Ed.), *Contemporary management of motor control problems. Proceedings From II Step Conference. Foundation for Physical Therapy* (pp. 99-127). Alexandria, VA: American Physical Therapy Association.

Horak, F. B. (1991). Assumptions underlying motor control of neurologic rehabilitation. In M. Lister (Ed.), *Contemporary management of motor control problems. Proceedings From II Step Conference. Foundation for Physical Therapy* (pp. 11-27). Alexandria, VA: American Physical Therapy Association.

Howle, J. (1999). Cerebral palsy. In S. K. Campbell (Ed.), *Decision making in pediatric neurologic physical therapy* (pp. 23-83). Philadelphia: Churchill Livingstone.

Jackson, J. H. (1932/1958). *Selected writings.* London: Staples Press. (Reprinted from *Selected writings of John B. Hughlings* [vols. I, II], by J. H. Jackson & J. Taylor, Eds., 1932, London: Hodder, Stoughter)

Lunnen, K. (1999). Children with multiple disabilities. 141-197. In S. K. Campbell (Ed.), *Decision making in pediatric physical neurological physical therapy* (pp. 141-197). New York: Churchill Livingstone.

Magnus, R. (1926). Some results on the physiology of posture (Cameron Prize lecture). *Lancet, 2,* 531-535.

Manning, J. (1972). Facilitation of movement: The Bobath Approach. *Physiotherapy, 58* (12), 403-408.

Martin, J. P. (1967). *The basal ganglia and posture.* London: Pittman.

Mayston, M. J. (1992). The Bobath concept: Evolution and application. In H. Forssberg & H. Hirschfeld (Eds.), *Movement disorders in children* (vol. 36, pp. 1-6). Basel, Switzerland: Medicine and Sport Science/Karger.

McGraw, M. (1945/1963). *The neuromuscular maturation of the human infant.* New York: Hafner. (Originally published by Columbia University Press, 1945)

Milani-Comparetti, A. (1967). Pattern analysis of motor development and its disorders. *Developmental Medicine and Child Neurology, 9* (5), 625-630.

Payton, O. D., Hirt, S., & Newton, R. (1977). *Scientific basis for neurophysiological approaches to therapeutic exercises: An anthology.* Philadelphia: F. A. Davis.

Quinton, M. (2002). *Making the difference with babies: Concepts and guidelines for baby treatment.* Albuquerque, NM: Clinician's View

Ritchie-Russell, W. R. (1958). Physiology of memory. *Proceedings of the Royal Society of Medicine, 51,* 9.

Ryerson, S., & Levitt, K. (1997). *Functional movement reeducation.* Philadelphia: Churchill Livingstone.

Schaltenbrand, G. (1928). The development of human motility and motor disturbances. *Archiv fur Neurologie und Psychiatrie, 20,* 720-728.

Schleichkorn, J. (1992). *The Bobaths: A biography of Berta and Karel Bobath.* Tucson, AZ: Therapy Skill Builders.

Sherrington, C. S. (1906). *The integrative action of the nervous system.* New Haven, CT: Yale University Press.

Sherrington, C. S. (1913). Reflex inhibition as a factor in the co-ordination of movements and postures. *Quarterly Journal of Experimental Physiology, 6,* 251-310.

Sherrington, C. S. (1947). *The integrative action of the nervous system* (2nd ed.). New Haven, CT: Yale University Press.

Stamer, M. (2000). *Posture and movement of the child with cerebral palsy.* San Antonio, TX: Therapy Skill Builders.

Valvano, J., & Long, T. (1991). Neurodevelopmental treatment: A review of the writings of the Bobaths. *Pediatric Physical Therapy, 3* (3), 125-129.

Van Sant, A. F. (1993). Concepts of neural organization and movement. In B. H. Connelly & P. C. Montgomery (Eds.), *Therapeutic exercise in developmental disabilities* (2nd ed., pp. 1-12). Hixson, TN: Chattanooga Group.

Walshe, F. M. P. (1921). On disorders of movement resulting from loss of postural tone with special reference to cerebellar ataxia. *Brain, 44,* 539-556.

Weisz, S. T. (1938). Studies in equilibrium reactions. *Journal of Nervous Diseases, 88,* 150-162.

White, R. (1984). Sensory integrative therapy for the cerebral-palsied child. In D. Scrutton (Ed.), *Management of the motor control disorders in children with cerebral palsy* (pp. 86-95). Philadelphia: J. B. Lippincott.

Woll, S. P., & Utley, J. (2001, January/February). Forced use–A handling strategy. *NDT Network,* 1, 4-6.

Index